Praise for
Healing Depression without Medication

"While there are dozens of self-help books on depression, Dr. Skillicorn has done a masterful job of explaining principles of neuroscience and how they work to create new neural pathways for healing depression. Neuroplasticity is the name of the game, and Dr. Skillicorn presents meticulous research about the need to look beyond 'diagnose and adios' medicine to help each individual develop his or her own customized program of activities and nutrition so that the brain can heal itself organically without dangerous medication. Whether you are a doctor, patient, or seeking help for someone you care about, you will find the help you seek in these pages."

—LAURIE NADEL, PhD, author of *The Five Gifts: Discovering Hope, Healing, and Strength When Disaster Strikes*

"In this well-researched and empowering book, Dr. Jodie Skillicorn demolishes the 'facts' surrounding depression, including the erroneous assumptions that it is caused by a flaw in the brain's neurochemistry and that pharmaceutical cocktails are the answer. Creating her own potent healing recipe of mindfulness, meditations, guided imagery, healing movement, nutritional advice, and much more, this is a book that anyone dealing with depression cannot afford to miss."

—CATE MONTANA, MA, author of *The E Word: Ego, Enlightenment and Other Essentials*

"If you think you need psych meds to cure your mood, think again. And read this book."

—CHRISTIANE NORTHRUP, MD, *New York Times* best-selling author of *Goddesses Never Age, The Wisdom of Menopause,* and *Women's Bodies, Women's Wisdom*

Healing Depression without Medication

Healing Depression without Medication

A PSYCHIATRIST'S GUIDE TO BALANCING MIND, BODY, AND SOUL

JODIE SKILLICORN, DO

North Atlantic Books
Berkeley, California

Published by
North Atlantic Books
Berkeley, California

Cover art and design by Howie Severson
Book design by Happenstance Type-O-Rama

Printed in the United States of America

Healing Depression without Medication: A Psychiatrist's Guide to Balancing Mind, Body, and Soul is sponsored and published by the Society for the Study of Native Arts and Sciences (dba North Atlantic Books), an educational nonprofit based in Berkeley, California, that collaborates with partners to develop cross-cultural perspectives, nurture holistic views of art, science, the humanities, and healing, and seed personal and global transformation by publishing work on the relationship of body, spirit, and nature.

The names and identifying details of patient stories have been changed to protect confidentiality.

North Atlantic Books' publications are available through most bookstores. For further information, visit our website at www.northatlanticbooks.com or call 800-733-3000.

Library of Congress Cataloging-in-Publication Data

1 2 3 4 5 6 7 8 9 KPC 25 24 23 22 21 20

This book includes material from well-managed forests and from recycled materials. North Atlantic Books is committed to the protection of our environment. We print on recycled paper whenever possible and partner with printers who strive to use environmentally responsible practices.

Contents

For Wade and Skye, who remind me daily
about the meaning of love, and
the importance of balance.

Acknowledgments

I am deeply grateful for all those who have helped me on this journey: First and foremost, my agent, Lisa Hagan, whose faith in my book made this adventure possible; my editor, Lisa Bess Kramer, who not only helped my sentences flow better, but offered assurance and encouragement at every step; North Atlantic Books, for taking a chance on an unknown author with a message, but no existing platform; Shayna Keyles, for delicately excising large chunks of my oversize manuscript, and offering an opportunity for discernment, letting go, and trust; Ebonie Ledbetter for her close attention to details in the final edits.

On the home front, this project would not have been possible without the love, support, and patience of my husband, Tom; my kids for keeping me balanced between play and work; my four-legged furry friends, for their companionship while writing, and insistent reminders to pause and pay attention to them; and my parents, who taught me (even though I did not always believe them) that I could do anything I set my mind to. Despite boxes of failed projects from the past in their attic, they never questioned that this project was possible.

I am indebted to the many teachers and healers in my life, too many to list, who inspired me and taught me that at the heart of all healing is the power of presence, connection, and listening.

I am grateful for my sister, friends, and fellow Chameleons, who believed in me and offered support, encouragement, and intentions throughout this process.

Lastly, there would be no book to write if it were not for all I have learned from my patients, who continually inspire me with their resilience, courage, and grace.

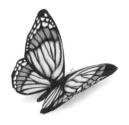

PART 1

The Insanity of Conventional Psychiatry

*To find health should be the object of the doctor.
Anyone can find disease.*
—A. T. STILL, DOCTOR OF OSTEOPATHY

*A reliable way to make people believe in falsehoods is
frequent repetition, because familiarity is not easily
distinguished from truth.*
—DANIEL KAHNEMAN,
THINKING FAST AND SLOW

Introduction:
The Unraveling of Truth

The hardest thing to explain is the glaringly evident which everybody has decided not to see.

—AYN RAND, *THE FOUNTAINHEAD*

"Look, Mommy, look," my daughter squeals as she rushes into my room clutching a letter from the Tooth Fairy. Fifteen minutes later she returns with a sly, wise smirk on her slightly less innocent face. "You're the Tooth Fairy, Mommy. I saw the letter on your computer. You have been Mom-busted!"

That unraveling of truth, that validation of a lurking unvoiced suspicion in one's gut, is how I felt after reading Robert Whitaker's book *Anatomy of an Epidemic*. The book challenged every dogma, every so-called truth about mental illness and how to treat it that I had learned in medical school and psychiatry residency. Imagine finding out that everything you had spent four long sleep-deprived years of residency learning was simply not true. Worse, imagine finding out that how you've been taught to "heal" people may actually be causing more harm than good.

The initial shock, anger, and despair I felt after reading the book shifted to an awareness of a deep inner knowing: I had recognized all along that this was not the way. I reflected back to my first days seeing patients on my own in the psychiatry residency clinic. My "new" patients were mostly old patients who were being handed down to me not only from the previous residents but the residents before them and before them. I remember wondering, even then: if medication and therapy work, why were these people not getting better?

This question became a challenge to dig into the research and find other healing options. I set about unlearning the knowledge I had acquired in medical school, and relearning yoga and meditation, which I'd been practicing for years. I obsessively read and attended classes in nutrition, mindfulness-based cognitive therapy, energy medicine, Emotional Freedom Technique (EFT), eye movement desensitization and reprocessing (EMDR), hypnotherapy, integrative medicine, Mind-Body Medicine, and auricular acupuncture. As I learned these skills, I continued to listen to patients' stories to find more clues and answers.

"Abnormal" Is the New Normal

Perhaps you are one of the tens of millions of Americans to visit a conventional psychiatrist or primary care doctor, and be quickly labeled with one of the ever-expanding lists of pathologies found in the psychiatric bible, the *Diagnostic and Statistical Manual of Mental Disorders* (DSM-5), which includes over three hundred disorders. With so many dysfunctions to choose from, I challenge you to take a look and not find one that fits you.

Many of these "illnesses" used to be considered normal responses to life's stressors, losses, and challenges, like grieving for the loss of a spouse, child, friend, or beloved pet for more than a couple weeks; feeling anxious when trying to meet too many needs at work and having no time for yourself; being diagnosed with cancer or some other chronic disease and feeling petrified, angry, sad, and stuck; not being able to focus on your schoolwork after your dad has been deployed to a war-torn country; not feeling safe at home with an abusive, alcoholic mom; feeling trapped in an unfulfilling relationship or job; wanting to disappear so as not to hear mom and dad arguing all the time; or just a whole host of other perfectly normal responses to life's unexpected, often unfair, twists and turns.

Although these emotions are perfectly normal responses to difficult situations, the new normal is to be labeled "abnormal" and "dysfunctional." The psychiatric community and their buddies the pharmaceutical industry have conveniently determined that we humans should not have to suffer with emotions like sadness or anxiety. Despite living in a world constantly vying for our attention twenty-four hours a day—with cable TV news, Facebook, and Twitter feeds instantly updating us about every catastrophe happening everywhere in the world—we should be able to focus and remain calm and happy at all times, or take a pill so that we can do so more easily.

Perhaps after being labeled with a "pathology," you were sent on your way with a prescription for one, or maybe two, medicines, which were handed over as casually as Pez candy from a SpongeBob dispenser. Perhaps you returned a month later for a fifteen-minute follow-up visit to see if that pill solved the presenting problem. If you were better, it would be assumed it was because of the medication, or medications, bestowed upon you with great authority. If you happened to be worse, it would be assumed that you need a higher dose or an additional medication—often to contend with the side effects of the first—or perhaps you did not take it correctly or "compliantly" enough. And sometimes, two Pez of different flavors must be better than one, right?

Actually, no. Despite all the talk about evidence-based medicine, research has consistently found that two antidepressants do not confer benefits over one, but do significantly increase the risk of side effects. Yet most psychiatrists continue to hand out multiple medications, because with only fifteen minutes to assess you, there's not much time to explore *why* you might be having these symptoms. It is easier to write it off to the widely propagated myth of a neurochemical imbalance. Seeking the *cause* for the imbalance and exploring what in your life may need balancing requires more time, attention, and listening.

Although there is ample evidence of frequent side effects from medications, it is rarely assumed that someone might be doing worse *because* of the medication. A 2014 analysis revealed that over nine hundred thousand emergency department visits a year occur after receiving a psychiatric or sleep medication. This is likely a gross underestimation of side effects, as most of the people suffering from side effects never visit the emergency department.

It is those people who do not visit the emergency department that often appear in my office, because they have heard I am a "holistic psychiatrist," and they, perhaps you too, are hoping for another way.

Another Way

Clinging to the familiar is a predilection of the human brain. Sometimes we see what we expect to see more clearly than what is actually in front of our eyes. A wonderful example of this can be seen in Daniel Simons's selective attention experiment, in which participants look at a video of a group of people passing balls to each other, and are asked to count the number of times those wearing white pass the ball. Before I spoil the experiment, please pause here and check it out on YouTube (www.youtube.com/watch?v=vJG698U2Mvo), so you can see for yourself how easily we can miss information right in front of our faces.

If you watched the video, chances are, if you were busy focusing on the ball, you may have missed the gorilla. Or perhaps you saw the gorilla and lost track of the ball. If asked in advance, I am sure most of us would assume that we could not possibly miss a man dressed in a gorilla costume walking through a small group of people, but I know I did the first time I saw it, and so did half of those tested. The point is, if we are focused on what we expect to see, we may completely miss the unexpected that is happening right in front of us.

So, what do overlooked gorillas have to do with psychiatry and depression? If researchers, physicians, and patients are myopically focusing only on the brain and neurochemistry, we become blind to the myriad interplaying variables below the neck and in the environment that may be influencing depression or other "mental" issues. What may look and feel like depression might be an illness or infection, chronic stress, a poor diet and nutritional deficiency, a hormonal imbalance, an abusive relationship or work situation, or a host of other problems not located in the head. Consequently, we end up asking incomplete questions and arriving at inaccurate assumptions, leading to ineffective and even harmful treatments. Even when more complete answers are elucidated in research labs, it can take seventeen to thirty years for this new information to infiltrate your doctor's office.

In my office, and in this book, I offer another way, based on the latest research. Instead of reflexively handing over a script, I take time to listen to your life story so I can better understand and help you understand how your particular symptoms might make sense and be an uncomfortable but normal response to your life circumstances.

Of course, I want to know about your symptoms and your particular flavor and experience of depression, anxiety, psychosis, or mania, but more importantly I want to know what was going on in your life when the symptoms began, what effect those symptoms had on your life then and since, what fears you now carry about any of those symptoms appearing and how you respond when they surface, what you believe about your illness and what you believe it says about you, and what your family believes about the illness and what it says about you. I want to know what you find meaningful and fulfilling in your life, what you believe in spiritually, what sort of balance you have in your life between work and play, and what you do to relax. I want to know about your relationships and the support you receive or do not receive, what you eat, what you do for exercise, what you do for play, what brings you joy. I want to know about your emotional life—what you are allowed and willing to express and how you do that, and what emotions are kept silent and buried, stewing beneath the surface.

These are not unique questions. These are the questions psychiatrists always used to ask before their jobs got reduced to fifteen-minute medication checks. Time, listening, and presence are at the core of all healing modalities, but they do not earn revenue for our medical system.

After gathering the pieces of your story, I attempt to weave the narrative of your life together with the latest research on the amazing neuroplasticity of the brain. We all have the capacity to rewire our brains to better focus, concentrate, and manage stress and emotions using tools you will learn in this book, like meditation, breathing, guided imagery, exercise, eating whole healthy foods, and getting outside in nature.

In my practice and in this book, I provide education about emotions and their intrinsic value in guiding you forward on your life path. I attempt to plant a seed that reframes your moods and emotions as *normal* messengers alerting you when life is out of balance, rather than pathologizing them as a threat to be feared and avoided.

I discuss the research showing the long-term physical and psychological consequences of the use of antidepressants, debunk the mythology of neurochemical imbalances, and educate you about a growing body of research, still largely ignored by the psychiatric community, that suggests that depression, and chronic disease, is often a result of inflammation. This inflammation is primarily caused by early childhood stressors and the accumulated unmanaged stress of daily life. If stress is a primary cause of what we call mental and physical illness, would it not make more sense and be far more empowering to learn how to manage stress ourselves rather than cover up its effects with medication?

Learning self-care skills empowers you for life and gets to the root of the problem, rather than making you dependent on a doctor and his or her prescription pad for your well-being. I hope to shift you out of a mind-set that you have been dealt a bad genetic card into the recognition that most mental and physical illness is more a matter of epigenetics—the interplay of your genes with the environment, which includes your beliefs, thoughts, emotions, behaviors, diet, and lifestyle—in other words, *changeable* factors. If this is true, as an ever-growing body of research indicates, then neither you nor I are passive players doomed to a lifetime of pills, but active participants in our own healing (or wounding). By collaborating in our healing process, we are removing the sense of powerlessness and helplessness that fuels anxiety and depression, and replacing it with a greater sense of control and self-efficacy, reducing the risk of mental illness.

In this book, I will share, with those I cannot see in my office, what I have unlearned, learned, and relearned about depression and how to treat it. In the first section, I will debunk the myth of the neurochemical imbalance and examine the effectiveness and risks of antidepressants. In the second section, I will present a more hopeful, holistic pathway for those seeking to avoid medication, or wondering if it is even possible to get off the medications you are already taking. Feel free to jump ahead to the second section if that serves you better. What I have discovered and compiled here are not new techniques but time-tested skills, tools, and lifestyle changes that healers have been using for thousands of years. In my studies, I have only rediscovered the simple truth that by balancing the breath, mind, body, environment, energy, and soul, people can not only get off and stay off medications but transform depression, heal, and thrive.

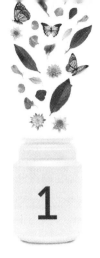

Debunking the Myth of Neurochemical Imbalance

There are two ways to be fooled. One is to believe what isn't true; the other is to refuse to believe what is true.

—SØREN KIERKEGAARD

A regal white tiger cub, Mohini, was presented as a gift to President Eisenhower and the National Zoo. At the zoo, she lived in a 12-by-12-foot cage with a cement floor and steel bars until a larger enclosure could be built for her. Once the new space—with acres of forest, hills, caves, and a pond—was complete, a large crowd excitedly gathered to witness Mohini's move. Sadly, when the cub was transferred to her expansive new home, she dashed straight for the corner of the enclosure and paced around a 12-by-12-foot space as if still in her former cage. Mohini remained in that corner for the rest of her life, oblivious to the possibility that she was no longer trapped and could now move beyond her narrow confines.

Many of my patients have suffered from depression and have been on medication for years, even decades, when they arrive at my office. When I first meet them and ask why they have come, I am often matter-of-factly told: "I have a neurochemical imbalance," or "I cannot function without medications." Many have been informed that the chemical imbalance in their brain is just like the dysfunctional production of insulin in someone with diabetes. Like diabetics, the person diagnosed with depression is told she will need to take medications for the rest of her life, to treat the disease and prevent a recurrence. This is what my preceptors, with great certainty and conviction, told their patients, and what I also used to tell mine. We doctors throw that information out routinely and casually. We ignore the emotional impact of such statements, which essentially declares that something is fundamentally wrong with you and your brain that requires medication forever to fix, or you will not be able to function. Wow! If that depresses you, no worries, because this prescription will help to numb the pain.

For far too many people, hearing this disempowering message repeated over time by physicians and the media has led to a firmly entrenched belief that they are fundamentally broken and trapped, without any options besides medications, in a cage of suffering created by a malfunctioning brain. Even when offered alternative explanations, some, like Mohini, cannot accept a different version of reality, especially for themselves, even when the newly offered reality is an improvement over the former reality. They remain insistent that others may suffer from depression for other reasons, "but I really do have a chemical imbalance."

In psychiatry, the assumption that mental illness is due to an inherent flaw in the brain and its neurochemistry has been the prevailing theory for more than half a century. The keystone to this theory is based on the backward logic that because antidepressants are assumed to be an effective treatment for depression, and we assume these medications work by changing the neurochemistry in the brain, therefore depression is caused by a specific neurochemical imbalance that is altered and corrected by the antidepressants. You may wisely note there are a lot of assumptions in that statement. Multiple studies also show that psychotherapy treats depression as well as medications, but we do not conclude that depression is caused by a deficiency in therapy. The problem with the chemical imbalance theory is that despite fifty years of research, there remains no evidence to validate it, and a long list of studies refuting it.

So, how can this be? To begin to understand how the majority of the population continues to believe a theory that evidence refutes, we need to look back at the dark, shadowy ghosts of psychiatry's past to see how we got here. Prior to the advent of psychiatric medications, the severely ill, trapped inside overcrowded mental asylums, were treated with a creative apothecary of treatment options that included the removal of body parts (teeth, tonsils, and the large intestines) in order to prevent infections from spreading to the brain; injections of horse serum; prolonged sleep therapy with heavy doses of barbiturates, opioids, or insulin to induce a semicomatose state; electroconvulsive therapy; and the lobotomy. Sure, these procedures turned patients into incapacitated zombies, but at least they were relieved of their presenting symptoms of agitation, psychosis, or depression, and the hospital floors were quieter and easier to manage. Although in hindsight, all these treatment strategies seem more insane—and sadistic—than the insane they were allegedly treating, it is critical to understand that at the time they were based on solid evidence and research, which were marketed to the public as safe and effective treatments.

Meanwhile, for the milder forms of mental illness, psychoanalysis ruled. From this perspective, mental illness in all its flavors could be treated with years of analyzing one's early childhood life experiences. Freud's psychoanalytic ideas enormously contributed to a heightened awareness of how our early experiences mold our unconscious motivations, fears, and desires that, in turn, powerfully influence our behaviors and perceptions.

By the 1950s, the U.S. government was attempting to figure out how to contend with the overcrowded, understaffed, and underfunded asylums, which were getting bad press for their horrific conditions. At the same time patients were being released back into the community, the accidental discovery of chlorpromazine, what later came to be thought of as the first antipsychotic, sparked the "psychopharmacological revolution."

Chlorpromazine acted like a "veritable chemical lobotomy," leaving patients sedated, detached, and disinterested. Psychiatric hospitals found it was perfect for quieting agitated and psychotic patients, and one has to imagine that this medication would be a massive improvement over ice picks or electric shocks. Psychiatrists, long considered inferior to other physicians, found the possibility of medication as a treatment option appealing: now they too could carry a prescription pad in their white jacket pocket, proving their medical prowess and increasing their financial worth. Pharmaceutical companies, with millions of dollars in sales, shared in the jubilation. Optimistic companies, researchers, and psychiatrists rushed to find new drugs. Surely if there were drugs for psychosis, one must exist for depression too.

Sure enough, while the drug iproniazid was being tested for tuberculosis, the researchers noticed it induced euphoria in some of the hospital patients. Psychiatrist Nathan Kline, jumping at the chance to test the drug on his depressed patients, glowingly described the medication as a "psychic energizer." The fact that these drugs were similar to amphetamines and induced psychosis, mania, and "behavioral disorders" in the majority of patients was conveniently overlooked. Researchers later determined the drug inhibited the enzyme monoamine oxidase, which prevents the breakdown of the monoamine neurotransmitters norepinephrine and serotonin, leading to higher available levels of these chemicals in the space between neurons, known as the synapse. This class of drugs became known as the monoamine oxidase inhibitors (MAOIs). It was assumed that the subsequent increase of the monoamines in the synapse acted to improve mood. This assumption formed one of the foundational pillars of the monoamine hypothesis, which evolved into the chemical imbalance theory.

At this same time of rose-colored dreams for the future of psychiatry, a Swiss psychiatrist, Roland Kuhn, discovered the drug imipramine. Unlike the stimulating properties of iproniazid, this drug was sedating in nature, bearing more resemblance to the antipsychotic chlorpromazine. Kuhn described imipramine as having "markedly antidepressant properties" that energized and motivated severely depressed patients, diminishing delusions and suicidal ideations. This miracle drug allegedly not only "cured" the chronically depressed in a matter of days but also converted a homosexual man back to heterosexuality, and resolved another man's impotence—clearly a multipurpose drug if ever there was one. Side effects like low blood pressure, blood clots, visual disturbances, increased agitation, mania, and increased risk of suicide were dismissed as "slight" or blamed on the patient's deviant "moral structure." Kuhn acknowledged that the medication was purely symptomatic, not curative, as the symptoms returned if discontinued. He also admitted that in some difficult cases, imipramine did not work until relationships and other life stressors were addressed first. Imagine that!

When Kuhn wrote this paper, the mechanism of action of the drug remained a mystery, but research later suggested that this new class of drugs—the tricyclic antidepressants (TCAs)—worked by blocking the reuptake of the neurotransmitter norepinephrine into the neurons. Thus, like the monoamine oxidase inhibitors, they were assumed to improve mood by increasing the level of monoamines available in the receptor.

What's interesting here is that these two drugs, the MAOIs and the tricyclics, both supposedly work by increasing levels of norepinephrine and serotonin, yet have opposite effects, one acting more as a stimulant and the other having more sedating effects. This inconsistency might make one question the specificity of the drug's effect, and wonder if some other unknown factor was responsible for the changes in mood.

Flash forward another decade and Kuhn was promoting the idea that this medication was a "specific treatment of depressive states" that "largely or completely restores what the illness has impaired." A not-so-humble man, Kuhn declared that because of the discovery of this medication, "medicine and science will be just that much different because we have lived." Fortunately, he never ended up in a psychiatric ward, or such grandiosity may have led to his being labeled manic and requiring medications.

Other psychiatrists and the media shared this enthusiasm. Psychiatrist Harold Himwich compared the medication to the "advent of insulin." The *New York Times* reported it could "reverse psychic states." These medications were no longer being touted as treatments but as cures; now psychiatrists actively and enthusiastically promoted the story that the medications fixed the brain by balancing its neurochemistry, even though actual evidence suggested otherwise.

Two review articles published over the next couple of years by pioneers in psychopharmacology research, Joseph Schildkraut and Alec Coppen, led to the birth of the monoamine deficiency hypothesis. Here's the crux of the theory:

1. Monoamine oxidase inhibitors and tricyclic antidepressants both appear to improve mood.

2. Both drugs increase levels of the neurotransmitters norepinephrine and serotonin in the synapses between nerves.

3. Previous reports suggested that drugs like reserpine, which deplete levels of these neurotransmitters, appear to induce depression.

4. Therefore, depression is caused by a deficiency of these chemicals (norepinephrine, serotonin, and dopamine), and elation is associated with elevated levels.

In both Joseph Schildkraut's and Alec Coppen's papers, they acknowledged the evidence was based on correlations and assumptions, the findings "inconclusive," and the observed behavioral changes may be due to yet unknown factors unrelated to neurotransmitters. Schildkraut sagely added that depression was unlikely to represent a single entity, but rather influenced by multiple factors, including the "roles of personality, environmental, and psychological factors." Those inconvenient details of the article were largely forgotten with time and marketing.

Let's take a look at each of the pillars of this theory and see what accumulating evidence has since revealed. We will begin by pulling the leg out from under reserpine, an herbal treatment for blood pressure, later used for psychosis. This drug works by decreasing levels of neurotransmitters in the synapse, so for the theory to hold, it should induce or exacerbate depression. Further research on reserpine revealed, however, that only about 6 percent of patients on reserpine developed depression, and later research suggested it actually acted as an antidepressant and improved mood. This alone should have destabilized the wobbly theory into oblivion decades ago.

Now, let's examine the evidence for a consistent pattern of a biochemical imbalance, which is at the heart of the story we are all told. For the theory to be valid, and for antidepressants to have a specific curative action on the brain, there should be a consistent pattern of monoamine levels for depressed patients as compared to nondepressed ones. Yet, despite fifty years of research, the evidence remains lacking and inconsistent. A 2008 review on major depressive disorder stated: "Numerous studies of norepinephrine and serotonin metabolites in plasma, urine, and cerebrospinal fluid, as well as postmortem study of the brains of patients with depression, have yet to identify the purported deficiency reliably."

The data remains consistently inconsistent. Whether depressed or not, about one-quarter of the population appear to have low serotonin levels, one-quarter have high levels, and the rest are in the middle. There is no "normal." Furthermore, there are drugs that act effectively as antidepressants that increase the neurotransmitters, and other equally effective drugs that decrease them. In fact, virtually any drug with any mechanism of action, including benzodiazepines, opioids, buspirone, stimulants, reserpine, antipsychotics, thyroid medication, lithium, and now ketamine, is as equally effective as those labeled as "antidepressants." How can the theory hold if both increasing and decreasing levels of monoamines can sometimes improve and sometimes worsen depression, and if medications with a wide range of actions all have identical effectiveness?

When the hypothesis was first theorized, only a handful of neurotransmitters were known to exist, yet we now know that hundreds of chemicals in the body function as neurotransmitters or "neuromodulators," including peptides, amino acids, and hormones, all of which constantly send messages back and forth from body to brain. Each of these chemicals act on receptors in the body and brain that are also constantly shifting and creating an intricate and vastly complex dance we have only begun to understand. To imagine that any simple medication could balance such a complex system is mind-bogglingly delusional.

What these inconsistencies seem to suggest is that no matter how long we keep seeking a neurochemical explanation, we are no closer to understanding the beast of depression. So, how can psychiatrists, other doctors, mental health providers, and the media continue to promote this theory when so much evidence exists to debunk it?

One simple reason is that when psychiatrists first give patients prescriptions, many get better, so the assumption is made that the improvement is because of something specific to the drug. Researcher Joanna Moncrieff compares the use of antidepressants to the use of alcohol to "treat" anxiety, social phobia, sleep difficulties, or depression. Although it may relieve symptoms, we can all agree it is not solving the problem. In fact, relying on alcohol to get through social situations prevents one from learning skills to manage such situations in the future.

Over time, it also exacerbates the anxiety and depression it was attempting to alleviate, while additionally increasing one's risk for other health issues. Likewise, just because antidepressants may increase monoamine levels in the brain does not mean the imbalance of these monoamines is the cause of the depression. In both cases, it is also possible that the "cure" may actually be creating greater dysfunction, making it even more difficult to recover.

Another obvious answer as to why this myth is so widely propagated is the direct-to-consumer (DTC) advertisements airing on television, published in magazines, and featured on the internet that keep suggesting how much happier we would feel if we just took a pill to balance our neurochemistry. The United States and New Zealand are the only two developed countries that allow pharmaceutical companies to directly advertise to the public. Spending on DTC advertising has increased from $12 million in 1980 to over $6 billion in 2016. Psychiatric medications are among the most heavily advertised drugs.

Misinformation is not just coming from marketing propaganda. Psychiatrists, other physicians, and mental health providers also continue to promote this invalid theory as truth. But why? Researchers Jeffrey Lacasse and Jonathan Leo collected responses from psychiatrists questioned about the chemical imbalance theory. One of those psychiatrists was Wayne Goodman, a former chair of the U.S. Food and Drug Administration (FDA) Psychopharmacological Committee. He referred to the neurochemical imbalance theory as a "useful metaphor" that he cannot bring himself to use with his patients.

Ronald Pies, a psychiatrist at Tufts University and former editor of the *Psychiatric Times,* courageously, although somewhat cavalierly, addressed chemical imbalance theory in several articles. He contended that psychiatrists have never taken the theory seriously: "In truth, the 'chemical imbalance' notion was always a kind of urban legend—never a theory seriously propounded by well-informed psychiatrists." He added, "In the past thirty years, I don't believe I have ever heard a knowledgeable, well-trained psychiatrist make such a preposterous claim, except perhaps to mock it." In another article, Pies referred to the theory as a "kind of bumper-sticker phrase that saves time, and allows the physician to write out that prescription while feeling that the patient had been 'educated.'"

Um, really? Well, count all my teachers in medical school and residency, most of my colleagues, other mental health providers, and myself as members of the not "well-trained" or "well-informed" club. That was the correct answer on many psychiatry exams. That is what medical students continue to learn. That is what the majority of psychiatrists I know continue to explain to their patients as the rationale for going on an antidepressant.

Here's what I remember hearing, literally hundreds of times: "I understand you may not want to take an antidepressant, but the fact is your brain is lacking certain neurochemicals it needs to function properly. It is no different than a diabetic who requires insulin to moderate her sugar levels. Because your brain is unable to function properly, it is likely you will need to take this medication for the rest of your life. For those who have had one episode of depression, you have a 50 percent chance of a relapse. If you have already experienced two episodes you have a 75 percent chance of relapse, and if you have had more than three episodes you have a nearly 90 percent chance of future relapses. But as long as you keep taking your medication to correct your imbalance, we can hopefully keep that from happening."

Let me take a moment to make a quick apology to anyone I personally said that to during my residency or my first couple of years in practice. I am so sorry that none of that is true.

I wish that all the well-trained, knowledgeable, well-informed psychiatrists "in the know" had bothered to tell the rest of us—along with the media, the public, and the FDA—the truth. To be fair, what I believe Pies was suggesting is that few psychiatrists would completely attribute depression to *just* a neurochemical imbalance. In theory, we are all taught to consider the social, psychological, and environmental components. But in day-to-day practice these other aspects are often just boxes to be checked off on the electronic medical records chart before a prescription pad is pulled out.

Daniel Carlat is another psychiatrist, author, and editor of a psychiatric newsletter who dares to talk about the flawed theories in psychiatry. When asked by a National Public Radio reporter what we know about antidepressants, he candidly responded, "We don't know how the medications work in the brain." Despite this gap in knowledge, he admitted to using the theory to explain the cause of depression to his patients, "because patients want to know something. And they want to know that we as physicians have some basic understanding of what we're doing when we're prescribing medications."

Yet another psychiatrist, Alan Frazer, offered a different rationale for his use of this disproven theory with patients. He suggested that the biologically based theory allowed patients to "feel better about themselves if there was a biological reason for them being depressed … and the drug was correcting it."

It appears that a big part of the reason many of us continue to believe a debunked theory is because the psychiatrists who are aware of the evidence, along with the marketing gurus at the pharmaceutical companies, think it is better to erase inconvenient truths and provide metaphors and "bumper stickers" to simplify complex ideas. These "knowledgeable" psychiatrists have passed this information on so effectively that medical students and psychiatrists-in-training continue to believe it, right along with you. Meanwhile, millions of antidepressants continue to be passed out routinely with deceptive explanations for why they should be prescribed. Yet how can anyone make an informed decision about how best to treat depression when given inaccurate information in the name of simplification and "feeling better" about oneself?

Although some psychiatrists may argue that a basic biological explanation alleviates stigma and self-blame, the vast majority of my patients tell me a different story. How does casting upon someone the harmful life sentence that your brain is fundamentally broken empower one to make changes in one's life? Many patients first heard these words as children. During our first session together, I suggest to patients that perhaps that belief is not true, and I present some of the evidence. I ask: What if your brain is not broken at all? What if the stressors in your life just reached a breaking point, and you lacked the skills to handle it at that time, under those circumstances? Many find even just this glimmer of possibility to be empowering and hopeful. Others reject this possibility at first, and some do forever, after being told another story for so long. Like Mohini, they remain trapped in their own cage of suffering.

Scant research has addressed the question of how different explanations for mental illness influence one's own perceptions about depression. In one interesting study, undergraduate students with current or past depression were given a sham "Rapid Depression Test," which was described as testing the levels of neurotransmitters to determine whether their depression was due to a chemical imbalance. Half of the group was shown data and graphs indicating that their levels were low, and their depression likely caused by a chemical imbalance. The other half was shown data revealing their levels were normal, and were told their depression was not due to a chemical imbalance.

The results were similar to what I see and hear with my own patients. Those who were told they had a neurochemical imbalance experienced greater despair, believing their depression to be more chronic and unmanageable. Believing they lacked the ability to regulate their own mood states, they were far more likely to seek pharmacological treatment over therapy. Worse, this false biological explanation did not diminish stigma or self-blame.

Hopelessness is a hallmark of depression, and we are delivering just that. Instead of seeking therapy and tools to manage emotions in the future, people are being handed mind-numbing medications that demotivate them to make changes in thinking, coping, and living—changes that might allow them to rise above their depressed states and flourish long-term.

The stories we tell have the ability to empower or depress us. We can tell people a false story about how they are broken, or we can educate people about the amazing ability of the brain to transform. The brain is anything but static. Nobel Prize–winning researcher Eric Kandel found that the brain changes in seconds. Connections within the brain are constantly being destroyed and rebuilt with every thought and action. If we keep sending the same signal, that path strengthens, creating a fast lane on a superhighway.

The classic neurology adage is "What fires together, wires together." The brain may be "temporarily broken," but it only stays broken if we believe it cannot change and keep feeding it the same message of hopelessness and brokenness. If we change the message, we change the pattern and we change the brain. If we continue to hear and believe the message that we are powerless to change our circumstances, we fail to see, let alone consider, other possibilities, just as we missed the gorilla walking by while focusing on the balls.

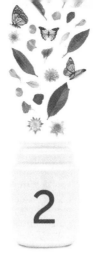

2

The Power of Placebo

The unfortunate reality is that current medications help too few people to get better and very few people to get well.

—DR. THOMAS INSEL, DIRECTOR OF THE
NATIONAL INSTITUTE OF MENTAL HEALTH

During World War II, anesthesiologist Henry Beecher became fascinated with the placebo effect after his clinic ran out of morphine and a nurse, preparing for surgery, confidently filled a syringe with saline water instead. After receiving the infusion of water, the injured soldier immediately calmed down and remained pain-free during the surgery. Although the Latin root of the word *placebo* means "to please," Beecher recognized the placebo had tangible benefits above and beyond pleasing the patient.

A compelling study by surgeon Bruce Moseley compared treatment protocols for osteoarthritis of the knee. Patients were randomly assigned to receive one of three procedures: surgical debridement, which involves cleaning out debris in the joint; surgical lavage, which rinses the knee joint with high-pressure water; or a sham surgery that involved cutting open the skin, simulating a surgery, and then suturing it back up. Follow-up care was the same for all three groups. These patients were followed for two years at periodic intervals to assess pain and function. The data demonstrated that "at no point" did either intervention group have "greater pain relief" or "improvement in function" than the placebo group. Amazingly, the group that received the sham surgery reported a greater ability to walk and climb stairs at two weeks, one year, and two years out, as compared to the group that received the costly standard treatment protocol of debridement. As you can see, "just" a placebo can be a powerfully effective healing tool.

Fears and negative suggestions also influence the body and brain, leading to a *nocebo* effect, from the Latin root meaning "I shall harm." My favorite nocebo case study illuminates the degree in which fear can shape our reality and physiology. In this story, a twenty-six-year-old male, referred to as Mr. A, entered a drug trial after being depressed for a couple of months following a break-up with his girlfriend. Mr. A started to feel better on the medication, but then got in an argument with his ex-girlfriend and impulsively swallowed the twenty-nine pills remaining in the bottle. Immediately regretting his decision, he called for help. Rushed to the hospital, he was documented as being drowsy, lethargic, and sweaty, with low blood pressure and an elevated heart rate. After four hours, a physician from the clinical trial arrived, and informed him and the hospital staff that the bottle contained "just" placebos. Mr. A was surprised, but relieved, and within fifteen minutes he was fully awake and alert, with normalized blood pressure and heart rate.

Researchers find both the placebo and nocebo effects pesky and messy, interfering with their data and results. Instead of trying to figure out what to do *about* the placebo effect, perhaps what we should be asking is what we can do *with* the placebo effect to facilitate healing, and what we can do to minimize the nocebo effect. When we offer hope, it is not just an act of support and kindness—it has healing properties. It is not inert; it is real, and it can be harnessed—not deceptively, but honestly.

A landmark study on patients with irritable bowel syndrome examined whether placebo would still work if patients knew it was a placebo. It turns out those knowingly given pills marked as placebos experienced the same degree of relief as those seen in the most effective medication trials.

I hope you can begin to see the immense potential of the placebo effect for activating the body's innate wisdom to facilitate healing. It works! Conversely, when we inform people that their brains or bodies are broken, that is exactly what happens.

What about Antidepressants

In the last chapter, we focused on the early antidepressants, the MAOIs and the TCAs, but psychiatry and our culture's perceptions about medications changed dramatically when Prozac arrived on the scene in 1988. Prozac was featured on the covers of *Newsweek* and *Time,* and ads appeared in everything from *Cosmopolitan* to *Reader's Digest.* The message? Depression "isn't just feeling down. It's a real illness with real causes," that "doctor's believe" may be caused by "an imbalance of serotonin in your body." The ads suggested that you did not need to be classically depressed and unable to function in order to benefit from medication, but merely "under the weather." It's safe. It's effective. Who wouldn't want to feel "better than well?" What could be more appealing than the possibility that happiness could be encapsulated within a once-a-day pill that could be taken with your morning coffee and newspaper?

Doctors were equally overjoyed, especially psychiatrists and overworked primary care physicians. When a patient cries while telling her doctor that she just broke up with her boyfriend, or her beloved dog died, or the overwhelmed mother complains of being tired, exhausted, and crabby because her husband "does nothing" to help out with the four kids and the dog—now there was finally something for your poor doctor to do to help, besides, you know, listening empathically and offering support. The marketing blitz to consumers and physicians paid off immensely. By 2006, antidepressants were the number-one prescribed medication in the country.

It did not take long for data to emerge that everything was not what it seemed in the Land of Happy Pills. Even though "educational" pamphlets passed out to patients in mental health clinics adamantly asserted the effectiveness of selective serotonin reuptake inhibitors (SSRIs), proclaiming, "Estimates are that eight or nine of every ten patients with depression can be helped by currently available antidepressants," the emerging data did not validate this lofty conclusion. In 1992 the first of many studies reviewing available data on the SSRIs was published. Roger Greenberg and colleagues analyzed twenty-two studies of antidepressant outcomes and found that although clinicians consistently reported significant effects, patient ratings showed no advantage for antidepressants beyond placebo effect. That is just one study and easy to dismiss, but plenty more followed.

In 1998 researcher Irving Kirsch thought depression and antidepressants might be a good place to investigate the placebo effect, since hopelessness is at the core of the "disease." He and his colleagues analyzed nineteen double-blind, placebo-controlled clinical trials involving over two thousand patients assigned to various antidepressants and other medications, including TCAs, SSRIs, benzodiazepines, lithium, thyroid medication, and barbiturates.

Shockingly, the data revealed that regardless of the type of drug and the mechanism of action, the placebo response accounted for 75 percent of the effect of all the medications. How could all these different medications have nearly identical effectiveness?

Kirsch pondered what all these medications might have in common. He could only come up with one answer—side effects. Nobody *wants* side effects, so why might they enhance the effectiveness of a medication? Imagine you are hopelessly depressed and enrolled in a placebo-controlled trial for a new antidepressant. Your hope is to get the real medication, not just the placebo. In theory, trials are blinded so that neither the participant nor the physician is aware of which pill one is receiving, yet studies have shown that doctors guess correctly whether a patient is on an active medication or placebo 87 percent of the time. Patients guess correctly 78 percent of the time. This means the idea of a truly blinded trial is more an ideal than a reality. Consequently, if you develop nausea, upset stomach, or another side effect, you are likely to assume that you are on the active medication. This boosts your hope for recovery, potentiating the placebo response.

Kirsch's findings led to another study, this time including 47 published and unpublished trials of antidepressants submitted by the pharmaceutical companies to the FDA. Obtaining all of the data is important, because many of the negative trials are buried in inaccessible archives and never submitted for publication, which leads to a vast overestimation of the effects of medications.

Based on this data, Kirsch found that the placebo effect accounted for 80 percent of the medication response and there was no clinical difference between the medication and placebo in terms of feeling better. The study also revealed that there was absolutely no additional improvement found at higher doses as compared to lower doses, contrary to current standard treatment practices in psychiatry. It wasn't just Kirsch getting these results. Other researchers, including those skeptical of Kirsch's results, conducted their own studies, arriving at the same conclusion.

You may be surprised to find out how little data is required to receive approval by the FDA. The agency requires only two controlled effectiveness trials showing a statistical advantage over placebo, and no obvious risk of harm. Drug companies can do as many trials as they want in order to find two successful trials. There is no need to show that the medication offers any clinical benefit. There is no need to study the long-term effects of a medication that someone may be prescribed for a lifetime. Most of the trials last only four to eight weeks.

Eli Lilly, for example, conducted eight studies on fluoxetine (Prozac) to get four with statistically significant results. GlaxoSmithKline (GSK) conducted nine trials for paroxetine (Paxil) to get two with positive results. Forest Laboratories submitted seven placebo-controlled clinical trials of citalopram (Celexa) to the FDA. Of those, three showed no advantage over placebo.

Based on these notably unimpressive results, as well as concerns about cardiac lethality observed in dog toxicology studies and carcinogenic effects in mice, Dr. Paul Leber, the director of the FDA Division of Neuropharmacological Drug Products, wrote a memorandum expressing concerns about the negligible advantage of citalopram over placebo. He stated, "While it is difficult to judge the clinical significance of this difference, similar findings for other SSRIs and other recently approved antidepressants have been considered sufficient to support the approvals of those other products."

So, based on the precedence of weak effectiveness data, and inadequately addressed safety data for other approved antidepressants, citalopram was added to the list, basically since it was no worse than the others.

You may imagine—and even hope—Kirsch's studies sparked a conversation. Although many psychiatrists clung to and continue to cling to their faith in medications despite the data, many researchers were unsurprised. One group of researchers wrote Kirsch, stating, "Many have been long unimpressed by the magnitude of the differences observed between treatments and controls, what some of our colleagues refer to as the 'dirty little secret' in the pharmaceutical literature."

Fortunately, science continues to ask questions and address concerns. Many critics suggested that perhaps Kirsch had not considered severity of depression; that possibly his studies had only been conducted on the mildly or moderately ill. To address this issue, Kirsch reanalyzed the data to examine the influence of severity of depressive symptoms on medication effectiveness. He discovered that, in fact, antidepressants offered no drug effect at all to those with mild to moderate depression, and only reached minor clinical significance in the most severe depressions.

How can this be? How can these drugs receive FDA approval without any meaningful benefit over a placebo? How can this information be hidden from the public and physicians?

A study published in the *New England Journal of Medicine* in 2008 offered some answers to these questions. For this review, data was once again obtained on all published and unpublished trials submitted to the FDA for the approval of twelve antidepressants. The study determined that basically half of the studies had positive results, while half were negative, meaning the drug performed no better and in some cases worse than the placebo—basically the flip of a coin. Here is where it gets interesting. Of the thirty-eight studies with positive results, all but one were published. Of the thirty-six negative trials, three were published that acknowledged the negative results; eleven were published with a positive spin, either entirely overlooking or majorly minimizing any negative data; and twenty-two studies were simply buried.

Furthermore, even in the positive studies, the effectiveness of the medications was magnified by about 30 percent in the journal articles, as compared to the actual results submitted to the FDA. This means that your physicians are getting misleading information. Ninety-four percent of the articles they might read are robustly positive, raving about the effectiveness of medications that have changed the face of mental health and the field of psychiatry. As the study's authors wrote, "Evidence-based medicine is valuable to the extent that the evidence is complete and unbiased."

One might imagine this article radically changed the prescribing habits of doctors everywhere. Unfortunately, no. I was in residency when this paper was published, and it was most definitely never mentioned, not even in a "Hey, you should at least be aware this is out there" kind of way. Maybe I am crazy, but this information seems incredibly important, and certainly helps explain the discrepancy between the actual data and the propaganda that is marketed as "research" to physicians and the public.

In 2009 the National Institute of Mental Health (NIMH) funded the largest study to date, evaluating effective treatment strategies for "real-world" patients, meaning complicated and messy ordinary people with multiple medical and physical complications. In most clinical trials these people are eliminated, as researchers opt instead for people with only one mental health diagnosis and limited physical issues. The goal of this six-year-long, $35 million Sequenced Treatment Alternatives to Relieve Depression (STAR*D) trial was to evaluate the management of TRD—meaning the majority of those who do not recover with only one antidepressant. Here was a chance for psychiatry to prove its value and the effectiveness of its standard treatment protocols.

The trial, true to real life, was biased toward medication management. All four thousand participants were initially started on citalopram. No controls were included in this trial, so it is impossible to know how placebo or therapy alone would have fared. It is easier to avoid asking questions that may lead to answers you are not prepared to accept.

The study was divided into four phases, followed by follow-up care for one year. Only one-quarter of patients recovered from depressive symptoms during the first twelve-week phase. Despite concerted efforts to keep people in the trial, including offers of free medications and $25 for showing up at appointments, another quarter dropped out in the first few weeks. In the next phases, those who did not recover were then randomly assigned to other treatment options, which included switching to other antidepressants or cognitive behavioral therapy (CBT).

The results? Regardless of the option chosen, only 12 percent recovered from depressive symptoms. Those getting therapy had the advantage of fewer side effects. What this means is that whether you provide therapy or literally any pill with any mechanism of action, the same percentage of people get better. The only thing all these treatments have in common is the offer of support and hope—this is the placebo effect in all its glory.

The results from the last phases of the trial were even bleaker. Ultimately, 92 percent of the patients who recovered in the first phase of the trial relapsed or dropped out within one year of continuing care, despite having access to the best care psychiatry could offer. The group that fared the best, but received the least publicity, were those receiving therapy. Only 8 percent of that group relapsed. Worse, it turned out that those who remained on medications, per official American Psychiatric Association recommendations, were *more* likely to relapse as compared to those who discontinued their medications. This suggests, as have other studies we will discuss in the next chapter, that these medications are not only minimally effective, but may actually worsen the outcome of depression. This data is depressing, but what is most disheartening is that the results have not changed prescribing patterns or medicine's delusional love affair with antidepressants.

The authors of the STAR*D trial chose to downplay the relative success of CBT. A few years later, however, another large trial, REVAMP, looked more closely at the possibility of augmenting medications with therapy for treatment resistant depression. In the study, twelve weeks of medication alone was compared to a combination of medication and CBT or medication and brief supportive therapy.

Once again, therapy-only or placebo-only options were not part of the study design, making inconvenient possibilities easier to avoid—the "don't ask, don't tell" policy for scientific research. The results, once again, found no difference in response rates regardless of treatment strategy. The paper emphasized that there was "no advantage" or "value" in augmenting with psychotherapy, ignoring the equal but opposite truth that medications offered no advantage over therapy in terms of effectiveness, yet resulted in many more short- and long-term side effects.

The value of combining medications to enhance depression outcomes, as is standard psychiatric practice, despite lack of evidence, was put to the test in the 2011 NIMH-funded CO-MED trial. Medication cocktails are the norm in psychiatry. Nearly 60 percent of patients are prescribed two medications in a typical psychiatric outpatient visit, while 33 percent are provided three or more. All too often I see patients who show up on five or more psychotropic medications. I once saw a patient who fell asleep several times during her initial evaluation. During one of Kathy's brief snoozes, I checked her medication list before waking her up. The list was a full page long and included multiple antidepressants, mood stabilizers, antipsychotics, benzodiazepines, narcotics, and sleep medications. How she opened her eyes and functioned at all is hard to imagine, yet none of her doctors had considered the impact all these medications were having on her body, her inability to function, her lack of energy, focus, and motivation, and her depressed mood.

In the CO-MED trial, just like in the STAR*D trial, it made absolutely no difference what medication or placebo combinations were offered; in each case, the same percentage of patients responded at twelve weeks and at seven months. What did differ was the risk of side effects—those on multiple meds suffered from more adverse events, just like Kathy.

Critics of the study suggested the doses of the medications had not been maximized, but when the numbers were reevaluated to look at those with the highest doses compared to those on lower doses, the results remained the same. The fact is that neither multiple medications nor higher doses offer any advantage, just a lot more side effects. Yet again, the profession of psychiatry chooses to ignore the evidence that does not fit into the preexisting dogmatic beliefs about what works and what does not. Polypharmacy remains standard practice.

What is amazing about all these studies is the consistency of the results. Study after study suggests that our "miracle" pills—whether prescribed alone or in combinations—offer negligible advantage over placebos, except in the most severe depressions. Countless studies point to the same conclusion. The drugs have no effect in mild to moderate depression and only reach significance in the very severe range. Yet over 70 percent of people started on these medications fall into the mild to moderate range.

The media heralded the most recent 2018 antidepressant meta-analysis with fanfare, declaring that the study offered conclusive proof that antidepressants work. The lead author, Dr. Andrea Cipriani, got caught up in the hype and stated to *Time* magazine: "We can say this is the final answer to the controversy." It is true the researchers spent six long years poring over published and unpublished data from 522 trials involving over 116,000 participants on twenty-one different antidepressants, yet the details boiled down to the same conclusions: antidepressants offer no clinical advantage except in the most severe depressions. Even the researchers acknowledged in the paper, if not to *Time* magazine, that the "certainty of evidence was moderate to very low," and that "estimates of treatment effect from our study are in line with previous reviews on the same matter." This is hardly radical or conclusive evidence proving these medications are highly effective, but merely more proof of their limited benefits and the power of propaganda to shift the story to a more positive narrative.

I could go on and on with countless other studies all pointing in the same direction. So, how can there be all this evidence that we simply ignore?

Let's step away from pharmacology and think about this simplistically for a moment. For my son's first science fair project, at age six, he wanted to determine the favorite food of his pet Red Niger *Uromastyx* lizard, named Tank. Wade's hypothesis was that Tank's favorite food was dandelions. Each day for a week Wade put different foods on a plate in different arrangements. Tank ate more peas than anything else, so Wade concluded peas must be Tank's favorite food.

Knowing Tank, we were all puzzled by this, because we have seen him nearly jump out of his cage to eat a dandelion. Later we realized that Tank only likes dandelions when they are bright, yellow, and fully opened. Yet Wade had done the experiment every morning before school, when the dandelions were still closed and brownish from their evening slumber. If he had done another experiment later in the day, the results would likely have been different. If he only published the data from the first experiment, positive for peas, and ignored the likely results from a second one, he would only have presented a piece of the story, and it would have been inaccurate.

Say we add another layer to this experiment. Let's imagine that the pea company sponsoring the costs of this experiment offers to pay Wade to continue his research on this topic. They even pay his way through college, offer him some educational trips to exciting locations, and give him all the chocolate and candy his sugar-craving heart desires. Even assuming Wade is a passionate, ethical scientist who seeks the truth over money, there is a good chance he might overlook other possibilities and explanations for the results, and keep doing the experiment in the same way, so that he continues to get more positive results that please the pea company, and that means more money from the pea company to conduct his experiments and buy more video games, books, and candy.

Now he's grown up, living in a nice house with a family of his own to support. One day Wade realizes what he has long suspected: maybe he missed a critical factor in his experiments. Maybe, in fact, the lizard not only prefers the free dandelions growing in his organic and pesticide-free backyard, but poor Tank is actually getting sick from the peas, which are not a natural part of a lizard's diet.

This not-so-young researcher now has a dilemma. To acknowledge that the previous results of his experiments were misleading and inaccurate could potentially mean not only losing his credibility in the research world but also his job, his house, his car, and security for his family. It might be easier to just ignore this "anomaly" and keep the information to himself.

Or perhaps he does come forward and, giving the pea company the benefit of the doubt, express his concerns about the information. Now the managers and executives of the pea company have a bigger, costlier dilemma. They too have families to support, and perhaps even bigger cars and houses to finance, thanks to their comfortable salaries. Now they too risk losing everything. It might be easier to just keep it quiet, until someone comes along who is willing to risk everything to expose the damage the peas are inflicting upon the health of the *Uromastyx.*

There is a good chance that out of fear, those who risk a change in status quo may go out of their way to discredit the whistleblower as a "crazy quack." Meanwhile, all this information is kept away from those in lower positions in the company. At the universities, herpetology professors continue to teach the dogma that peas are the food of choice for the *Uromastyx,* based on lack of any published information to the contrary. And the lizards continue to get sick.

With this elementary school illustration, I hope to demonstrate how easily one can get stuck in a particular way of seeing things and how multiple powerful forces work together to prop up the status quo. If my son chose to keep doing the experiments the way the pea companies requested, I cannot blame or judge him for choosing to buy more Pokémon cards and support his family, nor can I blame the pea company and their employees. My intent is not to *blame* anyone (well, maybe the executive of the pea company who had evidence from the very beginning that peas were harmful to lizards, and intentionally kept the information buried so that he could make his billions.) My hope, however, is to pull back the blinders so we can step out of the myopic, harmful reflex to solve every problem with a magical pea or pill, and be open enough to look at other possibilities.

In order to do that, however, we must recognize the consequences of blindly trusting the authorities and revered scientists of evidence-based medicine. We must see how money and power can distort the truth, and prevent contrary facts from reaching the pages of prestigious journals. We must understand how, even when these facts do reach the journals, the spin of marketing can dismiss and downplay them or point toward another collective villain so the truthful information gets ignored, overlooked, or forgotten.

Efficacy in Children and Adolescents

For a moment, let's step away from the adult and lizard world and look at the effectiveness of medications on the pediatric population, as many of you may have or know kids struggling with depression. Over two million kids are on antidepressants, even though two-thirds of all antidepressant trials have failed to show any effectiveness in this vulnerable population. The two most recent meta-analyses revealed that antidepressants offer little to no benefit. A 2016 review that included fourteen antidepressants and over five thousand children and adolescents demonstrated that of all these medications, only fluoxetine "*might* reduce depressive symptoms." The rest of the medications had no advantage over placebo whatsoever.

A 2017 review determined that none of the antidepressants offered any advantage over placebo, yet it found increased suicidality and side effects. Based on the benefits and risks of the medication, the reviewers concluded that therapy and other treatment modalities should be offered instead.

Unfortunately it is difficult to obtain data from pharmaceutical companies, and the printed data is often misleading. A 2004 review found that in every case, when only published data was examined, the medications appear to be minimally effective, but when unpublished data—at least what's accessible—is added to the mix, only fluoxetine has consistently shown any advantage over placebo.

How are over two million children being prescribed medications that appear to have limited to no benefit? Here is just one illustrative peek into exactly how this can happen. GSK conducted three clinical trials of paroxetine on children and adolescents in a failed attempt to get FDA approval for prescribing to this population. Of the three trials, one showed a mixed result, one showed that the placebo group did better than the medication group, and the last found no difference between paroxetine and placebo. This complete lack of effectiveness did not deter GSK from getting the largest of these trials published, to look as if it was an effective medication choice for children.

The trial, Study 329, was peer-reviewed and published in 2001 in the *Journal of the American Academy of Child and Adolescent Psychiatry* (JAACAP), the primary journal read by pediatric psychiatrists. Study 329 was lauded as being the largest trial on the use of SSRIs in the pediatric population, and it concluded that paroxetine is "generally well tolerated and effective for major depression in adolescents."

This is what your psychiatrist likely read or was informed about at a paid dinner, lunch, or spa program for physicians. Your pediatrician was likely informed of paroxetine's "remarkable efficacy and safety" by their helpful GSK pharma representative. Thanks to the marketing blitz, Paxil became the number one antidepressant prescribed in the United States, with sales of $340 million by the end of 2001.

The assertion that paroxetine is safe and effective is one of the most cited claims supporting the use of antidepressants in youth. The problem with this statement is that it is utterly untrue. The primary outcome measures the researchers intended to use all showed that paroxetine was no more effective than placebo. No worries; the simple way to resolve that problem? Create new outcomes that can be shown to be positive, and delete the negative outcomes from the article. Voilà! A successful study.

We only know about this evidence of "data torturing" because an internal memo from GSK was leaked to the *Canadian Medical Association Journal.* In the memo, the staff at GSK were cautioned to "effectively manage the dissemination of these data in order to minimize any potential negative commercial bias."

This sleight of hand is the norm in pharmaceutical research. One study found that the majority of trials shifted their primary outcomes to make the results appear more positive, and at least 35 percent of adverse events fail to get reported.

Why would physicians and researchers be willing to stake their reputations on false data? Just like the example of my son promoting peas instead of dandelions, 79 percent of the meta-analyses between 2007 and 2014 were written by authors paid by the drug companies. These "studies" were twenty-two times less likely to include any negative statements about the medications being evaluated. Short of accessing all the data (good luck with that one—it can take years, and even then, you are unlikely to get all of it), how is one to sort through all the bias in so-called evidence-based medicine?

A year after Study 329 was published, the FDA reviewed the data from the trial and concluded that "this trial should be considered as a failed trial." Yet, that same year, two million more prescriptions for paroxetine were written for youth in the United States alone, based on GSK's successful marketing campaign. In 2003, the FDA officially recommended that paroxetine not be used for children and adolescents with depression.

Three years after the paper's publication, a civil lawsuit for consumer fraud was filed against GSK that resulted in a $2.5 million fine and a requirement to post all study results on GSK's website. In 2012, the U.S. Department of Justice filed suit for submitting fraudulent information to Medicare and Medicaid. GSK pleaded guilty and paid a fine of $3 billion. Yet despite all of this, the number of prescriptions written actually increased by 3 percent.

Just as we saw with the neurochemical imbalance theory, if information gets repeated often enough, it gets accepted as fact, regardless of its accuracy. I completed my child psychiatry rotation several years after the FDA recommended against prescribing these medications to children. Once again, this information was never brought to my attention. Instead, my preceptor told me that paroxetine was the best choice for children with anxiety and depression. Although he did quiz me on which medications were FDA approved for depression, the fact that paroxetine was not on this list made no difference.

The fact that there was zero evidence for using paroxetine, and that there was an FDA statement against using it, made no difference.

This was partially because, despite the lawsuits and fines, the journal in which the article was published never retracted or corrected the article. The article remains accessible and citable as evidence for the use of antidepressants in this population. The lead author, Dr. Martin Keller, is the chief psychiatrist at Brown University and he was never disciplined or investigated in any way. In fact, he went on to be honored by Reuters in 2014 and 2015 as one of the "World's Most Influential Scientific Minds," because his papers are among the top 1 percent most cited by other research articles. The American Academy of Child and Adolescent Psychiatry (AACAP) also remained silent on the issue.

This may seem curious, as one would hope the health and well-being of youth might be their top concern, but things get murky when the organization receives $500,000 to $1 million a year from pharmaceutical companies. In fact, one of Study 329's coauthors, Dr. Karen Wagner, remains president of the AACAP as of 2019. The editor of JAACAP at the time of the publication, Dr. Andrés Martin, who has remained silent and unapologetic about the controversy, is also on the executive committee of the AACAP.

Meanwhile, millions of kids continue to be prescribed medications that evidence demonstrates do not work, and, as we will see in the next chapter, place youth at risk of serious harm.

I hope this glimpse into the secret workings of the pharmaceutical companies, the FDA, psychiatrists, and their organizations helps you to understand why the data we hear from our doctors is not necessarily factual. It is not because they are trying to lie or harm anyone, or because they are negligent in keeping up to date on the evidence. The powers at the top prevent accurate, accessible information from trickling down to the rest of us. Even when the evidence does become available, as in Study 329, or when lies get exposed, like in the memo leaked to the *Canadian Medical Association Journal,* there is such a deep abiding belief in the power of medications, and the stories that get repeated as facts, that any data to the contrary gets overlooked or denied. We are so busy counting balls that we fail to notice the gorilla walking in front of us.

3

The Cost of a Quick Fix

First, do no harm.

—HIPPOCRATES

Cheerful pharmaceutical reps bearing free food and sample medications, and happy people on pharmaceutical commercials, have lulled us all into believing medications can solve every problem. We are so busy paying attention to the soothing music, puppy dogs, cute kids, and beautiful smiling women in the commercials that we ignore the long, rapidly read list of potential side effects listed at the end of the commercials. Yet nearly a third of all drugs approved by the FDA between 2001 and 2010 were later determined to have significant safety issues, leading to a boxed warning or withdrawal from the marketplace. Worse, it took on average five years or longer before those safety issues were acknowledged and addressed.

Given the popularity of antidepressants, one might assume most people avoid side effects. Yet, depending on which study you look at, 60 to 84 percent of patients report the more common side effects, including nausea, stomach complaints, insomnia, forgetfulness, difficulty concentrating, fatigue, head-ache, dizziness, increased anxiety, dry mouth, sweating, changes in weight, and sexual dysfunction. Yet the average physician spends only 36 to 42 seconds discussing risks of commonly prescribed medications. Most of their valuable time is spent trying to convince you why you should take a pill.

For those who have been on medications for over three years, more severe side effects are often experienced, including 70 percent reporting moderate to severe withdrawal effects, sexual difficulties, weight gain, and feeling emotionally numb. Chronic use of the medications is associated with reduction in bone density and increased risk of fractures, increased risk for bleeding and strokes, a lowered seizure threshold, disruption of sleep architecture, and irreversible liver damage.

Nearly half of patients prescribed antidepressants discontinue them due to complaints of side effects or lack of effectiveness within three months. Three-quarters will discontinue within six months. A third will not tell their physicians they have discontinued. Of those who do inform their doctors of issues, many will be started on additional medications to manage the side effects of the first medication.

In fact, many antidepressant trials preventively put patients on sedatives to manage anxiety and other side effects from the antidepressant being tested. This is somehow an acceptable protocol, even though this information and other adverse consequences of the medications—including the majority of deaths and suicides—are partially or completely missing in 79 percent of journal articles and FDA reviews. You can be certain this data is not mentioned by the "informative and helpful" pharmaceutical representative offering free samples and coffee to your physician.

Sexual Dysfunction

To get a sense of how side effects get minimized or overlooked in trials, let's look at the stats on sexual dysfunction. This is tricky to sort out, because depression itself also leads to sexual dysfunction, and many of the other side effects commonly experienced on the medications. Without asking questions before and after starting a medication, it is difficult to determine the cause of side effects. Drug trials prefer to rely on voluntary reports about side effects instead of asking questions or providing a simple questionnaire. Yet how many patients are going to bring up sexual issues to their prescriber in a short visit? Besides, the participant may not attribute this or other issues to the drug, but rather to the depression or one's own inadequacy (also attributed to depression). Plus, many side effects do not show up for weeks after starting a medication, so it is unclear whether it is related to the medication or a new, unrelated problem.

How data is collected influences the results you will find. When a sexual dysfunction questionnaire is used to assess function before and after starting medication, data consistently shows that 75 to 90 percent of those on antidepressants experience sexual dysfunction caused by the medication. These results are drastically different from the statistics that arise when waiting for a voluntary, unsolicited report. It would seem that if drug trials are truly meant to ensure the public's safety, extensive side effect questionnaires should be required, and that information should be mandatorily included in the journal articles your physician might read.

Weight Gain and Diabetes

Weight gain is another example of a commonly overlooked side effect in antidepressants that few people are told about, and it is usually left out of the happy-go-lucky antidepressant commercials. How much weight, after all, can one gain in a standard four- to six-week trial? Some SSRIs actually lead to weight loss over the first few weeks, and then that weight and more is slowly regained and added on over time. Many doctors will blame the weight gain on the patient, not the drug. Yet 65 percent of studies have shown weight gain, sometimes by as much as fifteen to twenty-four pounds over six months to one year's time, depending on the specific medication.

A 2018 study found that antidepressants increased the risk of significant weight gain by 21 percent. Multiple studies have also shown that long-term use of these medications nearly doubles the risk of diabetes. More disturbing is the fact that this risk appears to be greatest in those under forty years old. Given that obesity, diabetes, and depression are intricately linked and lead to poorer health outcomes, I am not sure how adding twenty pounds helps with one's sense of health, energy, self-esteem, or recovery from depression.

Birth Defects

Women of childbearing age, the population most likely to be started on these medications, also happen to be one of the groups at highest risk of unintended consequences. For many women, by the time they know they are pregnant and tell their doctors, the critical moments of embryonic development, for which serotonin plays an essential role, have already passed. Too few doctors take the time to adequately address these concerns and offer safer alternatives before a potential pregnancy.

As you might imagine, the issue of potential birth defects is highly controversial, with a lot more concerns and questions than answers. Most SSRIs are considered category C drugs, which means that animal studies have shown potential harm, but there is still insufficient data to conclusively show potential damage to the human fetus. In 2005, the FDA mandated that paroxetine carry a category D rating, which means positive evidence of fetal risk does exist. In 2010, GSK, the maker of paroxetine, settled approximately eight hundred birth-defect lawsuits for $1.14 billion.

Zoloft's maker has faced allegations of covering up data linking its use with heart defects. As you might imagine, there are a multitude of variables involved in a healthy fetus and pregnancy, so it takes time, transparency, and access to data to accumulate enough evidence to confirm a link—not exactly standard practice for Big Pharma. So, while the results of studies remain inconclusive, 14 percent of pregnant women, and their offspring, continue to act as human guinea pigs while being assured the risk is negligible.

If you are a woman of childbearing age, here are a few studies to consider. A 2017 study examined the influence of antidepressants on fetal malformations in over eighteen thousand depressed women in Quebec. The researchers concluded that antidepressants increased the risk of potential fetal malformations. This was especially true of Celexa, which significantly increased the risk for musculoskeletal and cranial malformations. Consistent with prior studies, they found that paroxetine increased the risk of heart defects, and venlafaxine was associated with an increased risk of respiratory defects.

A 2015 study by the Centers for Disease Control and Prevention (CDC) assessed twelve years of available data, and concluded that birth defects occur 2 to 3.5 times more frequently among newborns of women treated with paroxetine and Prozac early in pregnancy. The study also confirmed links between Prozac and fetal heart and skull defects. With paroxetine they found links with brain, heart, and gut malformations. True, the risk remains statistically small, but when it is your child and not just a general statistic, is that a risk worth taking for negligible benefits when safer options exist?

One of the more common but significant risks is the potential of persistent pulmonary hypertension of the newborn (PPHN). This lengthy medical diagnosis basically means that the baby's blood continues to bypass the lungs after birth, as it had while in the womb, depriving the baby of oxygen. This is obviously no trivial matter. The link between antidepressant use during the third trimester and PPHN is strong enough that the FDA issued a public health advisory in 2006. Unfortunately, that warning got retracted in 2011, after another study questioned the link. More recent papers, however, found additional evidence confirming an association between taking antidepressants during the last trimester of pregnancy and a significantly increased risk of PPHN. But the FDA has yet to reinstate the warning.

Although far less serious, 20 to 30 percent of babies born to mothers taking antidepressants suffer from withdrawal effects, including agitation, abnormal muscle tone, insomnia, diarrhea, vomiting, and tremors. This is probably not how most of us imagine our baby entering the world. Bringing home an irritable baby with difficulty sleeping is unlikely to improve mom's sense of well-being—as if having a newborn isn't exhausting enough.

One of the most controversial topics around the use of antidepressants in pregnant women is the potential for increased risk of autism. A 2016 study gathered data from 150,000 Canadian pregnancies and found a startling 87 percent increased risk for autism associated with the use of all SSRIs during the second or third trimesters of pregnancy—even when taking into account a maternal history of depression. Even more shockingly, they found a 200 percent increased risk for women on Zoloft or paroxetine. Psychiatrists are quick to assure women that despite this data, the overall risk remains small, so there is no need for concern.

A 2017 meta-review of six meta-analyses sought to review the findings on this controversial topic. The results were remarkably consistent. All six studies found a significantly increased risk, although all but one acknowledged that the mother's mental illness might be the causal factor, not the medications. This familiar refrain is particularly (and conveniently) hard to disprove. It would be interesting to look at data comparing women with depression on antidepressants versus women receiving only therapy—both groups of depressed women utilizing different treatment options.

Anxiety and Akathisia

One of the more common side effects is increased anxiety. Documents disclosed during litigation reveal that Eli Lilly's own data showed that 38 percent of those given fluoxetine developed activation symptoms of anxiety, irritability, and inner restlessness, as compared to 19 percent on placebo. These high statistics do not account for the fact that many participants were given sedatives to subdue these symptoms. For some, this is just a slight, temporary exacerbation. But for those suffering from akathisia, the intense anxiety feels like an unbearable inner restlessness and agitation—kind of like having a horrible itch on the bottom of your foot that cannot be relieved. Only in this case, the itch is internal and everywhere, and you feel like you want to crawl out of your skin to escape yourself and this relentless turmoil. All too often these symptoms are mistaken for an exacerbation of the depression itself, and doses are increased or other medications are added, worsening the situation.

For some, this experience can lead to suicidal ideation or impulsive behaviors like cutting, or even violence. I know of one older woman who started taking an antidepressant after expressing sadness to her physician about her daughter's cancer diagnosis. Although she had no prior history of cutting or suicidal thoughts, a few days after starting the new medication, the woman cut her wrist so severely that she required surgery to repair damage to the severed ligaments. The medication turned a woman with no previous suicidal thoughts into a threat to herself, all because she expressed normal emotions that anyone would feel under similar circumstances.

Mania

One of the extreme ends of anxiety and activation is the development of mania, an excessively euphoric or irritable mood state, which may be accompanied by a decreased need for sleep, grandiosity, racing thoughts, frenetic activity, and sometimes dangerous impulsivity. In commercials, this is obliquely referenced with the statement: "Tell your doctor right away if you have changes in behavior." This is code for possible anxiety, agitation, panic attacks, insomnia, irritability, hostility, aggression, suicidality, impulsivity, and even mania. (This is straight from Paxil's packaging insert.) Although mania is listed on the labels of all antidepressants, this side effect is rarely mentioned by prescribers.

Paxil's label states that the medicine may induce mania in 1 percent of depressed patients and over 2 percent of "bipolar" patients (who may well have once been depressed patients given an antidepressant who developed mania and were then labeled as bipolar). Instead of attributing the mania to the medicine, it is cleverly reasoned that the patient must have had an underlying bipolar tendency brought to light by the medications. By this logic, people who develop a life-threatening rash from lamotrigine, or an anaphylactic reaction to an antibiotic (or even peanuts), or kidney failure from lithium, should be grateful that the medication has gratuitously brought to their attention their underlying skin, allergy, or kidney pathologies.

This raises the question: how many of the people diagnosed with bipolar disorders in this country are actually suffering from iatrogenic effects of the medications intended to heal their depression? In one study, evaluating five hundred psychiatric admissions over a fourteen-month time frame, researchers found that 8 percent of admissions were likely due to antidepressant-induced mania, with SSRIs accounting for 70 percent of those.

According to a study on the worldwide prevalence of bipolar disorders, 4.4 percent of Americans are labeled with this diagnosis, which is by far the highest rate among eleven countries surveyed. Are our treatments creating greater pathology for a subset of the population? This possibility is a question that urgently needs to be addressed.

Suicidality

In residency I was taught to tell parents, who were rightly concerned about the FDA warning of increased suicide risk for children and adolescents, that depression can lead to suicidal ideation and medications are needed and would help. The argument continued that "before the depressive symptoms disappear, your child may start to feel more energized. As the child is recovering, thanks to our effective intervention, your child may be at increased risk for this brief window of time, but we will be extra vigilant."

I don't know about you, but as a parent, my biggest fear for a depressed child would be the risk of self-harm or suicide. Depression passes with time. Suicide does not. Yet the data is quite clear for children, adolescents, and young adults up to at least the age of twenty-four: the medications double the risk of suicidality and aggression. The risk for adults remains controversial and less definitive, but the data suggests an increased risk for adults as well. What is clearest, and most troubling, is that pharmaceutical companies have known about this risk and attempted to bury it from the very beginning.

A disturbing article that appeared back in 1999 in the *Guardian* detailed some of the history and evidence of this risk. The article gathered many of the memos and documents released during litigation. To deal with the significant agitation and restlessness reported by a remarkable number of adult participants, the company started using sedatives in the trials to prevent this side effect. They removed patients with akathisia and suicidal ideations from the data. In fact, the use of the word *suicide* was not even allowed in the data. Instead Eli Lilly, and other companies since, set about cleverly coding with less threatening words like "overdose," "worsening depression," "emotional lability," or even "elevated liver enzymes" to indicate an intentional overdose of acetaminophen.

To ease concerns, Eli Lilly offered to conduct a meta-analysis—using one of their own scientists. Mind you, internal documents confirm that they were already well aware of this link a decade before the medication was released to the public. They had already conducted a meta-analysis comparing the rates of suicidality for those on fluoxetine and placebo and found the rates for those on fluoxetine were three to six times higher. This basically confirmed the facts that the new meta-analysis was designed to refute.

So what did Eli Lilly find in their new meta-analysis designed to alleviate inflated concerns about the safety of their product for children and adults? Although they had 27,000 patients involved in their drug trials, they only used the data set from 3,065 of those patients, a practice known as "cherry-picking." They excluded the 5 percent of patients with severe akathisia and 13 documented suicides. They also failed to mention that a large number of patients required sedatives to eliminate the potentially suicide-inducing akathisia they were trying to prove was not occurring. On the basis of this deeply flawed (dare I say fraudulent?) "research," the FDA determined there was "no credible evidence of a causal link" between the medications and suicidal behavior and thus no need for a warning label.

Other research, notably not conducted by Eli Lilly, revealed disturbing findings. One study found a four- to sixfold increase in risk of self-harm on fluoxetine. An interesting case study done at Harvard University in 1990 evaluated six patients with a history of depression who all became violently suicidal on Prozac. The suicidal thoughts began within days to weeks of starting or increasing the dose of the drug. "Coincidentally," in all six cases, the thoughts vanished upon stopping the drug.

A 1995 study in the United Kingdom compared suicide rates among individuals taking various antidepressants. They found a 3.5-fold greater risk of suicidality for those on SSRIs. A particularly frightening study reviewing all the deaths in the state of Maryland that had detected antidepressants in the blood at the time of death found that fluoxetine led to a threefold increase in violent suicides.

Although I have largely focused on fluoxetine here, primarily since it led the pack as the first of the SSRIs, the risk is increased in other SSRIs as well as serotonin and norepinephrine reuptake inhibitors (SNRIs). Multiple other studies continue to show increased risk among both the young and the old on medication. An interesting study examining high-risk periods for veterans being treated for depression found that the highest-risk period for suicide was, not surprisingly, after being released from the hospital, but the second period of greatest risk was after starting a new antidepressant. For the first four months, the risk of suicide was doubled—just like it is in the younger populations.

These days, all antidepressant packaging inserts, and even letters from pharmaceutical companies to prescribers, acknowledge a potentially increased risk for suicide for all patients. Somehow, though, this issue remains clouded in controversy and mixed messages.

Remember Study 329? The one that promoted paroxetine as "remarkably efficacious and safe" in the treatment of adolescent depression, even though they failed to get any positive data on the primary outcomes they were trying to test? This same paper noted a bothersome headache in one child as the only adverse event from the trial.

To be fair, the lead researcher, hired by GSK, did write in an earlier draft that "worsening depression, emotional lability, headache, and hostility were considered related or possibly related to treatment," but that section was removed from the final draft by the marketing department. In actuality, when the data was later reviewed by an outside researcher, those on the drug experienced a fivefold increased risk for suicidal events, a sixfold increase in gastrointestinal symptoms, and a fivefold increase in other psychiatric symptoms. All these extra "events" were carefully coded under different headings, simply not transcribed in the database, or filtered through clever statistics and shifting of outcomes. The stories go on and on.

You may wonder why the FDA does not inform physicians and parents that SSRIs double their child's risk of suicidality, and that Effexor increases that risk as much as ninefold over those taking a placebo. This seems like the very reason for the FDA's existence. Yet three-quarters of the agency's budget is funded by the very companies it is supposed to be overseeing. Between 1992 and 2016, Big Pharma contributed $7.67 billion to the FDA. In other words, the FDA's allegiance is, first and foremost, to their funders, and secondarily to the public they are hired to protect.

As a parent, and a psychiatrist, this horrifying information has and will continue to change my prescribing practices. I can think of no feasible reason for starting any kid on these drugs, and very few good reasons for adults either.

Treatment Resistance and Chronicity

So far, we have addressed the many short-term risks of taking antidepressants, but what do we know about the long-term consequences? Antidepressants disrupt our neurochemical balance throughout the body and numb the emotions. Is it possible that these factors may lead to a chronic state of low-grade depression, the very symptoms that propel so many people to start medication in the first place? The possibility that so-called antidepressants may act over time as pro-depressants, creating a treatment-resistant chronic state of depression, was first raised back in the early 1990s. Since then, a growing body of evidence has accumulated suggesting the medications themselves are leading to an epidemic of treatment-resistant depression (TRD).

In the early 1990s, TRD was reported in only about 10 to 15 percent of patients, compared to 40 percent in 2006. Prior to the advent of antidepressants, the vast majority of those with depression recovered without treatment and never experienced another episode. In fact, in 1964, Jonathan Cole at the NIMH wrote, "Depression is, on the whole, one of the psychiatric conditions with the best prognosis for eventual recovery with or without treatment. Most depressions are self-limited." Another researcher at the NIMH in the 1970s concurred, declaring that most episodes of depression "would run their course and terminate with virtually complete recovery without specific intervention." Today, however, depression is an entirely different beast. It is now considered a chronic disease with frequent relapses, despite a lifetime of treatment. So, what has changed?

The literature suggests that many people who may have an initial response to medications (or at least a robust placebo response attributed to the medications) over time become "treatment resistant"—a name that places the blame on the person and the depression. These people often tell me that their initial medication worked fabulously, pulling them out of dark hopelessness and despair almost instantly. Yet over time the medication "pooped out," requiring higher doses due to growing tolerance, and then "stopped working entirely." Since then, they describe living in a chronic state of low-grade depression that never goes away, constantly seeking that new miracle cure that will offer them the first medication's initial relief. They fear they are incapable of functioning without a medication to support them.

The good news is that a slow and gradual discontinuation of the medications often results in improvement. But the road off medications can be treacherous, as one is finally forced to face not only the emotions and lifestyle adjustments so long avoided, but also withdrawal symptoms. Many get scared and go back on the medications, only to be trapped by an increasingly intractable disease. Those who face the journey, however, find themselves reconnected with their emotions, their bodies, themselves, their loved ones, and the world around them.

A 2018 study followed a group of depressed people over a period of thirty years. They found that at all ages, and all points in time, regardless of the severity of the depression, those who remained on antidepressants had an 81 percent greater risk of having a severe illness at the five-year follow-up appointment than those who never started or discontinued the medications.

This is not breaking news. A World Health Organization study in 1998 examined the outcomes of depressed patients in fifteen cities around the world and found that those not on medications fared better. A 2004 study compared the frequency and duration of depressive symptoms among those on antidepressants versus those who were not. Those on medications over the previous year reported three times the number of new and longer episodes as compared to those not on drugs.

The even more dismal STAR*D study examined the outcomes of "real-life" outpatients with depression in a community setting for a year. This study compared those receiving treatment as usual (a basic ten-minute medication check) with the best modern psychiatry has to offer—the best doctors and resources. The results? In both groups nearly 97 percent of participants relapsed over the course of one year, despite having access to allegedly top-notch treatment. The good news is the standard of care in this country does not have any worse results than the best of care, which at least makes treatment of depression fair for all.

The researchers offered many possibilities for these lackluster results: poor compliance, not enough follow-up appointments, and a high proportion of socioeconomically disadvantaged patients. Near the end of the paper, they did acknowledge "psychotherapy was largely unavailable," suggesting, although not outright saying, that therapy may offer more than the best of psychiatric treatments. Nowhere in the discussion was the possibility raised that perhaps the medications themselves were leading to the poor outcomes.

In another study, researchers compared the naturalistic course of depression without medications to those on medications over a period of fifteen years. Eighty-five percent recovered spontaneously, without medications, within one year. The average time to recovery for the group started on medications was nearly twice as long as those not started on medication. The paper concluded that with an 85 percent recovery rate among the unmedicated, "it would be extremely difficult for any intervention to demonstrate a superior result to this."

Obviously, it can be argued that the group seeking medications may have suffered from more severe depression, yet other studies taking this into account arrived at the same conclusion. It is actually spooky how consistent the results are, yet they continue to be ignored since they do not conform with what we expect to see.

I could go on and on with other research pointing to the same conclusions, but I hope at this point you get the picture. It is clear from the data that the medications are not only failing to provide sustained benefits, but worse, they may be exacerbating the course of depression, changing it from an acute problem to an intractable, chronic one.

Scant research has been done on *why* this might be the case. As we saw in chapter 1, there is no evidence for depression being caused by a specific neurochemical imbalance, yet the medications induce a shift in this intricate balance and complex dance. Our bodies are designed to maintain homeostasis, so in the face of a force shifting our neurochemistry differently, the body will attempt to restore order. Research by evolutionary biologist Paul Andrews found that SSRIs may increase levels of serotonin four-hundred-fold within minutes to hours. The body is designed to compensate for this unnatural disruption by decreasing the synthesis of serotonin and reducing the firing of neurons in an attempt to restore equilibrium. After evaluating forty-six antidepressant studies, Andrews found not only that the risk of relapse was higher for those on medications than those on placebo, but the risk of relapse correlated with the degree in which the medications shifted the neurochemistry. In other words, the greater the disturbance to the system, the greater the risk of relapse.

Withdrawal

Few physicians mention the possibility of withdrawal symptoms that the majority of patients experience coming off their medications. All too often physicians dismiss these symptoms as just histrionics, or worse, attribute the symptoms to returning depressive symptoms. They may even blame the patient for defying medical advice and trying to live life without the medications—again, that reminder: you are broken and unfixable. Yet research demonstrates that these symptoms are the norm, not the exception, and cannot be written off as "craziness."

A recent study found that three-quarters of those who chose to taper off their medications experienced withdrawal symptoms; half of those were severe. The majority of patients required more than six months to complete the taper. Only 7 percent successfully discontinued in a shorter time frame. For a subset of people, weaning off medications can lead to debilitating symptoms that persist for months to years. Although all antidepressants can have this effect, Paxil, Effexor, and Cymbalta lead the pack in terms of severity.

The symptoms of withdrawal include depressed mood, irritability, anxiety, agitation, dizziness, cognitive difficulties, flu-like symptoms, electric shock sensations, tinnitus, diarrhea, constipation, confusion, headache, lethargy, emotional lability, insomnia, hypomania, "anger attacks," nightmares, muscle aches, and stiffness. But don't take my word for it; just check the insert of your antidepressant. Or check the Discontinuation Emergent Signs and Symptoms (DESS) checklist, developed in 1998 to track the forty-three possible symptoms that commonly arise upon discontinuing these drugs—despite assurances this does not actually happen. The insert advice is to taper slowly, and if symptoms continue, to simply go back on the medication. It sounds benign enough, but if you are suffering from symptoms that return with greater intensity than when you first initiated the medication, or new symptoms emerge during the taper, it is anything but harmless. It is a great business model, though, to market medications that are so difficult to get off that many people go back on them and, out of fear of experiencing the symptoms again, stay on them forever.

If you are reading this and already on medication, do not despair. In some respects, the survey on discontinuing psychiatric medications was highly encouraging and hopeful. Despite the emotional and physical challenges of getting off the medication, 82 percent were grateful for having done so. I continuously remind my dubious patients of this fact, as they suffer through the often-uncomfortable withdrawal process.

Since the reality of withdrawal symptoms is still contested by many physicians, it is no surprise that there is little research on how best to taper. Although some people can get off their medications within a few weeks, often the process can take months and even years. There is no one set path. Each patient must go at their own pace and comfort level, or fear will likely sabotage the process. My goal is always to return power to those who have been disempowered by the medical system.

The health-care system desperately needs safe, supportive spaces and understanding prescribers who can support the withdrawal process. Although we may be far from that reality here, in the Netherlands, the Ministry of Health, Welfare and Sport has created medication-free treatment wards where patients can be supported in coming off drugs. I hope someday we will have that same option in the United States. Meanwhile, all the tools we will learn later in the book to help with preventing and healing depression will also help manage withdrawal symptoms that may arise.

Emotional Numbing

"I feel numb," "I don't feel like myself," "I don't care about anything anymore," "I feel like a zombie" are phrases I hear repeated frequently. This disconnection from one's emotions and sense of self are one of the primary reasons patients come to me, desperate to get off their medications. People have told me they could not even cry at their mother's funeral, or feel joy at their daughter's wedding. A friend described how, for the week her seven-year-old daughter was on an antidepressant for anxiety, her daughter's previously colorful, creative drawings became just black and white. She literally lost the color in her young, formerly vibrant life.

Data about patients' experiences on antidepressants reflect similar results and sentiments. In a 2016 survey, not only did a third of respondents continue to feel moderately to severely depressed with suicidal thoughts, despite the medications, but the vast majority reported feeling "emotionally numb" and "not like myself." Feelings of indifference, emotional detachment, personality changes, and dampening of both positive and negative emotions were expressed by the majority of those on medications.

Emotions are an essential part of our being and understanding of the world around us. They act as messengers alerting us to what needs to be changed in our lives, and remind us what nourishes and enlivens us. To lose connection with our emotions is to lose contact with ourselves, the people we love, and life itself. This ability to connect is exactly what medications take from us. Instead of learning how to listen and respond to emotions, we learn to avoid and fear them. We become unmotivated, disempowered, disconnected, and dependent. The good news, as we will see in the second half of this book, is that it is never too late to find another path, to learn a different way of reacting and responding to emotions. It is never too late to change the narrative and reclaim our power and well-being.

Additional Risks

I want to point out just a few more significant concerns to consider when weighing the risks against possible benefits. Researchers have noted increased cardiovascular risks, including changes in heart rhythm, especially for older populations; in 2011 the FDA noted that this can be fatal. The medications also appear to decrease heart rate variability (HRV), which is not only a risk factor for cardiovascular disease, but also associated with worsening depression and anxiety—perhaps partially explaining the worsening outcomes for those on medications.

Though studies have been inconclusive, antidepressants may have carcinogenic effects for humans. In animal studies, over 70 percent of psychotropic drugs showed carcinogenicity, and a 2011 meta-analysis of sixty-one studies found an overall 11 percent increased risk of breast and ovarian cancer, with SSRIs showing greater risk than tricyclics. Additionally, antidepressants are linked to mental slowing and increased forgetfulness. One study looking at the risk of motor vehicle accidents before, during, and after the use of antidepressants found that use of medications beyond four weeks was associated with an increased risk of accident. This risk returned to baseline only after six months off the medication. Another study found a "robust association" between some strongly anticholinergic antidepressants like Paxil and the tricyclics and the risk of dementia, even twenty years after exposure. The risk increased with length of exposure.

Empowering Choices

By this point you may well be feeling overwhelmed by all the information and data. My goal in this chapter is not to add to your anxiety and stress, but to educate and empower you, so that you can make wise choices for your health and well-being based on facts. If you feel medications are interfering with living your life to your fullest capacity, and may be causing more harm than good, my hope is that this data validates your intuition and offers you information and support to seek another path.

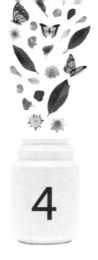

Getting to the Roots

To heal you have to get to the root of the wound and kiss it all the way up.

—RUPI KAUR, *THE SUN AND HER FLOWERS*

If depression is not a genetically based neurochemical imbalance fixable with antidepressants, then what exactly *is* depression? Sometimes what we call "depression" is really an emotional messenger at first whispering, then screaming, that we are stuck in situations not serving us, and what we need is not a medication but a change. Sometimes that change can be as simple as having someone to talk to so we don't feel so alone, or perhaps taking a new class or setting aside the endless to-do lists and adding moments of joy to your day. Other times, however, the change required might be more drastic. Maybe our body is calling for exercise and less time sitting in front of the TV. Maybe we need a new hobby, a new group of friends, or a new job. Maybe we need to escape our computers and cubicles and get outside in nature. Maybe we need to stop eating "chicken" nuggets and offer our bodies something nourishing and nutritious. Maybe we need to slow down, relax, and not fill every waking moment with activity and busyness. Maybe it's not medication that we need but a nourished, rested body and a curious mind so we have the energy and motivation to explore our surroundings and see what's beyond the confines of our self-created cages.

We can choose to make changes, but first we have to remember that we have the power and ability to do so. Ideally, doctors could offer help and support by reminding us of our body's tremendous capacity for change and healing. But, too often the labels and medications just create an even smaller, more confining cage. In order to create more space for change and hope, we can begin by thinking about our story differently. Instead of casting ourselves as victims of our biology and neurochemistry, we can recognize the symptoms we label as depression as a wake-up call to seek what is out of balance in our lives and perceptions, and recognize that we are strong and smart enough to open the cage door if given the right tools.

Humans desperately want answers and solutions. We want to *know.* We yearn to avoid the unknown, unlabeled states of being that make us feel uncomfortable and stressed out. Doctors can confidently pull out one of the three hundred tidy categories in the DSM-5 and offer a "diagnosis" and corresponding pill, and we can be assured that these unknown scary symptoms and feelings have a name and a solution. See? There really is something wrong with me! Just knowing this makes you—and your physician—feel better, at least initially. For our human brains, any answer is better than no answer.

In reality, these labels are arbitrary and often unreliable. Far too many of the decisions about what becomes a diagnostic code and what does not are more dependent on social, political, and financial (especially financial!) factors. Many of the psychiatrists on these panels have strong ties with pharmaceutical companies, which have strong vested interests in getting certain diagnoses into the manual so they can sell more drugs. It may sound conspiratorial, but it is, sadly, all too true.

Even Dr. Robert Spitzer, the task force chair of the earlier DSM-III, acknowledged in an interview that he had advocated for defining symptoms of depression and anxiety as "disorders" to push pharmaceutical treatments (controlled by psychiatrists) over equally effective psychotherapeutic options offered by psychologists and counselors. The task force chair of the DSM-IV, Dr. Allen Frances, acknowledged, "Alas, we have reviewed dozens of definitions of mental disorder (and helped to write the ones in DSM-IV) and must admit that none have much practical value.... Indeed, the concept of mental disorder is so amorphous, protean, and heterogeneous that it inherently defies definition." Later in the same paper, he points out that in reality a "mental disorder is what clinicians treat and researchers research and educators teach and insurance companies pay for."

The point of this is merely to recognize the many outside forces that have nothing to do with science that steer certain diagnoses into being. In the words of Allen Frances, "There is no scientifically proven, single right way to diagnose any mental disorder." These labels are not facts, but conceptual ideas created to organize and understand the messiness of life and human emotions.

All of this leaves us exactly where we do not want to be, with an unanswered question: What is depression, really? UCLA established a $525 million cross-disciplinary initiative that included neuroscientists, psychologists, economists, policy makers, and computer scientists all seeking to answer this question, but they concluded: "Depression is a real problem that's as old as humanity itself, yet we still don't even know what causes it."

Despite the ever-shifting explanations and possible treatments, the portrait of depression has remained remarkably consistent. As early as 400 BCE, Hippocrates described melancholia as a period of prolonged sadness and fear with "moral dejection, tendency to suicide, aversion to food, despondency, sleeplessness, irritability, and restlessness." Hippocrates wisely divided melancholia symptoms into those resulting from normal reactions to stressful circumstances and those that were "beyond due measure." For the next two thousand–plus years, these symptoms were viewed through the lens of an individual's circumstances. That changed with the publication of the DSM-III in 1980, when context was erased and depression was reduced to a list of checkboxes, almost identical to Hippocrates', although lacking the perspective of context.

The symptoms will sound familiar: depressed mood, diminished interest in activities one used to enjoy, change in appetite, change in sleep patterns, decreased libido, sense of restlessness or being slowed down, lack of energy, feelings of worthlessness or guilt, difficulty focusing, and suicidal thoughts. If you answer "yes" to five or more of these for a period of two weeks or longer, you are officially diagnosed and pathologized with the label of depression. Technically, according to the manual, other medical conditions and substance abuse have been ruled out. But in a ten-minute visit, who has time to dig beyond some basic lab work and a few questions into the long list of possible medication interactions and side effects, hormonal imbalances, allergies, gut issues, toxins, or nutritional deficiencies? There is most certainly no time to consider current or childhood life events that may have triggered this episode.

By the time of the publication of DSM-5 in 2015, even the possibility of bereavement and grief was erased as normal responses to life circumstances, and instead labeled as pathology. If you meet these criteria, you are simply diagnosed, likely offered medication, and informed that this is a chronic disorder requiring a lifetime of pharmaceuticals to regulate your alleged brain neurochemistry imbalance.

Despite the analogy comparing depression to diabetes that so many psychiatrists use to rationalize the prescription of antidepressants, depression is more like a fever than diabetes. Whereas diabetes is associated with abnormal responses to insulin, confirmable with bloodwork, a fever is a common symptom triggered by hundreds of possible etiologies. It is also one of the body's defense mechanisms designed to kill the offending bacteria or virus and rally the immune system. With a fever, some of us immediately rush to eliminate the symptoms with Tylenol, but sometimes the wiser course of action is to let the fever do its job in helping our body heal. A fever can, however, be indicative of a bigger issue that needs addressing.

The point is that, like a fever, depression does not have one cause, purpose, or treatment despite the common presentation of symptoms. So, we must take time to explore possible etiologies unique to each person. Some depressive symptoms may be due to current life stressors, losses, or traumas; others due to past events that deeply influenced how you perceive and react to the world. Some depressions may be due to physical hormonal imbalances or deficiencies. Some may be due to toxins in your diet, personal care products, or environment. Some may be due to toxic relationships, jobs, or perceptions. Most symptoms of depression are a combination of these factors, once again defying our desire for simple, cozy answers and solutions. The commonality among all these etiologies is some form of stress leading to a system overload or shutdown. Perhaps the symptoms of depression can best be described as our body's red-alert system informing us that the body and our lives are out of balance and need attuning.

Because the answer is unknown, and the story and meanings of depression are in constant flux and unique to each of us, we must sit in the uncomfortable but empowering answerless space where we can bring our own meaning to our symptoms. How we perceive our symptoms influences the outcomes drastically. We can choose to see ourselves as powerless, broken victims of our biology, as modern psychiatry informs us, or we can just as easily choose to view depression as a messenger calling us to find balance, connection, and meaning in our lives—nudging us to wake up and heed the call for growth and transformation.

The Influence of Childhood Adversity

One of the primary root causes for depression remains largely ignored by physicians. Dr. Vincent Felitti is trying to change this. Felitti is an internist who used to run a weight loss clinic, believing that helping people lose weight might lead to better health outcomes. After all, obesity is associated with just about all chronic diseases. Felitti tells the story of a woman he helped drop from 400 pounds to 132 pounds, and then in one week she gained back 30 pounds, and then continued to quickly gain all the weight back. Puzzled, Felitti asked the woman about the time in her life she had first put on weight. It turned out it was the same time her grandfather began molesting her. Further questioning revealed that she began to regain all the weight she lost at the clinic after a man at work had propositioned her. Just a coincidence? Felitti started asking his other patients similar questions. It turned out that hundreds had similar experiences. When Felitti presented his findings at a meeting, he was told by other physicians that these were just "fabrications" to provide an excuse for the patients' "lack of responsibility."

These stories radically shifted his perspective. Felitti started to recognize the weight as a protective defense. Over time, he came to realize that "most of our public health problems are unconsciously attempted solutions to personal experiences in childhood." Gaining weight may protect against unwanted sexual attention or physical abuse. Alcohol and drugs numb emotions and memories too painful to feel or discuss. It is not a lack of responsibility or motivation driving these apparently self-sabotaging behaviors, but a fear-based response meant to keep one safe.

In response to this information, Felitti created a ten-question survey about the most common early childhood traumas his patients had been reporting, in hopes of formally assessing how many people experience each one. When he initially presented his research proposal for approval to the Internal Review Board, they were concerned that even asking these questions might stir up "too much emotional turmoil." Felitti persisted.

The original Adverse Childhood Experiences (ACE) study gathered data from 9,500 members of the health maintenance organization Kaiser Permanente between 1995 and 1997. The participants simply checked off which of the listed traumatic events they had experienced in childhood. The questions were divided into seven categories, including emotional, physical, and sexual abuse; witnessing domestic violence; and growing up in a household with members who were mentally ill, suicidal, abused alcohol or drugs, or were imprisoned.

The study revealed shockingly strong associations between early childhood events and future emotional and physical health issues. What was perhaps even more surprising was the number of people experiencing these traumas. Even though this study was completed on a largely white middle-class population, Felitti and his colleagues found that 67 percent of the participants had experienced at least one trauma; a quarter had experienced two or more. A quarter of the population surveyed had grown up in a family with alcohol or drug abuse. Nearly that many had been sexually abused. Felitti discovered that the number of these events predicted the risk of future chronic diseases, including nine of the top ten most common causes of death in this country. In addition, the higher ACE scores corresponded with more risky behaviors like smoking, emotional overeating, alcohol and drug abuse, increased promiscuity, and sexually transmitted diseases, all of which further contribute to increased risk of future diseases. An ACE score of four doubles the risk of heart disease, cancer, coronary artery disease, stroke, and hepatitis, and quadruples the risk of chronic obstructive pulmonary disease (COPD). This data confirmed Felitti's observations in his clinic. Traumatic events are not "excuses" for "lack of responsibility," but the root of fundamentally altered physiology.

The link between childhood adversity, depression, and other mental health issues is even more staggering. A woman without any known childhood adversity (or at least any of the ones questioned about) has a roughly 15 percent chance of experiencing a depressive episode in her lifetime. For a woman who has experienced an adverse event, the risk increases to 25 percent. For those with two childhood traumas, that risk increases to 40 percent. For those with four or more ACEs, the likelihood of depression is increased by 460 percent and the risk of suicide by 1,200 percent. In fact, the risk of suicide increases by 60 percent for each additional trauma exposure.

The risks for other so-called mental illnesses are equally profound. There is an 800 percent increased risk of alcoholism and 500 percent increased risk of drug abuse.

Not surprisingly, given these statistics, higher ACE scores also lead to higher rates of prescribed psychotropic medications. A third of those with no childhood adversity are prescribed an antidepressant, and 16 percent are prescribed an anxiolytic—still a shockingly high number. Yet add one ACE, and the rate increases to 50 percent. Over 73 percent of those with three ACEs are on medications and 97 percent—yes, 97 percent—of those with four or more ACEs are on psych medications.

Worse, childhood adversity doubles the risk of developing so-called "treatment resistant" depression, which does not respond to the psychotropic medications that the majority of this population are prescribed. Is it possible that the medications are keeping this vulnerable population from facing childhood wounds and preventing them from healing? Maybe they are not "treatment resistant" at all, but rather a product of treatment-induced resistance. Maybe it is the outcome of attempting to close gaping soul wounds with a biochemical solution. Is it possible that conventional medical care is recreating the victimhood of childhood by informing this group of people that they are not resilient survivors, but broken and unfixable without the lifelong use of medications?

At this point, if you have experienced some of these early traumas, you may be feeling frightened, distraught, and overwhelmed by this information. After all, the past cannot be changed. The last thing I want to do is free you from the confines of your biology and neurochemistry, only to recast you as a victim of your childhood. This is only part of the story. Recognizing and acknowledging these early roots also offers hope, for if trauma can shift our physiology and epigenetics in one direction, the adaptability of the body allows for a shift in the opposite direction. Offering skills and tools that have been shown to change the structure and function of the brain, so that it is more adaptive to stress, is the goal of the rest of this book.

Perhaps you are thinking that some of these statistics could be explained more by a genetic link than an environmental one. A 2002 study that followed nearly two thousand female twins for nine years confirmed that the likelihood of depression was associated not with genetics, but rather a history of childhood trauma. The effects of unhealed trauma can lead to a vicious cycle, including the increased risk of suffering with anxiety, low self-esteem, and behavioral issues as a teenager. This further depletes self-esteem and social connection, leading to an increased likelihood of poor relationships and difficulties dealing with life stressors as an adult, which, in the presence of a current stressor, increases the likelihood of a depressive episode. This data challenges the genetic and biochemical models of mental illness, which imply the possibility of an easy pharmaceutical fix. Instead, it leaves us in the uncomfortable, messy space without simple answers or solutions.

The first of many studies examining the link between childhood trauma and future emotional and physical risks was done in 1998. Twenty years have passed, and these questions are still largely ignored by the majority of physicians, yet if we truly want to help people heal—not just minimize symptoms, but *heal*—these questions must be addressed.

What keeps these questions from being a part of all initial evaluations? In surveys, doctors have expressed fears of stigmatizing or offending a patient, viewing survivors as too fragile and emotionally unstable to handle the questions. Yet the data suggests that it is the physicians who are uncomfortable with the questions. A review of thirty studies exploring the risks and benefits of inquiring about abuse found that the vast majority of respondents experienced being asked and heard as validating and affirming. A 2017 survey of mostly lower-income families, in which more than half of those questioned had four or more ACEs, found the same results. And in one unpublished study, Kaiser Permanente found that simply by asking questions about childhood trauma, there was a decreased need for doctor visits.

The simple act of asking the question validates someone's experiences and allows them to feel heard and acknowledged, which can be healing in and of itself. Too often trauma is a secret swept under the rug (or numbed by a long list of medications). This creates a field of guilt and shame that permeates not only the individual's life but the entire family system, no doubt amplifying the risk of future disease. What remains buried only grows stronger and more entangled, with unacknowledged and unhealed trauma leaking out to future generations.

In 2018, Oprah Winfrey addressed the research on the link between childhood adversity and future health outcomes on the TV show *60 Minutes*. She pointed out that by asking about one's experiences, the question shifts from "What is wrong with you?" to "What has happened to you?" This is indeed the core question that needs to be addressed not only in therapy but in all medical fields. What if we approached our own self-sabotaging behaviors, and those of others, with this same curious, nonjudgmental stance? Sometimes, as Vincent Felitti noted when he was asked about mitigating factors that can help reduce the toll of early trauma, "the firmly held belief that I matter to someone" can boost resiliency. Sometimes it is just that simple.

Effects of Stress on Mind and Body

How do these early life experiences translate into future emotional and physical disease? Understanding a bit about this pathway brings us a step closer to understanding the etiology of depression for the majority of those diagnosed. The simplest explanation is that trauma creates stress. Chronic stress wears our bodies down, leading to gut dysfunction, impaired immunity, inflammation, and a maladaptive nervous system and brain, which all lead to disease.

To understand the effects of chronic stress, we first need to understand the basics of a normal, balanced stress response. Let's say you are faced with the proverbial tiger about to pounce on you, or, far more likely in the modern world, a car slams on its brakes in front of you. As you know, there is no thinking that happens in these situations. Our bodies simply react.

Sensory information is conveyed from our eyes, ears, and other senses to a primitive part of the brain, called the limbic system, where the information is urgently evaluated for a possible threat—you'll read more about this in chapter 7. Adrenaline is released within seconds, alerting the body to danger. The heart pumps faster; airways expand so we can get more oxygen to our lungs; our unessential blood vessels in the gut and skin constrict, so more blood can be pumped to muscles essential for our escape; and glucose is released to provide energy to fight, flee, or freeze.

Simultaneously, the hypothalamic-pituitary-adrenal (HPA) axis is activated, triggering a cascade of hormonal responses that culminate in the release of the stress hormone cortisol. This releases glucose into the bloodstream to supply enough energy to take action, and temporarily shuts down everything not immediately critical to our survival, including the frontal lobe of the brain, as well as the gut, immune, and reproductive systems. No need to analyze or plan for the future, digest your food, fight off a pesky virus, or reproduce if you might not live to see tomorrow!

Cortisol usually turns off the stress response once the danger has passed. But in cases of early and chronic exposures to stress and adversity, however, the repeated activation of the stress response leads to a hyperactive HPA axis, which becomes exhausting, energy depleting, and harmful to the body. The adrenal gland, responsible for secreting cortisol, tries to keep up with demand, but over time may become depleted and less able to respond.

Without cortisol to slam on the brakes, the system becomes increasingly dysfunctional. Repeated damage to neurons in the hippocampus (our memory center) may lead to difficulties with memory and cognition. Metabolism and balance of neurotransmitters become disrupted. Connections between various parts of the brain are weakened, decreasing its ability to communicate and function effectively. The prefrontal cortex, responsible for analyzing, planning, and controlling impulsivity, atrophies. The amygdala expands, becoming increasingly hypervigilant and reactive. Even neutral circumstances, facial expressions, and vocal tones now appear threatening.

Primed to perceive danger wherever we look, the world appears dark and menacing, further amplifying the stress response. The HPA axis and sympathetic nervous system become stuck in hyperdrive, inhibiting the parasympathetic nervous system and depriving the body of time to rest, digest, and heal. This leads to massive inflammation and a suppressed immune system—placing our bodies at increased risk for everything from colds to gastrointestinal issues, autoimmune diseases, cancer, food allergies, thyroid disease, diabetes, chronic fatigue syndrome, anxiety, and, yes, depression.

In fact, hundreds of studies demonstrate an association between depression and this maladaptive stress response, which leads to increased inflammation. Inflammation increases one's risk of depression, and depression amplifies the inflammatory response, which further wreaks havoc on the brain and body. Elevated inflammatory markers are observed in about a third of depressed patients. (Of course, we must be careful not to reduce all depressive episodes to just inflammation.)

All of this is further aggravated by the multitude of other stressors in our daily lives. It is important to understand that stress is not just the emotional strain caused by external circumstances of our lives that we typically judge as unwanted, but anything that causes a "nonspecific response of the body to any demand for change." This includes not only a conflicted relationship with your boss or spouse, or an imminent deadline for a critical unfinished project, but also the dream house you are about to move into, and the new baby on the way. It would include nutritional deficiencies in your diet; too much or too little exercise; exposure to foreign toxins in our processed foods, lotions, and soaps; the pesticides and chemicals in our yards, water, and air; too little or too much sleep; too much busyness; and not enough rest. Unfortunately, it also includes many of the medications that you may be taking for other symptoms and illnesses. According to a 2018 study, more than a third of adults in the United States take prescription medications that increase their risk of depression.

Other stressors include our catastrophizing thoughts about all the things that *might* happen in the future, or rumination and regrets about traumas and mistakes from our past. That includes worries stirred up by all that you have read in this chapter. Although it is wise to take action and find out more information, it does more harm than good to dwell upon possibilities. Our brain does not compute the difference between the disasters you imagine in your mind and actual events. All of these trigger a stress response. More alarmingly, these responses led to epigenetic changes that not only influence our own health and well-being but those of future generations.

One study of children found that chronic stress led to epigenetic changes on genes related to neuron and brain development and increased inflammatory responses, as well as epigenetic changes associated with increased risk for depression, substance abuse, diabetes, asthma, and cancer. A longitudinal study following kids from birth to age thirty-two found that children who experienced early maltreatment, such as maternal rejection, harsh discipline, and physical or sexual abuse, had increased risk of inflammation twenty years later.

What is more frightening is that the epigenetic changes and risks caused by the abuse and stressors literally get passed on to future generations. A fascinating 2018 study by Dr. Félice Lê-Scherban and colleagues explored possible links between the adverse childhood experiences of parents and the future health outcomes of their children. In this study, including over ten thousand adults living in Philadelphia, researchers posed the same questions asked by Felitti in his study, as well as some additional questions regarding traumas common to a more urban population. The researchers found that 85 percent of the parents had experienced at least one childhood trauma, and nearly one-fifth had survived six or more. They found that the more trauma experienced by the parents, the greater the risk for poorer physical and emotional health outcomes in their children.

Dr. Rachel Yehuda, a professor of psychiatry and neuroscience at Icahn School of Medicine at Mount Sinai, pioneered research on intergenerational trauma. Her research on Holocaust survivors revealed that their offspring, despite not personally being exposed to the trauma of their parents' generation, carried a greater risk for post–traumatic stress disorder (PTSD), depression and anxiety, and the other chronic health issues common to trauma survivors. This suggests, once again, that stressors prior to conception and during pregnancy can adversely influence the future health of the child.

What all this clearly demonstrates is that our parents' unhealed traumas become our traumas. Our traumas become our children's. Despite all this research and data, the deeply embedded consequences of these early experiences are mostly ignored. Abuse, neglect, and other social and environmental influences on our health, not prevented or resolved with pills, are relegated to the appendix at the back of the DSM-5. Without a diagnosis to validate this link, the emotional consequences are not reimbursable by insurance companies, because the symptoms are deemed not "biological." It should be painfully obvious by now that the results of trauma change the structure and function of the brain and nervous system, and also create a storm of inflammation leading to just about every diagnosable code in medicine. Perhaps it is time to move trauma to the front of the DSM.

Perception of Stress

Despite everything you have just read, it is essential to remember that for those who carry the enduring marks of traumas, and for those exposed to chronic levels of high stress, stress is not a demon to be vilified. If we believe that, we once again become passive victims—not of our genes and neurochemistry, but of our childhoods and experiences. A study at the heart of Kelly McGonigal's book *The Upside of Stress* offers the radically hopeful possibility that it is not stress and trauma that determine our health and well-being, but rather our perceptions and reactions to it. If this is true, we have the capacity to change how we think and react, thereby changing not only our relationship with stress, but our subsequent emotional and physical health.

In a 2012 study, Abiola Keller and colleagues followed the mortality rates of thirty thousand adults who had participated in a 1998 survey that asked about the level of stress experienced in the past year, and if the participants believed this stress was harmful to their health. Based on the results of the first question, the researchers found that those with higher stress had a 43 percent increased risk of dying. If that were the end of the story, that would indeed be depressing news, and perhaps unsurprising, based on the ACE studies we discussed earlier. After all, we most certainly cannot remove the stress from our childhood, and it is equally impossible to remove all stressors from our lives. But this is where the story gets interesting and hopeful. It turns out that higher stress only increases mortality if we believe the stress is harmful. Shockingly, those who did not believe stress was harmful had a lower risk of dying than those with far less stress.

Better yet, we do not have to be born a Pollyannaish optimist who can always seek a positive spin on the unpredictable twists and turns of life. We can learn to tend and befriend stress rather than resisting and resenting it. We can learn to perceive stress as an opportunity for growth rather than an enemy to be vanquished.

Sound impossible? Perhaps it is not as difficult as you think. Harvard University psychologist Dr. Ellen Langer devised a cleverly simple study, demonstrating how changing our perceptions changes our physiology. In this study, eighty-four full-time, mostly overweight female hotel room attendants were divided into two groups. One group was given a simple paper explaining the benefits of exercise and informing the women that their housekeeping work far exceeded the CDC's recommended guidelines for daily exercise. The other group was not given this paper or explanation. Both groups continued to work under their normal conditions. After only four weeks, the women who had been educated about exercise had significantly shifted their perspective of how much exercise they were getting on a daily basis, despite no actual change in work or exercise. In this short period of time, the informed women lost an average of two pounds and lowered their blood pressure by ten points. Their shift in mind-set changed their physiology. There was no such change for the other women.

In another study, two groups were subjected to a mock job interview in which the participants had to give an eight-minute speech, followed by a five-minute question-and-answer session. Some of the luckier participants received positive acknowledgment from the interviewers, while those less fortunate were faced with tough interviewers who provided only negative feedback. Sounds dreadful, doesn't it?

Before the interview, each group watched a video. The first group's video suggested that stress enhances performance. The second group's video promoted the classic message that stress is bad for you and should be avoided. Both groups were stressed by the interview, but the group that had been exposed to the possibility that their stress response may improve their capabilities in this stressful situation were rewarded with more positive emotions and a boost of the beneficial hormone DHEA, which is associated with decreased anxiety, depression, and chronic disease. This small pre-interview prompt shifted their perspective from seeing the situation as a threat to seeing it as a challenge and, in fact, the group that faced the hostile interviewers benefited from this shift in perspective most of all.

There is a sociological theory formulated in the 1920s by William and Dorothy Thomas, creatively called the Thomas Theorem, that states: "If men define situations as real, they are real in their consequences." If we define stress as a challenge rather than a threat, if we see an active job as a form of activity and exercise instead of seeing ourselves as a lazy couch potato, if we perceive depression as a wake-up call rather than a pathological destiny, the consequences are real and measurable. Only a decade ago, doctors were still informing stroke patients that it was impossible to regain functions of the brain, since it was believed that new pathways could not be formed in the brain as an adult. Theory became reality. Few stroke patients recovered since it was not considered a possibility. We now know this "fact" is simply not true.

Nobel Prize–winning neuroscientist Eric Kandel has demonstrated that the number of neuronal connections in the brain can double in just one hour of repetitive stimulation. How incredible is that? For most of us, most of the time, we continue to fire the same circuits activated by our same old beliefs and perspectives. We keep getting the same results over and over again, deepening the grooves of our familiar thoughts and patterns, laying down the same template, assuming it is the only possibility. "That is just the way I am," we say. But that is simply not true. If we choose to send different signals, open up new possibilities and new mind-sets, we create new pathways that trigger the expression of different genes, changing our bodies and physiology profoundly. Our entire body is changing constantly with each thought and action. The microtubules that provide the structure of our nerve cells die and are reborn every ten minutes. Given this marvelous miracle of neuroplasticity, consider the possibilities for change.

The labeling of depression as a chronic disease confines us to a cage of limited possibilities. Being told you need a medication to prevent a relapse creates a lurking fear, like the boogeyman hiding in the closet, waiting to attack if you let down your guard. This creates a pattern of fear and avoidance, which manifests as a state of chronic depression. It becomes a self-defining, self-limiting definition, shifting a passing mood or imbalanced stuck state into a chronic reality and constant threat. If patients can recover from massive damage caused by a stroke, does it make any logical sense that the effects of trauma and symptoms of depression cannot be reversed as well? That is true only if we believe it to be so.

Perhaps it is finally time to heed depression's wake-up call, alerting you that your body and your life are out of balance and need attuning. In the rest of the book, you will discover different possibilities for healing your stressed-out life. You will learn to modulate and reconnect with your emotional messenger system, which may be numbed by medications, drugs, alcohol, toxins, and excessive busyness, or it may be screaming so loudly you can barely move. Either way, you can restore sanity by learning to balance your breath, mind, body, environment, energy, and soul. Shifting even one pattern, however small, starts to create new pathways, new ways of being. You do not have to change everything at once to get significant results. You can go at your own pace and in your own order.

Our brains, behaviors, and reactions are all capable of change and adaptation, once we become aware of our choices and possibilities. Opening the door to new possibilities creates space for new realities. What if we choose to see the cracks of trauma and depression not as pathology, but the space through which light, healing, and new experiences may enter? What if just by reading what you have read so far, even if you do not yet fully accept all of it, you, like the housekeepers, have already shifted your mind-set and awareness, creating new connections in your brain and epigenetic changes in your DNA? Perhaps, without even knowing it, your healing has already begun.

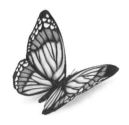

PART 2

Is There Another Way?

It is your time

to journey to the center of yourself;

to heal your life from past hurt,

in a way that is supportive,

intentional, and self-empowering.

It is your time to journey home.

—DR. KELLIE N. KIRKSEY,
*POETRY, PROSE AND
MISCELLANEOUS MUSINGS*

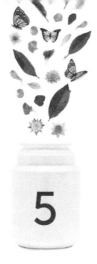

5

Call of the Imagination

We have not even to risk the adventure alone, for the heroes of all time have gone before us. The labyrinth is thoroughly known. We have only to follow the thread of the hero path ...

—JOSEPH CAMPBELL, *THE POWER OF MYTH*

Do you happen to remember the lovable, blue-furred Grover from Sesame Street? *The Monster at the End of This Book (Starring Lovable, Furry Old Grover)* was one of my kids' favorite books when they were little. The book begins with Grover panicking upon reading the title of the book, and fearing the scary monster that would appear at the end of his story. Terrified, he spends the rest of the book pleading and begging with the young reader *not* to turn the pages, so they will not get to the end of the book and have to face the monster. Grover desperately attempts tying the pages together with ropes, hammering the pages together with nails, and building a brick wall to avoid arriving at the end of the book and facing this unknown threat. When the end of the book finally arrives, the only monster at the end of the book is "lovable, furry old Grover."

Perhaps you too can think of a time in your life when you spent weeks fearfully dreading some future event, only to find out that when the event actually happened it was no big deal, or even if it was scary, you managed and survived. Perhaps you even felt uncomfortable, with a flurry of mixed emotions after reading the first section of this book, and finding out that everything you thought you knew about depression might not be true, and that there are no simple answers or solutions. Perhaps you have spent years, or even decades, viewing depression as a scary monster that could pop out at any moment, at the slightest twinge of sadness or discomfort. Perhaps the belief that you are broken and unfixable has kept you trapped in a nonexistent cage. Too often, our minds create monsters that do not really exist, especially if we have a history of trauma and met our share of real monsters.

One of the foundational skills you will learn moving through this book is the importance of checking in and noticing what emotions may be brewing under the surface. Acknowledgment helps tame emotions so that they do not become a threatening monster that you, like Grover, might desperately try to avoid. This allows emotions to move through, to flow along as they are supposed to, rather than getting stuck and inflamed.

A Journal for the Journey

Investing in a journal that calls to you, or just a simple notebook, is the first of many self-empowering tools I hope you will try as you move through this book. It is wise to remember and process your journey so you can learn from your mistakes and observe your progress and growth. It is so easy to forget. Our brains are wired to remember the bad times, and they easily overlook or forget progress and change for the better.

I cannot count how many times I have had patients tell me that they are feeling better than they have in years; that they never thought feeling this good was even possible. Then a few months later, some crisis strikes and they temporarily sink back into a depressive state, adamantly insisting that they have never felt better and never will. Often the initial impulse is to reach for a medication to make it stop, even though they originally may have come to me because medication was not working. I will flip through their charts and read back verbatim what they reported feeling a few months ago. Their own words serve to remind them, and you, that moods do pass, even though when trapped inside a dark one, it can feel permanent and impossible to escape.

A record of how you got through it last time creates a pathway you can follow so you can pull yourself out of the downward spiral of depression earlier this time. It will also remind you that the story your brain is telling you—that you have never felt good and never will—is simply not true.

Your journal can provide a reminder and feedback when times get tough, as they inevitably do for all of us. Journaling is perhaps the simplest and cheapest form of therapy as it can teach you about You—your reactions, perceptions, judgments, and assumptions. It can provide an outlet for pent-up emotions and frustrations. Writing for twenty minutes daily for a period of even just a few days has been shown to improve mood, decrease stress and anxiety, and even improve the immune system. It is one of many ways you will learn to release negative emotions and stress.

Imagine a pot of boiling water. If you put a lid on it, what will happen? Eventually, the pressure will build and the water will explode over the sides. But if you remove the lid what happens then? As you know, the water will settle. It is just so with anger, frustration, and sadness. We can repress, avoid, and deny our emotions, or we can acknowledge and feel them. One of many ways to do that is through writing about them.

WELLNESS RX: JOURNAL YOUR INITIAL IMPRESSIONS

Pause and take a moment to write down and reflect on what it would mean if your depression is not pathological, but an invitation for change and possibility. As best you can, write down whatever feelings, thoughts, and body sensations arise without censoring, just allowing whatever is there to be there. There is no need to worry about punctuation or grammar. The goal is to have a record of your experiences so that you can refer back to these writings. Just as it is important to remember history or we are doomed to repeat it, it is important to remember your own story as you move forward on this journey so that you can refer back and avoid falling down the same holes.

What would it look and feel like to frame your depression in this way? Simply notice what comes up as you consider this possibility. You may feel relief and hope. Notice that, and how that feels in your body. If you have been told for years or even decades that this is who you are—broken and depressed—it may feel scary and overwhelming to hear that this characterization may not be true. Identities are difficult to let go of even when doing so opens up new potential. You may feel resistant to the possibility; you may feel sad and angry for all the years spent under the influence of medications that may have prolonged your suffering. You have a right to that anger, and it needs to be acknowledged—ideally with kindness and curiosity, but that may take time.

You may insist that your medications saved you and you could not live without them. That is OK. It may be partially true. Remember, a placebo effect is very real and effective. Our belief in the power of medications and treatment changes not only our perceptions but physically changes the brain in a similar way to a real medication. For many, it can even cause some of the side effects we expect to have from the actual medication. Ask yourself: if the medication is working so well and the problem is resolved, then what draws you to this book? Just be curious about your response to that question, if it applies to you. These are all perfectly normal and acceptable responses, but they must be acknowledged or they can block the healing process.

We cannot control how we feel, only how we respond to those feelings. We can judge ourselves and our feelings, or acknowledge them with kindness and curiosity. This is the heart of mindfulness, which we will discuss later, but for now I encourage you to simply notice what comes up as you read these words and allow yourself to fully feel and acknowledge whatever arises as best you can. Now that you have your first recordings in your journal, set the intention to write down your experiences with all the exercises in this book.

Consider a Therapist

It is wise to gather guides and resources for additional support, so that you do not have to travel this journey alone. A therapist would be a useful companion in this process, to help you sort through the emotions that may arise, offer perspective, and provide support and guidance. Finding a therapist who is familiar with mindfulness and some of the other self-empowering tools in this book would be ideal, as he or she can support you on this journey.

I have included resources on my website for help in seeking a therapist. Decades of research have consistently shown that therapy with a trusted therapist works as well as medications at preventing and recovering from depression. The relationship between a patient and a trusted guide—whether that is a counselor, physician, acupuncturist, shaman, or any other healer—has, throughout time, always been at the heart of healing and undoubtedly plays a large role in amplifying the power of placebo.

Listen to your intuition, for the key here is a trusted relationship. If you meet a new therapist, no matter how highly recommended, and do not feel connected or listened to, or walk away feeling uncomfortable or worse, then trust that he or she is not the right guide for you and try again with another healer.

Inner Guides and Resources

Meanwhile, it is also important to begin building your own resources so that you are not completely dependent on others, and can start to discover your own innate power, strength, and abilities. One of the best resources available to you is guided imagery. Before reading further, I strongly encourage you to set aside fifteen minutes to discover and call upon these resources. I know: it is so much easier to just push on and keep reading and perhaps come back to this later. I am always guilty of this myself, so I totally understand. As a busy working mom, time is invaluable and can feel impossible to find, but part of this journey is realizing we can always make time for what we value. Think of all the time spent each day checking emails, Facebook, Twitter, watching TV, or just trying to decide which item on the endless list of chores you are going to tackle next. What if you put yourself and your healing at the top of today's to-do list? Perhaps it feels stupid or a waste of time, but maybe you could just be curious and see what happens. The choice is yours to make. Finding balance is essential for healing, as is being curious about your habitual responses, thoughts, and behaviors that may be getting in your way. Perhaps this is a perfect opportunity to pause and experiment.

WELLNESS RX: PEACEFUL PLACE

Find a quiet space where you will not be bothered for 15 minutes. Leave all distractions elsewhere. Place your journal and a writing instrument beside you.

Find a comfortable place to sit or lie down, and when you are ready, close your eyes. Notice your body in this moment. Feel your back against the ground or chair. Notice any areas of discomfort or tightness in your body, and see if you can adjust or move to make yourself more comfortable. Then take three deep breaths, breathing in through your nose and exhaling through your mouth, inviting tension to release with each exhalation.

Allow an image to come to mind of a place where you feel relaxed and calm. It may be a place you have been or just dreamed of going. It might be real or imaginary. It might be a beach, a mountain, a forest, beside a stream, or just curled up on a couch in a favorite room—wherever you feel drawn. Your mind may bounce between different possibilities, and that is OK. Now just allow yourself to settle on one of these places.

Look around and sense this space. Notice the light and colors, the time of day, the season. Feel the temperature of the air on your skin. Notice any familiar sounds, any familiar smells. Take the next few minutes to relax here. Your mind may get distracted with stories about what you need to do, but as best you can, just go back to this peaceful place, experiencing it fully. You may add or remove anything to make it feel more peaceful and comfortable.

As you rest here, notice how your body feels. Perhaps it relaxes. Perhaps relaxing does not feel safe yet. If this feels difficult or agitating, feel free to stop and try again later, or try with someone who can help guide and support you through it.

Otherwise, continue to spend some time here, giving your body a moment of rest and healing. Stay here as long as you like. When you are ready to leave, offer thanks for allowing yourself this time to begin your healing journey. Know that you can return to this space if you choose, anytime you feel the need for a break.

Take a few more deep breaths, and start to notice how your body feels after this brief respite. When you are ready, allow your eyes to slowly open, returning to this space. Notice your body and whether it feels more relaxed or if some new tension has appeared. Just notice and then open your journal and record this experience.

After reading through this exercise or other exercises in this book, you may use your smartphone or other device to record yourself reading this guided imagery exercise aloud slowly, or go to my website (jodieskillicorn.com) for audio files of the exercises.

The practice of imagery can be used as a tool anytime, anywhere for calming the nervous system. Imagery also offers us access to the unconscious brain and to our wiser selves. It steps away from the linear, logical brain that we habitually turn to for answers, yet often leads us spiraling downward with doubts and fears. Studies on imagery have shown the practice can help decrease symptoms of depression, anxiety, and stress, and improve immunity.

One of my favorite studies on imagery beautifully demonstrates the power of how changing our beliefs and perceptions changes how things physically manifest in the body. In this study, participants exposed to poison ivy imagined the plant to be harmless, and 84 percent of them were able to eliminate the histamine response that leads to the symptoms of itching, redness, swelling, and blisters. A reverse experiment was also conducted in which participants exposed to a perfectly harmless plant imagined it to be poison ivy, and guess what? Many broke out in rashes. This is the power of the imagination.

In another study on psychiatric patients in a hospital setting, one group was given a twenty-minute CD with guided imagery, while another was not. Those who used the CD experienced a significant decrease in depression, anxiety, and stress.

It is unfortunate that such a simple, inexpensive, yet effective technique is not a part of standard protocol to relieve stress and anxiety in psychiatric wards, hospitals, and even doctor's offices. Some hospitals, like the Cleveland Clinic, do use this technique with surgical patients because of its well-established benefits of decreasing anxiety before and after surgery, reducing post-pain and complications, and allowing the patients to return home sooner; other patients would benefit as well.

Research using imaging studies of the brain has revealed that by imagining a scene, your brain and physiology respond as if the scene is actually happening. A classic example of this is to imagine cutting a lemon. Imagine a kitchen counter with a cutting board. Just like you did in the peaceful place scene, imagine the lights and colors around you. Notice any familiar smells and sounds in the kitchen. Now imagine picking up a knife to cut the lemon. Imagine the sensation as you move your arm and make the cut through the center. Now imagine picking up one half and lifting it to your mouth. Imagine opening your mouth and preparing to take a bite and then, finally, biting into the lemon.

Perhaps as you did this, your body started to drool at the thought of food and then wince as you took a bite into the sour lemon. It is always fun to do this in a group and see all the facial expressions as people imagine taking that first bite.

The point is that although you are just using your imagination and not actually biting into a lemon, your mind and body respond as if it is actually happening. If you did this experiment while in a functional MRI machine, the visual cortex of the brain would light up as it envisioned the kitchen and the lemon. The auditory cortex would light up as you imagine and hear familiar sounds. The part of the brain that registers taste would light up as you bite into the lemon.

In one study, an exercise psychologist from the Cleveland Clinic Foundation in Ohio compared a group of people who worked out using a specific set of muscles to a group who lounged while imagining they were working out these same muscles. The results? Those who actually worked out showed a 53 percent increase in muscle strength, while the group that only imagined working out showed a 35 percent increase in muscle strength. The point, of course, is not that we should not be exercising, but rather to grasp the immense capacity of our thoughts and imagination to change our physiology—for better or worse.

Think about the implications of that. In the peaceful place guided imagery exercise, your body experienced a totally free mini vacation. You relaxed the body and activated the parasympathetic nervous system that allows your body to rest, digest, and heal. Conversely, when you are lost in thoughts about all the worst things that could happen to you, or trapped in fears that this depression will never end and you will never recover, your brain is responding as if that is actually happening. The stress response activates, the body tenses, your heart beats faster, and your breathing becomes more shallow and rapid.

Sometimes, however, if your life has been particularly chaotic and stressful, being relaxed can trigger fears of feeling vulnerable and unsafe. If that is the case for you, I strongly suggest seeking out a counselor to work with you for additional support and guidance beyond this book. With practice you too can train your brain to realize that relaxing is not a threat, but it will take a bit more time and repetition before those neurons rewire to allow that possibility.

If that is the case, do not get lost in more thoughts about how this will not work for you, but instead focus on what is possible. You can try dipping into a restful scene for a few seconds and just be curious what happens. Slowly work your way up to minutes as your body learns this is safe. Or, you can simply move ahead to the chapters on nutrition and exercise and start there. There is no right or wrong way to move through these exercises.

For the rest of you, I hope you were able to experience at least a brief moment of release. The more this skill, like anything else, is practiced, the easier it is to drop into these states for brief periods of time so you can take free breaks throughout the day to calm and regulate the nervous system.

Now that you have a place where you can momentarily escape to for peace and relaxation, let's try this exercise again. This time, we are going to add a few other resources to the scene. Remember, the goal here is to utilize the immense power of the imagination for stress relief and healing.

WELLNESS RX: GUIDES TO SUPPORT YOUR JOURNEY

Begin by returning to the peaceful place you visited in the last exercise, "Wellness Rx: Peaceful Place." Take the time to rest and notice how your body feels. Notice your surroundings. Breathe into the space.

When you are ready, allow an image to come to mind of a protective figure that can join you in your peaceful place. This figure may be real or imaginary, human, animal, or spirit. It may be someone you know or someone from a favorite book, movie, or painting. It should be someone or something that represents protective qualities, someone that's got your back and will look out for you and defend you. If you struggle to find anything, you can always just continue to relax in your peaceful place and try again later.

Allow yourself to feel the strength, protection, and support of that being within you. Know that you can call upon this protective figure whenever and wherever you feel the need for protection.

You may find it helpful to cross your arms in a hug over your chest and gently tap your arms back and forth, right, left, right, left in a rhythmic fashion to see if that helps relax and calm your body even more. If that does not feel soothing, just stop the tapping and spend a few more moments connecting with your resource and its protective qualities.

Now allow a nurturing figure to come to mind. Again, this may be a human, animal, or spirit, real or imaginary, but someone or something that represents nurturing and love. If you struggle to find anything, you can always just continue to relax in your peaceful place and try again later.

Allow yourself to feel this nurturing, loving presence. If you found the rhythmic tapping on your arms helpful, you may begin tapping back and forth. Stay here as long as you like in your peaceful place with your nurturing figure.

When you are ready, allow a new image to arise of a wise guide. Again, this may be anyone or anything that represents wisdom, guidance, and clarity.

Allow yourself to connect with this guide, noticing how this being looks and feels in your presence. You may want to communicate with this being, or any of the other guides. You may ask for a message or guidance and clarity about some issue worrying you. Perhaps you receive a response and perhaps you do not. Perhaps it is enough just to catch a glimpse of this being today, and over time you can gather more information. That information may come in different ways—it may be in words, but it also may be in the form of a color or sound or sensation or some other means of communication. Just be curious and open to possibilities.

When you feel ready to leave, be sure to thank your guides for joining you today and thank yourself for offering yourself this time to begin your healing journey. Know that you can call upon these guides any time you feel the need for protection, nurturing, or wisdom. Take a few more deep breaths, and start to notice your back against the chair or floor. Perhaps wiggle your toes and fingers to awaken your body. When you are ready, allow your eyes to open, returning to this space and this room. Just notice how you are feeling and then open your journal and record this experience.

Thank-you to Laurel Parnell for teaching me this resourcing technique in her EMDR training at Omega Institute.

Hopefully, you took the time to try out the exercise above. The critical part of your brain may balk at how such a simple exercise can help pull you out of depression, but remember your brain responds to your imagination in a similar fashion as when an event actually happens. Focusing on relaxing, protective, and nurturing scenes can relax and empower the body and begin to create a new circuit in the brain based on hope and possibility rather than helplessness and defeat. We can begin to heal the parts of ourselves that may not have received the protection and nurturing we needed growing up. The more we train this new circuit, the more it develops and the more easily accessible it becomes.

This is the power of neuroplasticity. Although psychiatrists continue to treat patients as if their brains are unfixable, this is simply not true. Our brain changes with every thought and action we carry out. When we focus on the negative, we strengthen that circuit; when we focus on hope and possibilities, another circuit gets activated. I think of it like a record player. If we keep playing the same song over and over, a rut develops, and we can get stuck. The only way to pass through the repetition rut is to pick up the needle of the record player and move it to another song.

There is a Native American story about a grandfather talking with his grandson about the two wolves that battle within each of us. There is the "Good" Wolf of love, hope, optimism, compassion, forgiveness, kindness, and joy, and the Big Bad Wolf of fear, hate, and resentment. The boy asks his grandfather, "Which wolf wins?" The grandfather responds, "It's whichever wolf you feed."

With every thought and every action, we can choose which wolf—which neural network—to feed and strengthen. Throughout this book, we will be learning more skills to nourish the Wolf of Hope. The Big Bad Wolf may howl in the background, slyly and deceitfully telling you that these are stupid exercises and change is not possible; others may be able to do this, but not you—you are broken and unfixable. What is the point in even trying? Fear is the language of the Big Bad Wolf. You cannot silence him, but you can choose not to heed, fear, judge, or feed his negativity. Ignoring him may initially cause him to howl louder, but remember, just by reading this book and choosing to try the Wellness Rx, you are opening to a potential for change. You are creating new connections and pathways in the brain and nervous system. You are feeding the Wolf of Hope.

The goal is to nourish the Wolf of Hope as often as possible. It's easier said than done, I know! Studies suggest that 25 percent of people who start a New Year's resolution will break it within one week, and less than 10 percent will follow through for the whole year. Yet not setting goals pretty much guarantees you will not follow through. So, what could you do differently to get more positive outcomes?

Consider shifting from resolutions to intentions. This may seem like mere word play, but the words carry slightly different tones that lead to different outcomes. The word *resolution* is defined as "a firm decision or determination," whereas *intention* is defined as a "decision based on purpose," or as Marilyn Schlitz, a researcher of intentions, defines it, "the projection of awareness, with purpose and efficacy, toward some object or outcome."

The most common New Year's resolution is to lose weight. This resolution starts with the premise that something is wrong with you and it must be fixed. Kind of judgy, no? A similar intention might be: "I make healthy, balanced food choices that lead to increased energy, strength, and vitality." Both can involve making healthier food choices and moving our bodies more, but one focuses on what is wrong, while the intention focuses our energy on what we want—to be healthy. Intentions seek to find the purpose behind the goal. Is health the target? Increased stamina and mobility for work and play? Be as clear and specific as possible. This may be a subtle but critical difference.

Resolutions require willpower, something that research suggests we ultimately all have in limited supply. Although willpower may lead to increased attainment of goals, it does so at the cost of stress and increased aging on the body. Intention, on the other hand, offers compassion for ourselves as we follow a higher purpose, which allows us to reach the same goal but with less stress. Sure, we may stray from our intent (most of us do) but we do not need to blame and judge ourselves for our failing, but rather recognize our efforts and gently evaluate how it might be avoided in the future—and then move on with our purpose still clearly in sight.

Western culture teaches us that toughness is a necessary ingredient to avoid straying from our determined outcome, yet the low success rates of resolutions do not validate this belief. Back in your school days, did you perform better in the class with the teacher that scolded and berated you for less than perfection, or the teacher with the same high expectations who offered support and encouragement? Research has shown that self-compassion and gratitude decrease the impulsivity and impatience that often break our resolutions. They gently guide us to persevere toward our purpose.

For many of us, self-compassion may seem like a foreign concept altogether. What would that look and feel like? As a starting point, imagine you have a friend who is upset and blaming herself for failing yet again, because she had resolved to avoid sugar and processed foods for a week, and four days later ate a whole pan of brownies. Would you reprimand her and unfriend her? Or would you offer support, kindness, and encouragement that old habits are hard to break and that it requires time, patience, and even failure to move past them and create a new habit? You might also remind her that she can keep beating herself up, which will likely only lead to more emotional overeating, or she can just start over. Although most of us would have no trouble offering that understanding and compassion to someone else, many of us struggle to offer that same small generosity to ourselves.

One simple technique I recommend for those moments when you are trapped in self-judgment is to gently place your hand over your heart and offer yourself the same kind words you would offer to a child or friend. As you do this, feel the contact of your hand against your chest and notice the movement of your breath and the beating of your heart. This simple act has been shown to stimulate the release of oxytocin, the "love hormone" that is secreted when mothers breastfeed or lovers touch. It is the hormone of trust and connection. This simple act also pulls us out of the self-critical stories in our head and back into our body.

Besides adding a dose of self-compassion, how we can establish an intention with the best chance of sticking? The following exercise is based on the wisdom of Lynne McTaggart, a journalist, researcher, and a Master of Intention, who has written several books on the subject.

The first step to setting an intention is moving into a receptive, meditative state. An intention will be easier to follow through with when it comes from the heart, not the head. We will start by using the skill you have already learned.

WELLNESS RX: SETTING YOUR INTENTION

Begin by sitting tall, but relaxed, and taking a few deep breaths in through the nose and out through the mouth. With each exhalation, allow the body to release and let go.

Now return to the image and feel of your peaceful place, immersing yourself fully in this place with all of your senses. Invite your nurturing presence from the previous exercise to join you. As you tune in with the feelings of love and support from this presence, imagine breathing in and out of the heart. Connect with the feelings, not the thoughts.

From this open-hearted space, you are ready to seek your intention: what your heart most desires to gain from reading this book and trying these exercises. Clarify this intention with specifics and frame it in the present tense as a positive statement. Instead of "I want to be free of depression," try, "I am filled with joy, peace, and vitality. I sleep through the night. I look forward with gratitude to what each day will bring." State your intention as if the transformation has already happened—as if the depression has lifted and zest for life has returned. Imagine what that would feel and look like with all of your senses.

Although your ultimate goal may be to feel contentment and happiness, you may need to establish smaller intentions along the way as stepping stones. If you are barely able to get out of bed in the morning, the bigger intention may feel far-fetched and unbelievable. Try starting with the simpler, more immediately obtainable intention of waking up energized and motivated. If, on the other hand, you have no energy because you are struggling to fall asleep and stay asleep, start there. "I fall asleep easily and sleep restfully throughout the night. I wake up fully refreshed and energized and ready to learn new skills so I may live life full of joy and vitality." Start where you are, with reachable goals that can empower and motivate you to reach farther. Be sure to write this intention in your journal.

As you progress through each chapter, continue to create intentions based on what you have learned and want to manifest in each area of your life. Whatever intentions you set, begin and end each day by imagining this intention fully manifested and how that looks, feels, tastes, and smells in your body. Write your intention down and carry it with you. Declare your intention with others so you will be held accountable. Draw a picture of what it would look and feel like once manifested, or create an intention board with pictures representing how you want to feel and what you want to bring into your life.

Notice any thoughts sabotaging your efforts that may be screaming, "This is stupid; this will never work; this isn't the right time; there's too much going on right now; this is a waste of time." Remember, these thoughts are not an enemy, but a scared part of yourself attempting to keep you "safe" by resisting change. Assure these thoughts and fears that you are safe, and these exercises will teach you skills that will protect and empower you.

As best you can and as often as you can, notice when you get stuck in dark, gloomy, critical, or catastrophizing thoughts that feed the Wolf of Despair. If you continue to focus on your failures and shortcomings, berating yourself for flaws and fears, that patterning gets stronger and your chances of achieving your intention diminish. Instead, intentionally choose to offer nourishment to the Wolf of Hope, Compassion, Gratitude, and Intention. If you can catch yourself stuck in negative thoughts, choose to focus instead on thoughts of hope, gratitude, and manifesting your intentions; those neural circuits will get stronger. When the dark thoughts arise, do not criticize yourself for having them—that just feeds the Hateful Judging Wolf again. Instead, acknowledge that the dark thoughts of imagined monsters are back, and then choose to offer additional sustenance to the Wolf of Hope and Optimism.

The act of holding an intention is a matter of moment-to-moment, compassionate vigilance regarding whether thoughts and actions align with your higher purpose. By setting these intentions and committing to trying and practicing the wellness prescriptions in this book for even five to ten minutes daily, you can slowly but radically rewire the brain to create new habits and lasting change.

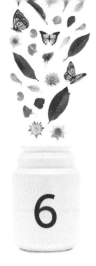

6

The Breath as an Anchor

Feelings come and go like clouds in a windy sky. Conscious breathing is my anchor.

—THICH NHAT HANH, *STEPPING INTO FREEDOM: RULES OF MONASTIC PRACTICE FOR NOVICES*

We all have tough days, sometimes because of major catastrophes, sometimes over minor annoyances. Just this morning, I was feeling energized and peaceful after meditating. I went downstairs to eat, and my daughter was lying on the couch whining, "I'm tired … My foot hurts … My head hurts … I'm tired … My foot hurts … My head hurts …" My son was beating the countertop with his spoon to the same annoyingly repetitive beat, while remnants of his breakfast sprayed across the countertop. The space I felt only moments before was rapidly disappearing.

I suddenly remembered that the woman who cleans our house was coming today, and as I glanced around, I saw dishes, cups, food, books, papers, dirty socks, and clothes on the floor, countertops, and everywhere around me. Ugh. I looked at the clock. Only ten minutes until we have to leave for school, and I haven't eaten, and what to do with this mess?

You may be thinking none of this is a big deal. This is not a crisis. You are absolutely correct. Intellectually, I knew this too. Yet my body failed to get that memo. My body was preparing for an imminent threat. My heart was racing, my stomach and chest tightened, my breathing shallow and restricted. I could feel anger churning just below the surface, and I was expending a lot of energy to stay calm and not explode. I packed my breakfast to eat later. I cleared what I could from the countertops. I threw the dirty clothes in the washer. I reminded my kids to brush their teeth and get their stuff ready for school.

My son decided he wanted a quick run on his new hover board. I wanted to scream, but suggested he save the hover-board jag for when he gets home from school. We were already ten minutes late. As I pulled out of the driveway, I realized I had a choice. I could churn all day and be ruled by my stress and emotions. I could passively decide this will just be "one of those days" and let it play out in a predictably negative way. I could add to it by judging myself for handling this all so poorly. Or I could choose to step out of my head and into my body, out of the recent past and into the present, by noticing my breath.

I started to breathe deeply into my belly. I noticed some judgy thoughts passing through my mind about how I should have been able to handle such minor problems with more grace and calm—I mean, I teach this stuff to others! Instantly, I felt my breathing tighten further at the self-criticism. I let the thought go and returned to the breath. As my breath deepened, my heart slowed down, my muscles released. I felt more peaceful and calm. I chuckled, remembering I am in the middle of writing the chapter on the power of breathing.

This is a perfect, everyday example of how quickly our minds and bodies catapult small, pesky, everyday life events into crisis mode, and how we can use the breath to downshift those emotions and reactions. Now I feel gratitude for the morning's cortisol rush and timely lesson. My perspective and physiology have shifted. This will be a good day.

Perhaps this sounds like a familiar morning to you. But what does this have to do with depression? If we cannot settle and clear space after minor irritants, how can we possibly manage the bigger stuff? Over time, as unavoidable stressors—big and small—pile on each other, what option do we have but to crawl under the covers and shut down, or find ourselves crying or exploding over spilled lemonade or whining children?

How does this happen? How does the brain create a mountain out of a molehill? To understand this, we need to take another look at the stress response. In my practice, I use Dan Siegel's hand model to visualize and simplify a complex process. To see this for yourself, form a fist with one hand, with four fingers folded over your thumb. You now have a handy-dandy model of half the brain. Your forearm represents your spinal cord. Just above the wrist represents the ancient, reptilian part of your brain known as the brain stem. This part of the brain is in charge of your breathing, heart rate, and making sure your basic needs get met.

The top of your fist, where the four fingers fold, represents the frontal lobe, the most evolved part of the brain that gives us the ability to time travel in our minds between past, present, and future. It allows us to analyze, and offers us the possibility of perspective and discrimination. It can also trap us with ceaseless chatter ricocheting around, distracting us from the present moment, sometimes creating catastrophes that will never materialize, and at other times repetitively and mercilessly beating ourselves up over mistakes, or tantalizing us by imagining how others must be judging us. Clearly this part of the brain is a blessing and a curse if we do not learn how to recognize and tame its creative storytelling.

The thumb in the middle of the fist represents the limbic system, where our emotional threat detector, the amygdala, and fear-based memory storehouse, the hippocampus, reside. The limbic system acts as Judge, deciding what is "good" and what is "bad," what we should move toward and what we should pull away from. This discrimination is based on past experiences, so if you have a history of trauma, abuse, or neglect, this system will be overly vigilant, always anticipating and preparing for the worst.

Based on this determination, the limbic system and brain stem together serve as the command center to activate the sympathetic nervous system and the fight, flight, freeze response. This primitive part of the brain is preverbal and cannot be calmed down with words, no matter how hard you or someone else tries. It speaks the language of the body and breath. When the body is relaxed and the breath is slow and deep, it acts as a limbic lullaby, shifting us from a state of high alertness to relaxed awareness. When the body is tight, or the breath is rapid and shallow, the limbic system interprets this as a threat, regardless of the magnitude of the stressor. The "threat" might be a car accident, a pending deadline at work, a comment from a spouse, or just a whining child and not enough time to eat breakfast.

Whether we are stressed due to an external event or an imagined catastrophe, the limbic system takes over and hijacks the frontal lobe, reducing the blood flow there by as much as 80 percent. Why? Imagine you are crossing the street when a turbocharged Ferrari turns the corner and is heading toward you. If your frontal lobe was in charge, it would be so busy analyzing the situation and trying to decide the pros and cons of each possible option that you would be run over and smashed before you ever took action.

To prevent this from happening, the limbic system is designed to shut down the analyzer and make an executive emergency decision to act, for better or worse. This is the best chance of survival when we're in real danger, but it makes for a lousy system when the enemy is in our own heads, or it is a ticker tape at the bottom of our TV screen informing us of the latest disaster that we can do nothing about, or a Facebook feed in which a friend makes a snarky comment and we—without tone or context—assume (based on the frontal lobe's interpretation) it to be malicious.

Because breathing is both unconscious and conscious, autonomic and voluntary, the breath offers us a means of communication with the limbic system. Our breath at any given moment is reflective of our emotional state. More importantly, it provides a pathway by which we can shift that internal state. By breathing slowly and deeply into the belly, we can activate the vagus nerve, which wanders up to the brain stem and limbic system to let them know we are safe. It is OK to relax, digest, and take care of the body's cleaning and mending duties, which are not essential during an emergency. Focusing on the breath also pulls us out of the unremitting gabfest in the cortex, bringing us back in touch with the body. We will learn more about this in the next chapter.

Teaching breathing exercises is where I start with everyone I see in my practice, whether they are coming for depression, anxiety, PTSD, bipolar disorder, or stress management. Being the one physiological process that is both unconscious and conscious, it is a fundamental tool for accessing information about our internal states, balancing the nervous system, and shifting our responses from automatic limbic responses to more thoughtful, evolved ones.

Better yet, it is free and, as long as we are alive, it is always available, accessible, and vitally important. We can survive without food for a few weeks and without water for a week, but we can only survive without air for a few minutes.

Despite the essential role of breath for life and survival, most of us are unaware of our breathing. We tend to take it for granted, unless we suddenly find ourselves panicked or gasping for air. Yet the breath is a common thread, marking not only the passage of our own lives from birth to death, but also the lives of all beings before us. Take the example of Julius Caesar, brutally stabbed to death on the marble floors of the Senate meeting hall on the Ides of March in 44 BCE. Sam Kean's book *Caesar's Last Breath* explored the mathematical likelihood that we might each be breathing a molecule from Caesar's last gasp of air. Crunching numbers, Kean suggests that the wind would have blown the twenty-five sextillion (25×10^{24}) molecules of his last breath around the entire planet within a period of two years, and proposes that "roughly one particle of Caesar air" will appear in your next breath. Obviously, there are a lot of assumptions here, but the basic premise is sound. It is fascinating to consider how viscerally intertwined we are with life around us.

The breath not only bridges life and death, past and present, internal and external, but also connects the conscious and unconscious, body and mind, emotions and spirit. Connecting with the breath, listening to its messages, and learning to breathe properly is the first step toward balancing your nervous system and creating emotional stability. It is the first step to getting unstuck and freeing yourself from the helplessness, loneliness, sleeplessness, and energy-depleting confines of depression.

On a simple, physical level the importance of breath as a source of fuel and energy is glaringly obvious, yet this is mostly overlooked in health care. An average adult takes about 16 breaths a minute, 960 breaths an hour, 23,000 breaths a day, and 8 million breaths a year. Each inhalation brings fresh air, oxygen, and energy into our bodies. Each exhalation releases toxins. Yet nine out of ten people breathe improperly. This affects every system in the body, resulting in fatigue, mental fogginess, poor digestion, poor sleep, impaired immunity, sluggish metabolism, and a buildup of toxins, which all lead to emotional and physical distress. By becoming more aware of our breath, and learning to breathe properly, many of these symptoms can be alleviated.

As we have seen, the breath also serves as a messenger and regulator of emotions. Becoming acquainted with our breath and how it shifts when we are happy, anxious, mad, and sad provides access to vital information about our internal states before they overwhelm us. You may notice when you feel anxious, your breathing becomes more rapid, shallow, irregular, and restricted and is confined to the upper region of the lung. On the other hand, when we are filled with joy, our breathing shifts into a slow, deep, relaxed breath into the belly. You will learn that by shifting the pattern of your breathing, you can shift your emotional state.

WELLNESS RX: NOTICING YOUR BREATH

In this exercise, you are going to explore your own unique breath as it is in this moment.

Find a comfortable, relaxed position sitting upright in a chair. Begin by placing one hand over your chest and one hand over your belly. Pay attention to the movement of your breath beneath your hands. You may find yourself trying to force a deeper breath, but for now just allow your breath to be as it is, without trying to shift or change anything. Feel the movement of the chest and belly as you breathe in and the movement as you breathe out. Follow the breath for the next few cycles. Perhaps your mind starts to wander. That is fine. That is what minds do. Simply notice the mind has wandered and return to noticing the next breath in and the next breath out.

As you follow the breath, begin to detect where you feel the most movement. Perhaps the hand over your chest is moving more; perhaps the hand over the belly. Just pay attention to the next few breaths and see what you discover. The point is not to judge, but simply to notice.

Now, move both hands to the belly and continue to follow the breath in and out. Perhaps you start to notice more movement in the belly just by fully shifting your focus there. Perhaps not. Continue to follow the expansion and contraction of your belly with each breath in and each breath out for the next five or six breath cycles, and see what you discover.

Begin to discern the difference between your inhalation and exhalation. After following a few breaths, you will start to notice that one is more restricted than the other. Perhaps there is a catch or hiccup somewhere in the breath. Follow the breath and see what you find. Once you have discovered whether you hold more tension in the inhalation or exhalation, break it down even further. Notice where in the breath the tension first arises. Perhaps you notice it is harder to breath in; pay attention to where that tension begins. Is it at the pause before you breathe in? Does it begin just as you start to inhale, or somewhere toward the middle or end of the inhalation? If you struggle a bit more with the exhalation, notice where that begins. Is it at the pause before you exhale? Does it arise just as you start to breathe out, or somewhere farther along in the exhalation? Observe with curiosity, as if you are conducting a science experiment on yourself and your breath, without any judgments or expectations.

Once you have figured out where the tension arises, begin to notice where it releases. Follow the next few breaths, watching the tension arise and release. The breath may start to shift. Perhaps the tension softens, stays the same, or even intensifies. Just observe.

Begin to notice the count of your inhalation and exhalation, counting one–one thousand, two–one thousand to the top of the inhalation, and then doing the same with the exhalation. Continue to do this for the next five to six breaths to get a good sense of your breathing pattern.

Once you have established your count, this is your starting point. One of the most common errors with breathing practices is attempting to breathe so deeply to somebody else's count that you actually create more tension in the body. The key is to begin where you are and slowly build from there. Let's say you discovered your breath is two counts in and two counts out. Add two-count pauses at the top and bottom of the breath. Breathe in for a count of two or longer, holding at the top of the inhalation for a count of two, exhaling for a count of two, and then pausing at the bottom of the breath for a count of two. Simply notice what happens as you intentionally shift the habit of the breath.

If your breathing pattern was, for example, a count of two in and a count of three out, simply add the two-count pauses at the top of the inhalation and bottom of the exhalation. In your case, you would breathe in for a count of two, hold for a count of two, exhale for a count of three, and hold for a count of two.

Continue your pattern for the next five to six breaths, noticing your experience. If you observe yourself straining and trying too hard, back off and try a shorter count. If you notice your breath deepening, try lengthening the breath in and out.

When you are ready to move on, remove the pauses in the breath and just allow your body to breathe as it wants to breathe, noticing how it feels. Observe the count of the breath now. Perhaps it has deepened. Perhaps not. Check back in with the point of tension you discovered earlier on your inhalation or exhalation. Notice if that has shifted or softened in any way. Notice how your body feels, having taken time to explore this breath that you may have taken for granted for so many years. Perhaps you feel calmer, less tense. Perhaps the restriction in the breath released. Perhaps the breath deepened. Perhaps you feel frustrated because you "didn't get it right" or it was difficult to stay focused on the breath this long. If that is the case, notice how the judgment feels in the body. See if it is possible to just acknowledge the judgment with kindness.

The goal is to simply notice your breathing patterns and even your reactions to the exercise. This is just a starting point. Like everything else in life, paying attention and shifting our breathing patterns requires practice. Now take a moment and write your observations in your journal, so you can look back and observe your progress over time.

As you went through this exercise, you may have noticed that you breathe into the chest. Thoracic breathing is common with anxiety and depression. Breathing into the upper lungs creates tension that sends a message to the limbic system, alerting it to some unknown threat. You might be sitting on your favorite reclining chair, perfectly safe, yet your brain is interpreting the shallow, tight breaths in the chest as a signal of a pending threat. You may wonder why you feel anxious, and then judge yourself for feeling this way when there is no "appropriate" reason. As we will see in the next chapter, that judgment causes more restriction and keeps the pattern going.

By breathing slowly and deeply into the belly, rather than the chest, air flows into the lower lobes of the lungs, which provides six times more oxygen to the body. This will also activate the vagus nerve, which wanders up to the brain stem and limbic system to give the "all clear" signal, brake the sympathetic response, and turn on the parasympathetic system, allowing the body a much-needed moment of rest.

You may have noticed that you started off breathing into the chest, but as you brought your awareness to the belly, you could feel more movement there. That is the idea. The mere act of shifting our attention and awareness can shift the pattern of breathing. If this did not happen for you, that is perfectly OK. Sometimes deeply ingrained patterns simply take more time and practice to shift, but it is entirely doable.

Next, you shifted your attention to the difference between your inhalation and exhalation, to see if one felt more restricted than the other and where in the breath you felt that restriction begin and where in the breath it released. I do not believe there is any research on this, but what I have found in practice is that the way we breathe tends to reflect how we approach life. Some people inhale easily and fully, but feel restriction on the exhalation. They tend to be quick to take chances and try new activities. They may more easily accept love and help from others, but they have difficulties letting go of past hurts, betrayals, and judgments about themselves and others.

Others get stuck on the inhalation, but exhale with ease. They may struggle to find motivation or courage to try new opportunities and reject the support and help of others, but more easily let go of past grievances.

It may offer insight to consider how this may or may not apply to you, your breathing pattern, and your life story. What never ceases to amaze me while working with others is that by becoming more aware of our breathing patterns, we start to shift the long-held beliefs and approaches to life that are keeping us stuck.

You may even have noticed that in the short time you explored the areas of resistance in your breath, some of the tightness relaxed or released. Awareness is key to making shifts. We cannot change that which is buried or hidden.

Next, you examined the count of your inhalation and exhalation, and later added pauses at the top and bottom of the breath. Depressive symptoms often manifest as shallow, restricted breaths into the upper chest. Research has shown that the optimal breath, which reflects a well-balanced nervous system, is somewhere between four to six breaths per minute, or a five- to seven-count breath in and out. Most people have a far more rapid breath than this, which means that an unnecessary alert signal is being constantly sent to the brain, keeping us unnecessarily on guard and stressed. Adding a pause between breaths serves to shift the brain stem out of old, ingrained habits of breathing.

Many of us intuitively recognize the power of the breath, and may even advise others to take a deep breath when stressed. In yoga classes and therapist offices, we hear this all the time. Some people, however, feel more tense after trying to force the body to inhale and exhale for a count much longer than their normal, short, shallow breathing. Often patients will tell me they have tried deep breathing when stressed out, but "it just doesn't work." I will ask to see how they have been taking deep breaths. They will take a deep inhalation high into the chest, shoulders shrugged up to the ears, neck tight and strained. I will mimic this posture so they can see the tension this creates. Vertical breathing is anything but relaxing! A deep, full breath is indeed what we are striving for, but we must breathe correctly, starting where we are and slowly deepening and expanding from there, to avoid unnecessary tension.

The brain stem, like us, can fall into deeply ingrained routines and patterns that may no longer be serving us. Conscious breathing helps us break free of unhelpful habits and create new ones. Learning to shift the rhythm of our breathing offers us the ability to calm the limbic system and balance our nervous system so that it is less reactive to anything and everything. Then, we can more adeptly pull ourselves out of unnecessary emotional turmoil.

This skill is central to stress resilience, or the ability to recover and rebound from life's challenges. Resilience can be measured with HRV, which reflects the variability in our heart rate from beat to beat. To better understand this, pause for a moment to notice your own pulse.

Gently place a couple of fingers over your wrist or neck to find your pulse. Notice your pulse as you breathe in and out for a few rounds. Can you observe a difference in the pulse between the inhalation and exhalation? Do you notice your heart rate increasing slightly as you inhale and slowing as you exhale? The increase of the heart rate as you breathe in activates the sympathetic nervous system. As you breathe out, the parasympathetic system gets turned on and the heart rate slows. The breath keeps these systems balanced.

The heart, respiratory function, and autonomic nervous system are intimately linked with every breath. A healthy heart is flexible and adaptable to second-to-second changes, based on activities and emotions. An unhealthy heart loses that flexibility and becomes rigid and resistant to change, leading to a low HRV. Depression, anxiety, PTSD, and even attention deficit hyperactivity disorder (ADHD) are all associated with low HRV, as are many other chronic diseases. Breathing at a rate close to your resonant rate of three to six breaths per minute can increase your HRV tenfold. This increase in HRV is indicative of improved overall health and balance of the mind and body.

Spiritual practices have recognized the power of a slow, deep breath for thousands of years. In fact, in many ancient cultures the word for breath is synonymous with the word for spirit. In this sense, restricting the breath diminishes our spirit. Descriptions of the use of breathing practices, or *pranayama,* for healing date back to at least 700 BCE. *Pranayama* is a Sanskrit word that translates as "control of breath." Ancient yogis in India, *qi gong* masters in China, kahunas in Hawaii, martial artists, and even the Russian Special Forces have long recognized the power of the breath to bring greater energy, attention, and vitality to life. Buddhist monks in deep meditation breathe at a coherent rate of six breaths per minute. The chanting of the Latin Hail Mary also leads to a breath of six breaths per minute. It seems we keep forgetting and having to relearn what ancient mystics and healers have known for thousands of years.

The key to benefiting from deep breathing is to breathe correctly, which is something few of us do in a world where we are often slouched over computers and glued to cell phones, where we are taught to suck in our bellies to be slimmer, and we are in a constant rush to do more and more and more.

You do not have to disappear to a hermitage or cave for months, years, or decades to benefit. A study found that even a one-day retreat focused on controlled breathing relieved emotional distress from job burnout among mental health professionals. Don't have time or resources for that? Research has shown that just one breathing practice can significantly reduce blood pressure, improve oxygenation of the body, and increase HRV.

The ancient yogis believed that we all take a certain number of breaths in our lives. If we breathe more rapid, shallow breaths, that end will arrive sooner. The Framingham Heart Study, which has followed more than ten thousand participants over a thirty-year period, and the Buffalo Health Study both found the same results: our breathing patterns predict longevity. If you didn't try the breathing exercises yet, perhaps you are now inspired to try?

When stuck in a deep depression and barely able to get out of bed, living a longer and healthier life may not be particularly motivating. How might these breathing practices help you better manage depression? Randomized controlled trials show that slow, deep breathing decreases symptoms of stress, anxiety, anger, and depression. It improves mood, energy, motivation, attention, and overall quality of life. One study compared the effects of yogic breathing practices to the antidepressant imipramine and to electroconvulsive therapy. By the fourth week of the trial, breathing was equally efficacious as the antidepressant, but without the side effects—or the price tag.

Psychiatrists Richard Brown and Patricia Gerbarg have studied and written about various breathing practices in their book, *The Healing Power of the Breath*. Along with teaching breathing and yoga practices to health professionals, their patients, and military veterans, they have offered their breath, body, and mind techniques to ease anxiety in survivors of natural disasters and trauma. In one study, they taught these skills to 183 survivors of the 2004 tsunami in Southeast Asia, most of whom showed signs of PTSD. Over a period of six weeks, participants' PTSD scores dropped by 60 percent and depression scores decreased by 90 percent. Those on the waiting list did not show improvement.

They found similar results when they brought these healing tools to people who survived the 2010 earthquake in Haiti, 2005's Hurricane Katrina on the Gulf Coast, and genocide in Rwanda and Sudan. If a pill provided those kinds of results, everyone would be taking it. These amazing outcomes prove what ancient healers have long known, that conscious breathing is a powerful healing force that we all have access to, regardless of resources or circumstances.

WELLNESS RX: BASIC BELLY BREATHING— CALMING THE NERVOUS SYSTEM

Here is a shortened version of the most basic of calming breaths that can be used anytime, anywhere to quiet the nervous system. Sit tall but relaxed in a chair noticing your breath as it is in this moment. Then intentionally bring your focus to the breath in the belly, perhaps laying your hands there to keep your focus. Remember not to force the breath, but keep it even and relaxed, allowing it to deepen at its own pace.

Notice the belly expanding in all directions as you breathe in, rising like a small balloon. Notice the slight pause at the top of the inhalation before you start to release and breathe out. Notice the belly deflate, moving inward toward the spine as you exhale. Continue to follow the ebb and flow of the breath, breathing in and out. Your mind will likely start to wander, as our minds love to do. Simply notice where your mind has gone and kindly and intentionally shift your focus back to the breath ... again ... and again ... and again. Record your observations.

Beginning to notice the patterns of your breath at different times offers you a barometer into your internal state, so you can intervene before your system goes into full-fledged red-alert panic mode or simply shuts down in over-whelm. Check in with the breath and notice its flavors and variations as you move through the day. Perhaps even set a timer hourly to remind yourself to notice your breath as it is, and then take a few deep breaths to prevent stress-ors of the day from building up like unmopped floors covered with layers of grime. You may want to set an intention to notice your breath whenever you transition from room to room or shift activities. I always take a few cleansing breaths between patients, so I do not carry any emotional charges from one person to another. I often start my sessions with a few minutes of breathing so that both the patient and I can clear space together and find a moment of calm, clarity, and connection.

Although the belly breath is perfect for destressing and calming the mind and body, at times we may require more focus or energy. Different breathing patterns shift our physiology in different ways. One breathing practice that is highly beneficial when your mind is running all over and cannot be still long enough to even focus on simple belly breathing is called alternate nostril breathing. This practice helps balance the right and left hemispheres of the brain and calm the nervous system. Even Hillary Clinton promoted this practice during her book tour as a way to alleviate anxiety. I am guessing she might know a thing or two about managing stress. Since balance is the key to health, let's take a few minutes to try this one out.

WELLNESS RX: ALTERNATE NOSTRIL BREATHING—FINDING BALANCE

For this exercise, you will be using your right thumb and ring finger to block off alternating sides of the nostrils. You can support the elbow of your right hand against your chest as you do this or rest your index and middle fingers between your eyebrows—whichever feels more comfortable.

If you are congested in one or both nostrils, rub in gentle circles about halfway down the nose on the bony shelf on either side of the nose. This may alleviate some of the pressure and open up some space. You could also try gently pulling the skin away from one side of the nose while you attempt to breathe through the other side.

To begin, use your thumb to block off the right nostril. Inhale through the left nostril slowly. At the top of the inhalation, block off both nostrils using your ring finger and thumb. Pause for a moment, then release your right thumb and take a slow, easy breath out through the right nostril. Breathe in through the right nostril. Pause at the top, blocking off both nostrils. Release the ring finger and exhale through the left nostril. Repeat this cycle five to ten more times. As best you can, breathe slowly and deeply, keeping your focus on the movement and sensations of the breath. When you have completed your rounds of breathing, release your arm to your side and take a few deep breaths into the belly. Notice how your mind and body feel and write down your observations.

This exercise has several variations, depending on how you are feeling and what you need most in the moment. The variation you just learned is beneficial for balancing the hemispheres of the brain and calming the nervous system.

If you are feeling fatigued and in need of more energy and focus, you could try breathing in through the right nostril and out through the left, and back in through the right and out through the left. This activates the left, linear, logical, analyzing side of the brain.

If you are feeling anxious, jittery, agitated, or cannot turn off the incessant chatter in your brain, you could start with a few rounds of breathing in through the left and out through the right. Then complete a few cycles of the alternate nostril breathing to provide more balance. Left nostril breathing activates the creative, intuitive right side of the brain.

In as little as six to eight weeks, setting aside twenty minutes a day to focus on the breath can change the structure and function of the brain. The amygdala becomes less reactive, and the frontal lobe less easily hijacked. This starts to shift the early wiring of childhood adversity and trauma. It offers us greater stress resiliency, increased flexibility, and adaptability to the unavoidable stressors of life. It is getting to the roots of this beast we call depression and, ultimately, the messiness of being human.

Wherever you are reading this right now, why not just pause for a moment, notice your breath, and take a few deep breaths into your belly? While you are at it, perhaps you could set an intention to set aside twenty minutes tomorrow to begin to see for yourself how this one simple practice can change your days, weeks, months, years, and life for the better.

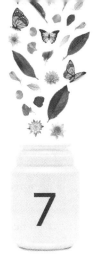

The Mind as Master Storyteller

I have been surrounded by troubles all my life long, but there is a curious thing about them—nine-tenths of them never happened.

—ANDREW CARNEGIE, *AN AMERICAN FOUR-IN-HAND IN BRITAIN*

"Follow the yellow brick road," Dorothy is told by the Munchkins, and by Glinda the Good Witch. So off she goes, dancing along the yellow brick road in ruby-red shoes. Dorothy is told, and so believes, she must follow the yellow brick road to the Emerald City to find the all-powerful Wizard of Oz who can help her get back home. Along the way, she meets her friends the Scarecrow, the Tin Man, and the Lion, who are each unhappily stuck in their own tales of woe about their perceived inadequacies. Life would be better "if only" they had what they thought they lacked—a brain, a heart, more courage, the power to return home.

By facing their fears, through the adversities they experience together, Dorothy and her friends uncover their innate gifts. The Scarecrow, despite "lacking a brain," keeps coming up with good ideas that save them. The

Lion, despite "lacking courage," continuously faces danger to protect his friends. The Tin Man, despite "lacking a heart," is a sensitive soul who cares deeply for his friends and other living creatures and must hold back his tears to avoid rusting. Dorothy learns she had the power within her all along to navigate her way to Oz, face danger, motivate her friends, and ultimately return home.

Their perceived inadequacies were all fictional stories in their heads, and the Wizard did not have the power to help any of them. They had to find their own intelligence, heart, courage, and power. On their journey, they learned they were smarter, braver, more loving, and more powerful than they had imagined. You may argue that it was the magical shoes that transported Dorothy home, but shoes are just shoes unless we give them power and meaning. Any good witch understands the power of belief and expectations. Wicked witches understand the power of fear to control others. You may argue that the adventure was all a dream. But does it matter? As we learned in chapter 6, our brain does not know the difference between what is real and what is imaginary.

When people talk about "depression," they are stuck, like the characters in the *Wizard of Oz*, in their own convincing tales based on perceived failures and deficiencies. "I am broken and only a medication and a doctor can piece me together." "I can only be happy once I have been fixed, once I find what I lack, once I am thinner, once I am braver, once I have a job, once I get out of this marriage, once I find a loving soul mate, once I have a child, once my child is grown." The list of conditions for happiness goes on and on and on, always keeping the possibility of happiness far in the future. It is often this thinking pattern, and the resulting emotions and behaviors, that keep us stuck in unhappiness. Perhaps you, too, are looking for the Wizard to fix you, not yet believing you have the capacity, by changing old patterns and habits that are no longer serving you, to heal yourself.

The point is not to cast blame or judgment on yourself for falling into this trap. Dorothy would never have found her way home if she dejectedly disparaged herself for falling for the illusion of Oz and insisted "How could I have been so stupid?" It was, after all, facing the challenges of Dorothy's journey to

Oz that taught her valuable lessons. What if your adversities and journey with depression are challenging you to wake up and seek your own innate powers and gifts?

The human brain is a master of storytelling. Preferring to avoid uncertainty, the stories of the brain lack the complexity and ambiguity of literature, choosing to stick to common patterns, casting everything into labels, categories, simplistic explanations, and often faulty assumptions, so that information is quick and easy to access: This is good. That is bad. This is right. That is wrong. I am right. You are wrong. Along the path to depression, this story often shifts to self-denigrating categories that include: I am wrong. I am broken. I am weak. I am a failure.

Growing up, we also develop a long list of "shoulds," taught to us by our families, culture, and past experiences. It *should* be this way and not that way. A lion should be scary and fierce. A wizard should have power. An average everyday kind of girl like Dorothy should need a good witch or a mighty Wizard to find her way home. I should feel happy. I should not feel sad, unless, of course, I have a good reason, and even then, I should keep it to myself. I should be stronger. I should not be so weak.

In reality, none of our thoughts are inherently good or bad, right or wrong; they are just thoughts and stories the brain creates. Stories only gain power and become threatening if we automatically believe our negative thoughts, judgments, and assumptions to be true. The discrepancy between how things are and how we would like them to be, or think they should be, only creates more suffering. Learning how to notice our thoughts as stories manufactured by the brain, not facts or truths, frees us from becoming ensnared by the negative stories we spin that can lead us down the funnel of depression. Even while reading this paragraph your thoughts may be arguing, coyly trying to convince you of the veracity and importance of your negative stories—but those arguments are just more thoughts.

What we perceive as "good" or "bad" depends on our limited perspective and on the story we choose to tell. Life is what it is. Sometimes life can be tough and painful. Terrible things certainly happen. We need to acknowledge the feelings that arise, but adding additional blame and judgment to the experience—getting trapped in stories about the story—only adds to the suffering. If we can pause and step away from the stories, step out of instant reactivity and judgment, we can broaden our perspective and find clarity that will allow us to decide if there is something we can or should do about the situation.

Perhaps it is best to let things be and to remain open and curious as to how the experience will unfold. What if we learned to step away from the narrative altogether, and just gently acknowledge whatever arises as it arises without the stories, labels, and judgments?

The mind's ability to time-travel into future possibilities and remember the past can be a great gift—enabling us to create literature and art, construct offices and cathedrals, study physics and history—but it is also an enormous burden. Unlike the gazelle that successfully runs away from a tiger, shakes her body to release all the stress hormones, and then peacefully returns to grazing in the grasses, we often continue to dwell upon our experiences and cloud ourselves in fearful anticipations and brooding regrets.

The gazelle is not blaming herself for not seeing the tiger in the tall grass earlier. She is not blaming her friend who did not warn her sooner. She is not cowering in terror that the tiger now knows she is here and might return. She is not wondering "Why me? Why not the narcissistic gazelle with the longer antlers?" She is not wondering why the world is so unfair and filled with so many cruel predators. No. She shakes off the fear in her body and returns to the present moment, which is perfectly safe.

Sure, that lion or another predator may appear at any moment, but she is not going to waste precious time and energy worrying about that now. There is grass to eat and water to drink. There are other gazelles with whom she can romp and play. What is done is over, and what might happen next she cannot know. She is content right here, right now. We have much to learn from the gazelle.

As the Buddhist monk Thich Nhat Hanh says, "Peace can only exist in the present moment." Shame, blame, and regret for past actions lead us reliably toward depression. Fears about possible future catastrophes lead us down the overly treaded path of anxiety. The anchor to this moment, as we learned in the last chapter, is stepping out of the stories in our heads, and into the breath and the body. This is the essence of mindfulness.

Antidote to the Wandering Mind

Mindfulness is a word that pops up everywhere these days, from the cover of *Time* magazine to the titles of more than seven hundred research articles published in 2016 alone. It is being embraced by yogis, engineers, techies, therapists, athletes, artists, and even politicians like Tim Ryan, a congressman from Ohio, who is not only advocating that it be taught in schools, but is also teaching it to willing political colleagues, after experiencing its powerful effects on his own life and well-being. (We could sure use more politicians like that!)

Mindfulness is not, as some believe, a passing fad that requires sage, crystals, or expensive meditation retreats. Mindfulness is compassionately and nonjudgmentally paying attention to this moment as it is—not as we might like it to be, not as it "should" be, but just as it is, without stories and judgments attached. It is not a religion, although most religions have mindful practices. What is prayer, after all? Assuming you are paying attention to the prayer and not lost in thoughts about something else, "Prayer is, at root, simply paying attention to God," according to theology professor Ralph Martin.

The touching of Rosary, Mala, or prayer beads as well as dancing, chanting, and poetry are all forms of mindfulness, ways to focus the mind away from its storytelling and back into the present moment. It is not some exotic concept, but one that we all have experienced at some point in our lives.

Can you bring to mind a moment in your life when you were fully engaged in an activity, fully in the flow, and lost all sense of time? Perhaps you were running, dancing, writing, singing, playing an instrument, reading, or just watching a beautiful sunset, or listening to the rain or ocean waves crashing on the shore. In those moments, all worries about the future and regrets about the past vanish. You are fully present. That is mindfulness. The trick is to learn how to train the mind to spend more time there and less time lost in the worries and ruminations of the wandering mind.

In the broadest definition, all the exercises you have already tried in the last two chapters are aspects of mindfulness. We will continue to build on what you have already begun to experience and learn. By becoming more aware of the thoughts and stories of the mind, we can recognize them for what they are and choose to step away and give them less power.

WELLNESS RX: A TASTE OF MINDFULNESS

This exercise requires a yummy treat and about ten minutes of your time. Chocolate is my preference, but you could try this with another type of soft candy or a raisin. Once you have picked your treat, set it aside for a moment and just settle into a comfortable position, sitting on a chair or the floor. Elongate your spine, sitting tall. Feel your feet on the ground beneath you. Begin to notice your breath. Feel the air moving through your nostrils, throat, chest, and belly. No need to change anything; simply notice your breath as it is in this moment.

Slowly, intentionally reach for your treat of choice. Notice the movement of the body. Notice any sense of anticipation or impatience to grab. Pick up the object and hold it in your hand for a moment. See it with the fresh, curious eyes of a child. Notice the weight and feel of the object in your hand.

Slowly, carefully open the wrapper, noticing the movement of the fingers and the sound of the wrapper. Hold the substance in your hand and explore the object from different angles, noticing the shape, texture, and color. Notice any ridges or markings. Observe how your mind may be wandering, labeling, or judging. "What is the point of this?" "How is this going to help with depression?" "This is just a piece of chocolate." Just notice the thoughts as thoughts, and kindly return to your investigation of this new, exotic edible. There may be a sense of urgency to go ahead and eat it, or, having held it in your hand for so long, there may even be a sense of revulsion. Just gently notice whatever arises.

Bring your hand up to your nose and notice the aroma of this object. Inhale deeply, fully taking in the smell. Perhaps you notice saliva forming in your mouth, or the gurgling of your stomach.

Slowly and deliberately move your hand toward your mouth, paying attention to the movement of your arm and hand. Take one small bite, but do not swallow yet! Notice the sensation as you bite into the substance; notice the flavor as it first meets the taste buds; notice the desire to swallow or move faster. Move the substance around in your mouth, allowing it to melt, noticing the feel and taste. Now, finally, swallow the bite. Observe as it moves down the throat. Pause for a moment and just tune in again with the breath.

Repeat these steps with another bite, taking time to mindfully slow down and notice your experience.

Once you complete the exercise, jot a few notes in your journal about this experience.

Thanks to Maureen Sloan and Dr. Jane Eckert for introducing me to this exercise and leading me to attend mindfulness-based cognitive therapy training with Zindel Segal.

You may be wondering, what does eating a piece of chocolate have to do with depression? Some may argue (including me!) that chocolate itself is an antidote to unhappiness, but even if that is true, it is certainly a short-lived one. Perhaps while savoring the chocolate, you noticed how difficult it can be to remain attentive to one focal point, and how often your mind became distracted with some other thought, label, judgment, or worry. The brain always wants to wander. It has the attention span of a three-year-old child, always asking why, why, why, but never being still long enough to listen to the answers.

Most of the time our brains are on autopilot, mindlessly wandering from thought to thought, lost in the maze of our contemplations. When we are constantly rushing to move on to the next thing and the next, we miss what is going on right in front of us. Once again, we fail to see the gorilla because we are busy counting the balls. Perhaps you have had the experience of driving to work, school, the grocery store, or some other familiar place and realizing that you have no idea how you even got there. You were so busy replaying a conversation from yesterday, or figuring out how you were going to get everything done tomorrow, that you missed the whole ride. Fortunately for us, our brains know the route and keep us safe while we daydream. Unfortunately, we miss a lot of our lives lost in these trances.

Perhaps when you are depressed, it does not feel like a loss to miss out on periods of your life. But what if these stories created by the Master Storyteller are keeping you depressed? If you are lost in thought about everything that was ever wrong with your life, relationships, and job, how nothing will ever work out, nobody will ever understand you, you will never find a job you enjoy or somebody who appreciates you. Do you think these perceptions are helping to pull you out of your depressed mood, or sinking you farther and farther into the abyss of despair?

Remember, our brains do not discriminate between the real and the imagined, so as you drift off into stories of gloom and doom, your body responds with heightened vigilance, preparing for fight, flight, or death. Now your brain is on high alert, looking for danger. Suddenly, the neutral expression on your spouse's face becomes a disappointed scowl; a flippant remark by a friend becomes an intentional insult; the beep of a horn reminding us the light has turned becomes an attack; a whining kid becomes a critique about your parenting skills. You get the picture. These perceived attacks amplify the sense of urgency, disconnection, and despair, leading to more negative thoughts, and so it goes, on and on and on. Thoughts, emotions, body sensations, and behaviors are all linked, fueling and feeding each other. Most of the time this happens outside our awareness. Paying full attention to our breath, thoughts, emotions, and body sensations anchors us back in the present moment, breaking the vicious cycle of sustained unhappiness.

Although we can all get trapped in this cycle, research reveals that those with a history of depression can get entangled in this web far more easily. The founders of mindfulness-based cognitive therapy (MBCT) were tasked with finding an alternative solution to preventing relapses of depression, other than with a lifetime of prescription medications. Scouring through research, they discovered that those most likely to relapse have a tendency toward depressive rumination. This is a fancy phrase for the inner chatter in our heads we have been discussing.

They found that for those with a history of depression, the thoughts, emotions, body sensations, and behaviors linked to past episodes get wired together into an intricately woven tapestry of depression. Tug on any one thread and multiple threads start to unravel and get entangled together in a hopeless mess. A stray thought about an old regret unwinds a twinge of sadness, entwined with more memories of past depressive episodes, failures, and losses. Now the sadness merges with more thoughts and feelings of hopelessness, helplessness, despair, and fear. Familiar, repetitive tunes begin to play in the mind like a rut in a record player. "Here I go again." "This will never end." "What's the point, anyway?" The body responds to the old tune and emotions in an equally familiar pattern. Perhaps your chest tightens around your heart, your throat may constrict, your posture caves into itself, the body feels heavy and fatigued. All the while, the brain attempts to figure out what has gone wrong, what did I do, what can I do? Why is this happening? Now add in the sprinkle of self-blame and judgment to top off the dessert of gloom.

Perhaps your particular melody has a more anxious, depressive feeling, a state particularly common among those with a history of abuse or emotional neglect. Your anxious thoughts about the future and ruminations about the past trigger the amygdala to sound the alarm alerting the body to imminent danger. The body goes into a state of fight or flight, the heart races, the breath becomes rapid and shallow. You cannot sleep, and become increasingly agitated and restless. You fear this will never end. Meanwhile, your brain is struggling to find an answer, digging up more and more evidence of past shortcomings, further fueling the flames. Trapped in your misery, you may start to avoid others, thinking you need to preserve your energy for the "essential" things—going to work, cooking meals for the kids. You put the activities you love to do on hold.

That doesn't exactly make you feel better, does it? The intent is not to judge, but to recognize that although a familiar melody stuck on repeat may feel like reality, because you have heard it so many times, the tune is a storytelling narrative, not a fact. With mindfulness, we can learn to focus on the present and allow the song to play quietly in the background.

Once you become conscious of the cognitive, emotional, and physical soundtracks associated with your depression, you have options. You can return to playing the same sad song, but is it serving you? You can intentionally lift the needle out of the well-worn groove. You can tune in with the breath and enjoy a few moments of silence, a reprieve from the Master Storyteller's charismatic pull. You can ground yourself by noticing what you hear, touch, or smell in this moment as another means of getting back in the body. You can choose a different song: perhaps a more upbeat and hopeful one. You could offer yourself kindness for getting trapped in the same old rut and, better yet, congratulate yourself for consciously noticing that you were trapped this time.

WELLNESS RX: NOTICING YOUR STORIES

The goal of this exercise is to become more aware of your personal soundtrack. Set a timer so that you do not get sucked into a whirlwind of thoughts and lose your way. If you do, you can always use your breath to lead you back to the present moment. Close your eyes and notice your breath.

Intentionally shift your focus from the breath to your thoughts. Observe the focus and content of your own thoughts just as you would listen to dialogue in a TV show, movie, or play. Notice how they appear out of seemingly nowhere and pass by, if we do not attach to them, just like clouds in the sky. Observe, but do not engage. If you notice you are getting sucked into a story, return your focus to the breath for a few seconds and then observe again. After a minute has passed, shift your focus to the breath.

Write what thoughts you noticed in your journal. If you did not notice any, that is fine. Start to keep a list of thoughts you observe passing by, during this exercise and throughout the day. Common thoughts in depression that may arise include, "I am broken," "I am worthless," "I am unlovable," "I am not enough," "I am all alone," "It's hopeless. Nothing will help me."

Thanks to Zindel Segal and MBCT training for teaching me this exercise.

The goal here is to start to become aware of our recurrent narratives, especially the ones that lead us down the path of depression. This allows us to witness thoughts as just thoughts. They are not facts. They are not you. They just pass through. Many are old familiar tunes you have been hearing for so long that you assume they are accurate facts. If you do not recognize your stories, you cannot free yourself from their lure. The act of noticing is the first step toward freedom. Acknowledging a thought as just a thought, a story as just a story, offers all of us enough space and distance to pause and step away. This is the practice of mindfulness.

Benefits of Mindfulness

Mindfulness, like depression, has many forms and expressions. It is a skill, a practice, a way of being, a way of relating to the world, and also now an evidence-based treatment for depression. Zindel Segal and his colleagues developed MBCT as an eight-week group therapy specifically designed to address the root causes of relapsing depression. The focus of the group is to teach mindfulness as a means to step out of the ruminating mind by anchoring oneself nonjudgmentally with the breath, emotions, and body sensations of the present moment.

Multiple papers by different researchers have all concluded that MBCT reduces depressive symptoms and halves the risk of relapse in those who have suffered three or more previous episodes. In other words, it appears to help even the so-called "treatment resistant" folks, without the side effects of medications. MBCT has been shown to alleviate anxiety; decrease rumination, negative thinking, and judging; increase awareness of emotions and body sensations; decrease emotional reactivity; and improve sleep, concentration, and overall well-being. It offers a broader sense of perspective and an expanded sense of self. If a pill offered all of that, wouldn't we all be on it?

The practice of mindfulness has been shown to balance the autonomic nervous system, decreasing sympathetic arousal and increasing the parasympathetic response. As we learned in the last chapter, in as little as eight weeks of daily practice, twenty minutes a day, imaging studies show that mindfulness changes the structure and function of the brain so that the amygdala and limbic system are less reactive to stress. Long-term meditators develop enhanced connections between the limbic system and cortex, so there is improved communication that diminishes the likelihood that the cortex will be hijacked.

Most of the research suggests that practicing meditation for twenty minutes daily offers an optimal balance of effort and reward. One study has shown that even one eight-minute session of focused attention on breathing can decrease mind wandering and distractibility, improving memory and focus.

Obviously, the benefits of a single eight-minute practice are not sustainable. Like exercise, the results are dependent on consistent practice. As many of us know all too well, just having a membership to the gym does not improve our physical fitness. We must show up and work out. Showing up once a month is better than not working out at all, and we will undoubtedly feel better momentarily for having done it, but it will have limited long-term benefits in terms of building muscle mass or endurance. We are far more likely to stick to anything if it is part of our daily or weekly routine.

No matter how much muscle you may build up lifting weights for the weeks you showed up, in as little as a week after you stop lifting, your strength will slowly start to diminish, and your motivation disappears even faster. One of the surest ways to lose motivation is to get trapped in the all-or-nothing story line. If we don't have time to go to the gym for an hour, there is no point in going, so we might as well just find a spot on the couch in front of the TV for the night. We forget that a five-minute walk around the block is better than not moving at all. Parking a little farther away from the grocery store adds exercise to our days. It is just so with mindfulness.

Counteracting years of mental habits with new neural pathways takes cultivation and care. All too often, patients I have not seen in months, sometimes even years, will show up at my office in a state of distress and despair. I will always ask what they have been doing to nurture themselves. Inevitably, I will hear that they had been feeling better and had stopped practicing breathing and meditating, stopped using the very tools that had pulled them out of depression in the past. Often just that reminder and a new-found commitment to returning to their practice, whatever form that takes for them, is enough to pull them out of the old rut.

WELLNESS RX: ORCHESTRA OF SOUNDS

For this exercise, set a timer for three minutes. Find a comfortable space indoors, or better yet, outdoors, if possible. Sit or stand. Feel your feet on the ground beneath you. Close your eyes and observe your breath.

Begin to notice the sounds around you. See if you can sense the sound not just with your ears, but with your entire body, as if

---

your skin is a giant antenna bringing in the sounds from near and far, beside you, in front of you, and behind you. Soft sounds and loud sounds. Notice the sounds of your own breath and body. As best you can, listen to the tone, melody, and rhythms of the sounds without labeling them. There is no need to strive to hear sounds; just be open to receiving. Gently notice any stories, labels, or judgments that arise and return your focus to the sounds.

When your alarm goes off, return for a moment to focusing on the breath. Notice how the body feels. Slowly open your eyes and take a few moments to write down what you noticed and felt. Perhaps it was frustrating and difficult to focus. Perhaps you felt more expansive and open. Perhaps you were annoyed by a particular sound, like the ticking of a loud clock, or perhaps you were swept up in the symphony of life and lost all sense of time and place. Thank yourself for taking this small moment to explore the workings of your mind and senses.

Perhaps the greatest gift of the practice of mindfulness, whether we are focusing on a piece of chocolate, our breath, or the sounds around us, is its ability to put us back in the driver's seat of our own lives. The hallmark of depression is a sense of hopelessness and helplessness, amplified by "helpful" doctors informing you that you are permanently broken, absent pharmaceutical intervention. You feel you no longer have control over your own destiny. You are at the mercy of the "dis-ease," the physicians, the pills—or at least that is what the mind tries to convince you.

There is an analogy I love to share with patients, which I borrowed from Susan Orsillo's and Lizabeth Roemer's book *The Mindful Way through Anxiety.* Imagine you are the driver of your own bus. You have a goal and destination in mind. In the back of the bus are a crew of unruly teenagers, representing the thoughts, judgments, and doubts in your head. They are loud, whiny, demanding, and sometimes even threatening. You are heading home, toward your deepest values and desires, but the teenage bus riders want to go to Oz for an evening of distractions and illusions.

You have three choices in this moment (parents know these choices all too well). You can be pulled off course and go to Oz. The voices are so loud and belligerent. It is so much easier to just give in and heed their demands, even though you know this is not in your best interest. Alternatively, you could stop the bus and attempt to placate the bullies, but to no avail; now you are going nowhere. Your third option is to drive toward your desired destination. You hear the voices, screams, and threats, and may feel anxious, annoyed, frustrated, or even fearful of what they might do, but you choose to breathe into the fear and tightness in your chest, the anger in your throat, and you keep on driving.

You remind yourself that thoughts are just thoughts. They only have power if you feed them. You notice your breath is fast and rapid in your chest, and you start to breathe into the belly. You feel your hands gripping the steering wheel, and slowly relax them. The voices of the kids become a distant blur of noise—still there, but in the background, not the foreground. You notice the landscape outside your window: the trees, the birds, the road signs, the scattered clouds passing through the vast expanse of blue. You roll down the window and feel and hear the breeze, softening the now muffled shouts receding farther into the background. You are on course. You, like Dorothy, are going home.

If feeling more empowered, emotionally stable, and stress-resilient is not incentive enough, mindfulness has also been shown to decrease blood pressure, reduce pain, improve immunity, and reduce the risk of heart disease, stroke, and Alzheimer's. Mindfulness can also slow age-related atrophy of the brain, alleviate PMS and menopausal symptoms, and improve psoriasis, and if that is still not enough, it has also been shown to extend your lifespan.

You may wonder dubiously how one skill can possibly affect so many aspects of one's life. If you remember from chapter 5, the common underlying root for depression and so many other physical and emotional issues is our reactivity to stress, and the subsequent inflammation. Mindfulness rewires the brain's response to stress, decreasing inflammation and its deleterious effects on our bodies and minds. Given these potential benefits, I bet you can find eight minutes in your day to begin to improve your mood, health, and well-being.

If your mind is spinning some creative tale about why you cannot find that time, or why it will not work for you, or how you will never be good at mindfulness so why even try, gently remind yourself, and your storytelling mind, that these are just more thoughts, not facts. Then take the driver's seat, roll down the windows, turn on some upbeat motivating tunes, and start driving toward what you desire.

What Mindfulness Is Not

Mindfulness, which is often practiced through meditation, is not a powerful wizard in a pointy moon-and-star-patterned hat offering us a path to pure happiness all the time. Meditation is a practice that allows us to become more aware and open, to see our tales of woe and blame as stories. It is an opportunity to see our quirks and foibles from a place of curiosity and compassion, rather than from a place of self-denigration.

As you focus on the breath, the mind will travel. It is what minds do. Each time you become aware that you have drifted, and return to your chosen destination, this is a success. You are no longer lost on autopilot. You are in the driver's seat. You can choose to step out of doing, analyzing, judging, and trying to fix things into a state of awareness and presence.

You may find this awareness leads to calm and peace. This is a fairly common and pleasant side effect, but not the goal. The intention is awareness of whatever arises, even thoughts, feelings, and sensations that are not pleasant. If we use the practice to eliminate and resist thoughts, emotions, and sensations we do not desire, we have just found another means of avoidance and resistance. What we resist persists. Trying not to think about something or not to feel an emotion only fuels the flames, like a pot of water on a stove. If we keep the lid on the pot and avoid disturbing thoughts or feelings, the water will eventually explode over the sides. If we remove the lid, providing space and air, the water calms to a simmer. If we remove the pot from the heat of our ruminations, the water settles even more.

It is easy to fall into the trap of thinking we know what meditation should do, or how we should be after practicing meditation for a long time, and then berating ourselves for "failing" the practice. I heard author and meditation teacher Susan Piver speak on the podcast *Ten Percent Happier* with Dan Harris, about her own experience. She told a story of how she had been practicing meditation for many years and had just completed her first book. She had a meeting with the publisher, who told her the book was terrible and unpublishable. Piver was understandably devastated, and blamed herself for not being able to handle the situation better after so many years of meditation.

That inner critic gets the best of all of us at times. Fortunately, a friend and fellow meditator passed by and took Piver to lunch, where she poured her heart out and expressed her frustration that she was not coping better. Her friend kindly reminded her that the point of meditation is not to feel less, but to lean in and fully feel the emotions of the moment so they can be released and freed.

The goal of meditation is not to be holier-than-thou stoic but to feel and experience the full range of emotions while noticing the stories that arise with the emotions—the unfulfilled expectations, the self-blame, the shoulds—and recognize them for the old narratives they are, fueling the fire, keeping it burning. In other words, if you are sad, it is OK to feel the sadness. What is unnecessary and counterproductive is to get sucked into a whirlwind of thoughts and stories about the sadness. Why am I sad? Nothing happened. There is no good reason to be sad. Why am I so weak? Why can't I handle things better? Soon you, like Dorothy, are swept away in a tornado of negative thoughts, which makes things look and feel worse and worse.

The yellow brick road that can lead you home comprises acts of kindness: stepping out of the thoughts and into the breath and body, gently noticing areas of tightness and tension and breathing into them, noticing thoughts of blame and judgment and acknowledging them as old familiar thoughts but not truths. Your brain may want to argue with you—the mind hates to lose an argument—but those are merely more thoughts.

Tara Brach is a revered psychologist and meditation teacher who has written several wonderful books on mindfulness, and she offers a free podcast. In one episode she spoke of the process of dying cloth the color indigo. With each dip of the cloth into the blue vat, the material turns the subtlest shade darker. Initially, the color is barely visible, but with each subsequent dip, the color intensifies and deepens.

WELLNESS RX: MINDFULNESS OF DAILY ACTIVITIES

Now it's time to bring nonjudgmental, compassionate awareness into the "real" world. It could be mindfully noticing the feel and temperature of the water on your back as you take a shower; bringing full awareness to your first two bites of breakfast; noticing transitions between sitting and standing or as you move between rooms or spaces; taking a few breaths at red lights or while waiting in lines; noticing movements and sensations of your body as you wash dishes, brush your teeth, or fold laundry. Pick at least one activity and set the intention to be fully present each and every time you engage in it this week.

Similarly, each time we return from the frantic storytelling of the mind, back into the present, we slowly, deliberately saturate our lives with color, meaning, and joy. Our thoughts and emotions color the world around us. As we continue dipping the cloth of our lives with attention and kindness, the colors intensify.

Intentionally seeking moments throughout the day to dip into presence, with attention and kindness, will shift your world from the shades of gray, in which Dorothy was enveloped when bored by her life in Kansas, to the deeply saturated colors found in the Land of Oz. Mindfulness is a powerful tool against the self-defeating hopelessness and gray cold freeze of depression. It is at the heart of all the other skills and lifestyle changes we will discuss in future chapters, because it is not just a skill and a tool, but a way of approaching, perceiving, and being with life.

Pauses to tune in to the breath, emotions, and sensations of this moment become your own richly colored yellow brick road, guiding you away from the tornado of your thoughts and back into the driver's seat of your own life. Each dip into the dye of awareness and presence provides a path home.

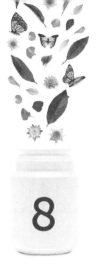

8

The Body as Navigator

The body says what words cannot.

—MARTHA GRAHAM

Angie's head was throbbing as she sat across from me to meditate for a few minutes at the beginning of our session. I encouraged her to lean into the sensations with curiosity, using the breath as cushion, support, and anchor. As she focused on the breath and explored the tightness, she envisioned a Frankenstein-like head, with two big boulders of red volcanic rock on her forehead getting bigger and bigger, heavier and heavier, weighing her down. She felt disconnected from her body and the world around her. As she continued to breathe into the heaviness, she gained a broader perspective, radically different from what her thinking mind defined as reality. She started to relax, but her thinking mind desperately wanted to make sense of her experience, and she tightened again.

The thinking mind and the sensing body have two different vocabularies, and the harder Angie attempted to translate, the worse her head throbbed. I gently reminded her to step out of the stories and return to the breath and the sensations.

As she breathed in and out of the pain, her perception expanded. She began to have awareness of her thoughts and the part of her observing the thoughts. She recognized that her thoughts were part of her, yet also separate from the body and mind. She attempted to put her experience into words. "My brain has all these thoughts, but they are separate from me. It's confusing because they are in my head, but not part of me. Everything makes it seem like it is mine, but the brain in my head isn't what belongs to me."

Angie continued to breath in and out of the sensations, and the pain intensified as she struggled again to make sense of her experience, fighting off waves of fear stirred by this uncomfortable uncertainty. It felt like nothing fit. "Everything is too big or small. Everything is tight and being squeezed." Angie felt herself trying to shrink to squeeze into the narrow, confining space of the thoughts pressing in on her. Her shoulders, neck, and jaw tightened and her brow furrowed in a whirlwind of thoughts and resistance to the pain and fear.

I encouraged her to step back into the sensations of the body and let go of the story about it. As she continued to focus on the breath and the sensations, space started to open. She saw a tiny crack in the massive boulders of her forehead through which she could walk. This took her into an open space, billowy and filled with light. Form disappeared. "It feels like being the air and being in the air," she said.

This is a perfect description of the space available to us when we step out of the confinement of our heads and thoughts. The word for suffering and distress in Sanskrit is *dukha,* which literally translates as "obstructed space." *Sukha* is the Sanskrit word for happiness, or "unobstructed space." As Angie brought curiosity to her fear and body sensations, and stepped out of the story about what was happening, she entered a spacious place of peace and expansiveness, a place of *sukha.* This is the wisdom of the body and the tranquility that can be found there, if we can summon the courage to lean into the sensations of the body rather than ignoring, resisting, or running from them.

I know this may sound abstract and even "woo-woo." Trust me, every time Angie has these experiences, a part of her finds them looney and illogical too. "It's crazy, isn't it?" she often asks. She has seen images of objects and places she has never heard of, let alone seen before, yet these are entirely relevant to helping her navigate her current circumstances and feelings. Our bodies possess wisdom our thinking mind cannot access.

The Buddha understood long before modern science and physics that the body and mind are distinctions that do not actually exist. Research by modern pioneers of Mind-Body Medicine, like Dr. Candace Pert, confirms that the body and mind are inseparable. Pert referred to this inseparable network of information and energy as the "bodymind." She wrote in her book *Molecules of Emotion,* "Mind doesn't dominate body, it becomes body—body and mind are one … the body is the actual manifestation, in physical space, of the mind."

Still, most of us walk around much of the time as if we are bobble-head dolls with "ginormous" heads tenuously attached to a body that holds us up. We have been taught "I think therefore I am" since René Descartes in the early 1600s. It is no surprise we start to think our body's sole purpose is to hold up the head and obey all its orders.

In reality, far more information is sent from the body to the head than vice versa. Yet, many of us fail to notice the body until something goes wrong, and then we quickly seek a solution to make the "problem" go away, usually with a medication. We hush the messenger. Perhaps it would be wise to notice our bodies before that happens, to lean in, to observe, and listen.

WELLNESS RX: NOTICING THE BODY

For this exercise find a quiet, comfortable place to lie down. Know that the directions in this exercise, and all the others, are suggestions. Always listen to the cues in your own body.

Begin by noticing your body in this moment. Feel where your back is making contact with the floor and where it is not. Feel the texture of the ground beneath you. Observe your breath. Bring your attention to the belly for the next few breaths, allowing it to fill like a balloon as you breathe in, and deflate as you breathe out.

Now, allow your breath to breathe itself; no need to control it. Shift your focus to your hands, lying palms-up beside your body. Start to notice any sensations in your hands at this moment. Feel the texture of the surface upon which they rest. Notice the temperature of the hands. Check in with the fingertips. You may notice a tingly sensation in one or more fingers. Maybe you do not feel any sensations. It is OK. There is no right or wrong here.

No need to judge. The intent is to simply notice your own experience as it is, right here, right now.

At any point your mind may start to wander. Simply observe, and mentally note, "thinking," "judging," "worrying," "planning." Congratulate yourself for having noticed your mind wandering, and return to whatever sensations you may or may not notice in the hands.

Now, let go of your focus on the hands and start to move up your arms—the lower arm, elbow, and upper arms. If it is easier to do this one arm at a time, take the time to do this. If you need to make changes that feel more comfortable to you, honor that, but see if you can, for just a few breaths, first acknowledge and notice the sensations of discomfort before automatically reacting and "fixing." If you start to feel restless or anxious, notice that, and see if you can feel the sensations and the emotions and let it all be there for a few breaths before automatically pulling away and avoiding the experience.

Shift your attention into the shoulders, back of the neck, and base of the skull. What do you observe? Perhaps you notice tension in the shoulders. Explore it. You may want to imagine breathing in and out of the tense spaces, allowing the breath to provide support and nourishment. Perhaps the movement of the breath creates some space there. With each breath in, offer kindness to the areas of tension. With each exhalation, imagine releasing some of the tightness. Be careful not to set expectations. The intent is not to change anything but simply to notice with kindness and curiosity.

Observe the back, sides, and top of the head. Observe the sensations of the forehead. Notice the space between the eyes where many of us furrow with tension. See what happens if you imagine breathing into this space. Observe sensations of the eyelids and eyes. See if you can notice the space behind the eyes. Bring your awareness to your nose. Notice which nostril has a freer flow of air in this moment. Feel the air above your lip as you breathe in and out. Notice the sensations of the cheekbones and jaw. Observe where you are holding your tongue. Allow it to rest at the bottom of the mouth and see how that feels.

Follow the movement of the breath into the throat. Become aware of the sensations there. Notice the sound and feel of the air as it passes in and out of the throat.

Follow the breath into the chest, becoming aware of the movement. Notice any areas of tension or tightness. You may want to breathe into those spaces, offering support and release.

Follow the breath to the abdomen, becoming aware of the expansion and contraction of the belly in all directions with each inhalation and exhalation. Observe the sensations within the belly. Sense the organs and the space around the organs. Notice areas of tightness or discomfort. Notice how each movement of breath may or may not change those sensations.

Draw your attention into the pelvic area, feeling any sensations. Notice the movement of the breath even here, feeling the rise and fall of the pelvic bone.

Move your focus downward into the upper legs, knees, and lower legs. Feel where the legs touch the ground beneath you and where there is space. Move into the ankles, feet, and toes. Notice sensations in the tips of the toes, bottom of the foot, and heel. Perhaps you are starting to feel restless, or bored, or sleepy, or ready to finish this and move on to the next item on your to-do list. If this is the case, just observe the thoughts telling you there are more important things to *do*. Notice how that influences your breath and body. Note to yourself, "thinking," "judging," "planning," and simply return to the sensations in the feet. Use the feel of the foot as an anchor back into the body and out of the mind.

Direct your attention up the back of the legs to the sacrum. Feel the ground beneath you. Observe the motion of the sacrum with the breath. Perhaps you notice the sacrum pressing toward the ground as you exhale, and curving slightly upward with the inhalation. Notice the sensations that arise with these motions.

Continue to move your focus up into the lower back, middle back, and upper back. Notice any areas of tightness or tension and breathe into those spaces. Notice how the movement of the breath causes the back to expand and contract.

Spend a few more moments tending to any areas calling for attention, perhaps a tight shoulder, neck, or back. Just notice and acknowledge.

Draw your attention back to the belly, to come full circle and end where you began. Breathe in and out of the belly, allowing it to fill like a balloon as you inhale, and deflate as you exhale. Notice how your body feels now. Perhaps it is more relaxed than when you started. Perhaps you feel growing tension and anxiety to get moving. Notice your thoughts. Perhaps they have quieted down or perhaps they are screaming to move on. No judgment here. Just observe.

Thank yourself for the time and care you offered to yourself and your body. Now slowly open your eyes. Then take a few minutes to jot your observations down in your journal about your experience with the body scan. Were there any particular areas of tightness that called out to you? Any sensations you were surprised to discover? How difficult was it to stay focused? Did focusing on certain parts of the body stir memories you may not have recalled for a long time?

Thank-you to Maureen Sloan and Dr. Jane Eckert for first teaching me the Body Scan and leading me to seek further MBCT training with Zindel Segal.

How was it to spend time noticing the body? Did it feel uncomfortable and scary, like strange and unfamiliar territory, or refreshing and surprisingly familiar, like a childhood friend whom you have not seen in decades?

You may be wondering what paying attention to the body has to do with healing depression. Research suggests that depressive symptoms are associated with reduced awareness of the body, and that therapies focusing on body awareness result in reduction of depressive symptoms. Why might this be the case? The body serves as another anchor, like the breath, to pull us out of the tornado of negative thoughts and stories associated with depression. Learning to sit with uncomfortable sensations, rather than resisting them, empowers us to lean into discomfort rather than pull away—an important skill for emotional resilience.

Connecting with our bodies also offers us access to the felt experience of our emotions and a different way of relating with them. Exploring the sensations of the body teaches us how to experience the breath, the body, and our emotions, rather than thinking about or reacting to them. It enables us to feel pain in the chest without immediately assuming we are dying of a heart attack, or discomfort in the abdomen without assuming the appendix is about to burst; to see a blemish on the skin without concluding it is cancer. It creates space between the sensation and the reaction. It allows us, like Angie, to find the crack in the boulders leading us to a place of spaciousness and light. It grants us access to our emotions so they can be acknowledged, felt, and passed through, rather than getting stuck and buried within us.

Becoming aware of our bodies and emotions offers us choices. Awareness puts us back in the driver's seat. Listening to the body, and the emotions expressed through the body, offers us an inner guidance system, our own portable, always accessible GPS, unique to us and our needs. It is never out of range, no matter what remote places we may travel. Like all other guidance systems, however, we must learn how to use it. We must learn which signals point us toward our desired destination, and which ones signal that it is time to stop and recalibrate a different route.

The body speaks through the language of emotions. Emotions act as messengers linking mind and body, "translating information into physical reality." They form a bidirectional network keeping the body apprised of second-to-second changes, sorting through the thousands of signals constantly being picked up. Emotions act as a compass, pointing us toward what needs our immediate attention, and keeping us informed as to internal and external changes in weather.

The blue sunny skies of happiness inform us that our needs are being met. We are meeting our nutritional and emotional needs—at least for this moment. Gray cloud cover may obscure the blue skies at any time, but that is OK, because we cannot fully appreciate or understand happiness without its relationship with sadness, just as our understanding of light is relative to our experience of darkness.

The word *emotion* derives from the Latin word *emovere*, meaning "to move out." This is what emotions are supposed to do—move through and out of us, just like the ever-changing weather and clouds in the sky. Clouds always pass. The gloomy skies of sadness inform us of loss—whether it is a person, a situation, or even an old idea no longer serving us.

As we all know, even positive changes—a new house, a new relationship, a new job, or the end of a terrible relationship or job, come with loss or regrets of what came before. The more resistance we feel toward the overcast skies, the darker the clouds seem to appear. Perhaps storm clouds are moving in with lightning and thunder? Fear keeps us alert for possible threats—often, as we learned, imaginary ones. Anger moves us toward action for ourselves or others.

Like the clouds in the sky, our emotions and thoughts pass through, offering information that may or may not be based on facts. Sometimes, despite dark ominous storm clouds floating overhead, it never rains. Unlike the weather around us, we have control over how long we are stuck in our internal thunderstorms. Or, at the very least, by learning to read the nuances of the emotional signals in the body, we can access raincoats and umbrellas so we will no longer be caught in bad weather unprepared and without shelter.

WELLNESS RX: NOTICING THE BODY'S RESPONSES

In this exercise, you are going to bring to mind something that stirs up a few storm clouds—not threatening or scary ones yet, but something that stirs up some angst as you think about it. First, ground yourself by taking a few deep breaths. Now allow yourself to intentionally bring a difficult moment to mind.

Close your eyes and bring your awareness to your emotions and your body as you hold on to that thought. If it becomes too intense, just return to the breath. If you can keep the thought in mind for a bit longer, notice how your body and emotions respond to the thought. Notice your posture. Notice your breath. Are you breathing in the upper chest or the belly? Is the breath shallow or full? What emotions are stirred up with the thought? Note the emotions: "There is sadness." "There is anxiety." "There is despair." "There is frustration."

Observe and be curious how that emotion is expressing itself in the body. Notice where you hold tension in your body. Check in with the face, head, throat, neck, and chest—all areas where we commonly hold emotions and tension. See if you can breathe into the areas of tension, not trying to change or get rid of anything, just acknowledging the emotions and sensations with curiosity and kindness. Observe if anything shifts as you breathe into the sensations. Perhaps they intensify, soften, or even disappear. Perhaps nothing changes. The intent is to simply notice with as much acceptance as you can offer in this moment, to lean in rather than avoid or resist.

If the emotions feel too intense, bring your full attention to the movement and sensation of the breath in the belly. Let the thoughts be in the background. Observe as you breathe in and breathe out. Continue this for a minute or so and then check back in with the sensations of the body. Do they feel the same or different from when you were focusing on the negative story about yourself? Perhaps the thoughts about the difficult situation intensified the emotions and restricted the body. Maybe your body slumped over, shrinking in on yourself. Maybe you felt your face furrow into a grimace or frown. Perhaps by shifting your focus to the breath, you created a little more space, a little less tension. Maybe you even sat up taller.

Now shift your focus back to the breath in the belly and bring to mind a moment of contentment or something for which you feel gratitude. Notice how that feels in your body. Observe your posture, your energy. Notice areas that had been tight and see if there is a shift. Allow your experience to be whatever it is.

Can you feel your muscles relax a bit, or perhaps a subtle sense of spaciousness and lightness? Although we are all quick to notice pain or discomfort, it can take a while to notice the subtler sensations and shifts in the body.

You are learning a new way of leaning into and being with the body, the emotions, and the breath. You have to honor the timing of your own journey. Tuning into the body with awareness enables you to shift your relationship with emotions and thoughts. This is the essence of mindfulness. Take a few moments to record your experience in your journal.

Tending and Befriending Emotions

I dreamed the other night that my son was crying and sad because a friend had been unfairly accused of some minor infraction and lost recess privileges at school. At first I too felt sad, but this shifted to righteous anger that his friend had been unfairly targeted. I walked into the school carrying all of these unexpressed emotions. The head of the school noticed my distress and asked what was wrong. By this time I was choking back tears, but explained what my son had just told me, and that both he and his friend were sad and frustrated. She proceeded to tell me, "It's OK. Feelings give flavor to life. Without them life is drab, boring, and meaningless."

Even though this message came through a dream, the head of the school was right. Feelings not only give flavor, color, and meaning to life but they guide us. Without them we are like a ship without a rudder, staying afloat, yes, but aimlessly moving through the water. We do not feel the waves below us or notice the awe-inspiring sunrises and sunsets. We fail to notice when the weather changes and we need to change course, or if there is a hole in the boat that needs to be mended. Without emotions, or when we are numbed to them by medications or other means of avoidance, we stay in jobs, relationships, and situations longer than necessary. We just keep bailing the water out of the boat rather than fixing the problem.

Feelings yank us out of our comfort zone and alert us when something needs to change. Life with emotions is uncomfortable and messy, but necessary and unavoidable. The trick is not resisting and fighting the feelings—that's what gets us stuck and leads to depression and anxiety—but rather to notice and "befriend" the feelings with curiosity. The pain can be physical or emotional. Ultimately, in the "bodymind" they are linked together and inseparable.

Learning to lean in, rather than pulling away or running in the opposite direction, offers space. The harder we resist and pull away, the more intense pain and emotions become. It is like the Chinese handcuffs you may have played with as a kid. The harder you pull to escape the cuffs, the tighter they get. If you release the resistance and move your fingers toward each other, the tension releases. It is the same with our emotions. If we can "stop, drop, and breathe," as my daughter likes to say, we can release the sense of being strangled and entrapped by the emotions, and provide ourselves enough space to be curious about what is happening, and breathe into it.

I encourage patients to think of their intense emotions as they would a two-year-old child who has been physically or emotionally hurt. Imagine a two-year-old falls and scrapes her knee. In one scenario, the anxious mother rushes over asking, "What's wrong? What happened? Are you OK?" The child cries harder, her hurt buried under a barrage of questions.

A second mom stomps over and tells the girl: "Stop crying; stop being a sissy. You are fine. Just brush it off and get over it." The girl cries louder. Now she is not only physically hurt, but also unacknowledged and scolded. Over time, she will indeed learn to be silent and suck it in, but in the process, she learns that her emotions are not valid or allowed to be expressed. They are to be buried and pushed through. This is the equivalent of putting the lid back on the pot of boiling water. Sooner or later it will find a way to release tension, often spilling over unexpectedly.

A third mom, on the playground of life, calmly walks over, hugs her daughter, and offers a kiss to the scraped knee. The girl jumps up and returns to playing. What the fallen child needs is simple acknowledgment, something many of us were never offered or taught as kids. In the same way, when we are feeling sad and down, we need to acknowledge those hurt, angry, or frustrated parts of ourselves. All too often, we blame and shame ourselves and our emotions for arising, which only intensifies the internal emotional response.

As we have seen, different emotions are expressed in different places in the body. When I ask where people feel pain in their bodies, those thinking about the pain rather than feeling it often point to their head; those filled with sadness point to their heart; those aching to express unwanted emotions point to their throat; those torn by indecision or fear point to their stomachs; and those feeling powerless and out of control point to their diaphragm. As the modern dancer Martha Graham said, "The body never lies."

Once the emotion is located in the body, we can step out of the story by noticing the sensations of the emotion in our body, and breathing into the tightness. This often softens the intensity. But as soon as we add expectations of a certain outcome to the mix, we add stress and pressure to the system, much like the mom scolding the two year old. The intention is only to be open and curious, to lean in rather than pull away.

Sometimes emotions get stuck in our bodies in what may seem like odd places. To give you an example of how this might play out, meet Ann. She hurried into my office for her first visit with a grim, determined expression, declaring her desire to "be fixed." She had a lifelong history of anxiety and depression with chronic passive suicidal ideation. She remembered being a four-year-old and riding her tricycle down to the train tracks with a wish to die.

With her sixty-fifth birthday approaching, she was determined to figure out what was wrong, and she thought a type of therapy called eye movement desensitization and reprocessing (EMDR) might be the answer. She was disappointed by my suggestion to first start with some basic breath training, so she could learn to sit with her emotions and modulate intense arousal before we started EMDR. Despite my periodic suggestion to try to approach her breath with curiosity and playfulness, not as a problem that needed to be solved, her face was set in a stern grimace of disapproval that she was not "doing it better."

Struggling to breathe through her nose, I suggested rubbing some acupressure points near her nose to open up the nostrils. As she rubbed these points, a deep sadness instantly passed over her face. I asked her to locate the sadness in her body. She felt it in her chest and throat. I encouraged her to breathe into the sadness with curiosity to discover more about it. She described a round, solid ball of sadness in the center of her chest. I suggested she breathe into it with as much kindness as she could, imagining that her breath could cuddle and support that ball of sadness.

As she did this, the tightness softened and a new sensation arose behind the ridge of her eyes. She became aware of a "big tiredness." Her tight, rigid body sagged, and her face looked older and exhausted. I asked her to imagine breathing in a healing, energizing light. As she did this her body straightened and face softened. "It's gone. The sadness and tightness are gone."

There was a long pause as she puzzled over this experience. "So breathing in with kindness? That's it?" she asked. I nodded. Her face sank into despair and disappointment. I asked her to notice where she felt the emotions. She waved her hands over her throat, now visibly tightening. She breathed into it, feeling the sadness and dismay dissipating. Her face softened and her breath became smoother and deeper. As I pointed out what changes had already occurred in just an hour, she nodded, grateful for the awareness, but also discouraged that this was not the quick easy fix for which she had hoped. She could not avoid or get rid of undesired emotions. Healing is a process that begins with acknowledging what feelings arise as they arise, and breathing into them with kindness. "So that's it, huh?" she asked again.

"Yep, that's it," I agreed.

Smiles, Frowns, and Slouches

For Ann, a release of stuck energy around her nose shifted a long buried emotional state. On a day-to-day basis, there are simple ways to adjust our bodies to boost our moods. In one classic study on the relationship between the body, mind, and emotions, researchers had college students place a pen in their mouths in positions that either facilitated or inhibited a smile while they watched cartoons. Those whose mouths were manipulated into smiles found the cartoons funnier than those prevented from smiling. The smile stimulated brain activity associated with positive emotions. A similarly designed study, which measured stress responses and heart rates, found that all those who smiled—whether they were aware of the smile or not—experienced lower stress responses and lower heart rates when faced with a stressful task than those with neutral expressions.

Other research has explored the influence of posture on mood. In one study, thirty depressed, hospitalized patients were asked to sit in either an upright or slouched position, while presented with an assortment of positive and depressive words. When later asked to recall the words, those slouched in the chairs primarily recalled the negative words, while their upright peers remembered the positive and negative words equally.

The body and emotions are in constant bidirectional feedback. Our facial expressions and how we hold our bodies in any given moment influence our emotional state, and our emotional states affect how we hold our bodies. We cannot choose our emotional states, but becoming more aware of our bodies offers us another empowering tool to shift the messages from the body that influence our moods. Take this moment to pause and notice your posture and facial expression. See what happens if you sit or stand a bit taller and lift the corners of your mouth into a gentle, nonforced smile. Notice how this small attunement feels in your own body in this moment.

Think about the implications of this in your day-to-day life. What if you started paying attention to your body, posture, and facial expression throughout the day? How might your daily mood and life change in a week, a month, or a year? Make this your own experiment and journal your results.

Our bodies, emotions, and life are our teachers, if we only learn to pay attention. Now it is your turn to see for yourself how quick check-ins with your breath, thoughts, body, and emotions can shift you out of whatever stuck place you may be experiencing in this moment.

If you are lucky enough not to feel stuck right here, right now, please notice that. Our brains are wired to fixate on what is wrong and to ignore all the many things that are right. Part of the healing journey is not to toss these skills aside when things are feeling OK, but to pay full attention to the moments when we feel good too. Both are worthy of our acknowledgment. We must remember to feed the Wolf of Hope as often as we can.

WELLNESS RX: BREATHING SPACE

Set aside a few minutes to clear space when feeling pulled by ruminating thoughts, powerful emotions, or painful body sensations.

Begin by paying attention to your posture, sitting or standing tall. Bring awareness to your feet planted on the ground. Notice your breath.

Check in with the **thoughts** passing through your head, and note "thinking," "planning," "judging," whatever is there, simply recognizing it as a thought, and just a thought.

Quickly scan through the **body**, noticing what sensations may be calling out for your attention. Observe any areas of tightness or discomfort and breathe into them in acknowledgment.

Notice what **emotions** are present in this moment and gently note, "There is sadness," "There is stress," "There is frustration,"

"There is anger," "There is fear." By labeling the feelings, we give ourselves a bit of space around the emotion.

Now, bring your full attention to the **breath** in the belly, using it as an anchor to this present moment. Notice the movement of the belly as it fills and expands, contracts and releases. If your mind wanders, simply notice and gently return your focus to the breath again.

Broaden your focus, sensing your whole body breathing, feeling your whole body's aliveness as you breathe in and out, your entire being expanding and contracting. Notice what calls out for your awareness and breathe into that. If there is a painful body sensation, breathe into that with curiosity and kindness. If a difficult emotion is center stage, lean in and breathe into that. If repetitive thoughts scream for your attention, recognize them as just thoughts passing through. Notice how your body feels as you expand your awareness.

This exercise is based on the Three-Minute Breathing Space Practice from my MBCT training with Zindel Segal.

Learning to tune in and listen to the body's wisdom bestows upon us responsibility and power. We are not at the whim of the body, but a cocreator of its state of well-being. We must accept stewardship. Our thoughts have physical consequences expressed through the body. We can feed our bodies fear, negativity, and blame, or fuel our bodies with acceptance and nourishment. We can repress and resist our emotions, or acknowledge them with kindness. We can fixate on negative thoughts and stories that perpetuate our stress, or notice them as just passing thoughts and choose to place our focus elsewhere.

We can no longer blame dis-ease on "bad luck," but we also cannot blame ourselves for causing our illness, for "failing." That is just another story and an attack on ourselves and our choices. Remember, the key here is to meet the body, emotions, and thoughts with kindness, even when—especially when—we catch ourselves failing to be kind to ourselves. More self-blame and judgment only continue to stir the pot and feed the Wolf of Despair.

There is an ancient Buddhist story about King Sakka and the Demon. Once, when Sakka, the king of the gods, was away from his palace, an angry demon climbed onto the king's empty throne. As the guards angrily and fearfully yelled at the demon, he transformed into a fierce fire-breathing beast. Fortunately, the wise king returned to the palace at this time. Seeing the demon on his throne, the king greeted him kindly and respectfully with outstretched hands, offering him food, drink, and a comfortable chair. The demon shrank in size and disappeared, just like the Frankensteinian boulders in Angie's head and the hurt from the child's scraped knee—with acknowledgment and kindness. Sometimes, as unbelievable as it may seem, stepping from obstructed suffering to unobstructed space and happiness really is this simple. "Crazy, isn't it?"

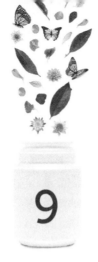

9

Moving the Body

All that is important is this one moment in movement. Make the moment important, vital, and worth living. Do not let it slip away unnoticed and unused.

—MARTHA GRAHAM

Inertia and fatigue pulled me like a giant magnet deeper and deeper into the couch cushions. Seven sixth-grade boys would be sleeping at our house after a night of trick-or-treating. They were already wired high on sugar, camaraderie, running, and the thrill of an Ohio State football victory, and then, just before bedtime, they started talking excitedly about girls.

As you might imagine, it was a loud, late night with little sleep for any of us. I awoke the next morning feeling crabby and fog-brained with no motivation to do anything except sit and stare at a wall. Fortunately, my dog, Bean, pleaded with eager puppy eyes to go on his morning run, so I mustered together enough energy to put on a coat and head out the door. The cool air felt invigorating as Bean took off at a run, pulling me along behind him. Within minutes my tired, achy body started to feel more energized and alive, despite the lack of sleep. This is the power of fresh air and exercise, but, oh, the effort to get started and pull ourselves out of sedentary ways.

The average American spends about eight hours a day engaging in stationary activities—watching TV or a movie, talking on the phone, sitting at a computer, sitting in a restaurant, sitting in meetings, sitting in a car, sitting in church … lots and lots of sitting. We all know we *should* be exercising, right? We turn on the TV and headlines scream "Sitting Will Kill You" and "Is Sitting the New Smoking?"

The research behind these headlines concludes that our sedentary lifestyles increase our risk of obesity, cardiovascular disease, diabetes, cancer, death, and, yes, depression. In fact, the National Health and Nutrition Examination Survey found that lack of physical activity doubles the risk of depression. Ugh. One more thing we *should* be doing that we just don't have the energy for.

The last thing anyone wants to do when they are depressed is exercise. After all, if you cannot even get off the couch to take a shower, how on earth do you find the motivation to get yourself to the gym for a workout? I hear you. I know that even without depression, when I get home from a typical day at work and then feed the kids and take them to their activities, the last thing I want to do is put on my tennis shoes and go outside for a walk, even though I know that is exactly what I need.

Fortunately for me, Bean hopefully wags his tail for his evening walk every day, refusing to accept "not today" as an option. For me, not letting someone else down—canine or human—is my call to action. We all need to find what drives us. I also know that my mood plummets if I go more than a couple of days without activity, and I always feel more energized and happier once I muster the motivation to get up and go. With each passing sedentary day, the pull of inertia grows stronger and stronger.

For many of my patients, one of the biggest hurdles to moving is the old stories they carry about what exercise means. Perhaps you have a childhood memory of gym class and boring calisthenics, or maybe you were the kid who always got picked last for team sports and learned to avoid "exercise" altogether, preferring to grab a book or a spot on the couch for some finger calisthenics, as you thumb through the pages or channels on the remote.

Exercising does not mean you have to do one-handed push-ups like GI Jane, or pump up monstrous biceps like Arnold Schwarzenegger. Maybe you are more like Bridget Jones and cannot even get off an exercise bike without falling on your butt. But I would be willing to bet that there is some form of movement you could find that might not only appeal to you but also boost your mood. We get too easily stuck in ideas of what exercise "should" be. But playing with kids is exercise, cleaning is exercise, washing the car, mowing the lawn, walking the dog, hula-hooping, jumping rope, dancing, or even shaking are all forms of exercise.

Shaking? Yes, shaking. It happens to be one of the oldest forms of mindful movement and healing. Bradford Keeney's book *Shaking Medicine* documents the use of this powerful tool, which dates back to the San people of the Kalahari over a hundred thousand years ago—talk about a time-tested healing strategy! Shaking is practiced by people all around the world, including the Quakers of New England, the Indian Shakers of the Pacific Northwest, *qi qong* masters of China, or the modern American trend of Buti yoga.

My first experience with whole-body shaking was with Dr. James Gordon's Mind-Body Medicine workshop. Imagine a dimly lit conference room with over a hundred health professionals spread around, shaking to loud tribal drum music. Sounds weird, right? For me, it initially felt awkward, then invigorating, then exhausting, and finally, liberating. I felt an immense yoke around my neck and shoulders release and vanish. The tightness had become such a part of my being that I had been unaware of its presence until it released.

Since then, I have taught shaking in my own groups, and have witnessed people burst into long-held-back tears, beam with long-forgotten smiles, and look wide-eyed and incredulous after some long-buried tight space releases and opens.

You may be thinking, *Um, I think I'll skip this exercise; it sounds way too strange for me,* but part of shaking is freeing energy and shaking out stale ideas, limitations, and fears. These same stuck places are also associated with depression, so, why not give it a try?

WELLNESS RX: SHAKING, YES, SHAKING

There is no right or wrong way to shake. There were no detailed instructions painted on the cave walls a hundred thousand years ago, so let go of any expectations or judgments.

Set a timer for eight minutes. If you have access to some fast drumming music, turn it on. If not, silence works too. In the second part of the exercise you will be dancing, so pick out your favorite dancing song and get ready to turn it on after you shake.

Start by planting your feet on the ground about hip distance apart, with the knees slightly bent and relaxed. Feel the floor beneath your feet, offering support and grounding. If you cannot stand, sit or lie on the ground. Check in with your body in this moment. Notice the internal weather. Observe any areas of tightness. Notice the breath, emotions, and thoughts. Acknowledge the inner critic, and set the intention to be curious and open to whatever arises. Maybe there is a growing sense of openness and willingness to try something new. Honor that with awareness and a smile.

Whenever you are ready, begin to shake, at your own speed, in your own way, allowing your legs to gently bounce up and down, keeping your heels planted on the ground for support and balance. Notice which parts of the body start to spontaneously shake, and which remain more resistant to movement. Experiment with adding in different parts of the body and seeing how that feels. Can you move your arms a little more? What if you lift and release or roll your shoulders? Allow the neck and head to move up and down, side to side, or to spiral. See what your body calls for. Move your hands and fingers. Can you move your belly, chest, and hips side to side, front to back, or in figure eights?

Experiment with how different movements feel. Notice what areas are tighter and looser in your body. Try shaking faster and slower. Just play. Keep checking in with your body and its sensations. You may notice thoughts telling you to stop, or insisting you are too tired to continue. Try to just listen but not shift course from your intention. If you are tired, try slowing down or moving more gently for a brief reprieve.

Often fatigue is the sign of resistance, fear, or stuck energy trying to free itself, so if you can, keep moving! If uncomfortable emotions arise, can you allow the movement of the body to help them move through, instead of resisting and stopping? Each time we allow ourselves to sit with physical or emotional discomfort and lean in, rather than back away, we build resilience. If there is actual pain, then honor the body and stop. Continue to move, feel, and observe your body in this moment.

After the timer goes off, turn on a favorite song and dance. Keep your eyes closed and allow your body to move however it wants to move. You might notice that even when nobody is watching, the inner critic of the mind is skeptically judging. Keep dancing and let your body move anyway. Do not let the inner critic change your intentions.

When the song ends, stand tall and still for a few minutes with your feet planted on the ground, noticing the breath, the body, and the emotions. Congratulate yourself for taking this time to try something that may be new to you.

Jot down some notes in your journal about this experience. What was your initial reaction to the exercise? How did that change once you began? Did you notice any places of tightness or restriction? Did those change as you continued to shake? Were there points when you wanted to stop? Did you get detoured or stay on course? Did you notice any judgmental or critical thoughts? Did any emotions or memories arise?

Thanks to Dr. James Gordon's Mind-Body Medicine training for introducing me to this form of dynamic meditation.

If you are feeling edgy, angry, or sad, just shaking for a couple minutes can move some of the stagnant energy. Try it out in different situations and notice what happens. Perhaps the exercise even shifted your perceptions of what exercise is and is not, and cleared space for new possibilities and motivation for moving your body.

So, why might it be worth your time and energy to clear this space and find motivation to move your body? According to neuroscientist Dr. Wendy Suzuki, exercise is the most "transformative thing you can do for your brain."

Suzuki's early research focused on memory formation in the hippocampus, a part of the brain that diminishes in size with stress, depression, and other mental illnesses. After one particularly long day in the lab, which followed years of other long days in the lab, she had a moment of insight in which she realized she was spending so much time in the lab, she had no social life, was gaining weight, and was "miserable."

To break out of her rut, she went on a white-water rafting trip, only to discover that she was the weakest person on the raft. Determined never to be the weakest again, she started exercising and immediately noticed changes in her body, mood, and ability to focus. These internal discoveries changed the course of her research.

Suzuki's studies and her personal transformation led to exciting findings on the healing potential for exercise. Her research demonstrates that just one aerobic workout increases levels of dopamine, serotonin, and norepinephrine, and offers one of the best ways to regulate and improve mood and attention, for up to two hours after exercise. Acute exercise also changes brain waves, increasing alpha and theta waves, which are associated with increased relaxation, decreased anxiety, and improved neuroplasticity of the brain. Exercise also increases the production of our body's natural opiates and cannabinoids that likely contribute to the runner's high many experience.

More astonishingly, over time, exercise, like meditation, changes the structure and function of the brain. It doubles the formation of new cells in the hippocampus, improving memory, but also protecting the brain against future neurodegenerative effects of aging, stress, and life. It increases the connectivity of the brain, enhancing functionality and regulation.

Decades of research has confirmed over and over again that exercise is as effective at treating depression as medication or therapy. It makes sense, right? If sitting up taller and smiling sends a message to the brain that enlivens one's mood, imagine what a walk in the park or an aerobics class might do?

Researchers for the Standard Medical Intervention and Long-Term Exercise (SMILE) studies conducted several randomized controlled trials on depressed adults that compared aerobic exercise, antidepressants, and a combination of the two. The exercisers did some form of aerobic exercise for forty-five minutes three times a week. At the end of four weeks, all the groups had improved about equally. At the ten-month follow-up, however, 70 percent of the exercisers had improved or recovered from depression, versus only 48 percent in the medication-only group. More curiously, only 45 percent of those in the exercise-plus-medication group improved. Differences in relapse rates were just as dramatic: 8 percent of those in the exercise group relapsed during the ten months, versus 38 percent in the medication-only group and 31 percent in the combo group.

Why might this be? We cannot say for sure, but the results certainly correlate with the data we reviewed in chapter 3 about the negative long-term effects of medications. The results suggest, once again, that medications may be interfering in the healing process or exacerbating the chance of relapse. The authors proposed, and I would concur, that while exercise empowered the patients and offered a sense of self-efficacy, the medications negated the immense power of hope and mastery.

Exercise "works" equally on men and women, young and old. Although mood improves after only one workout, to gain a steady, consistent improvement in mood, one must exercise regularly for nine weeks or longer, much like medications, meditation, and therapy. The reasons why exercise is so beneficial remain a topic for investigation, but research suggests that the increased availability of neurotransmitters, endogenous opiates, and cannabinoids play a role, along with decreased rumination and increased sleep and self-efficacy. Basically, exercise enables the body to access its own internal pharmacy and wisdom.

Studies have compared aerobic exercises like running, brisk walking, and aerobic classes to anaerobic exercises like weight lifting, and found them equally effective. What matters is that your body moves. The exercise that is going to work "best" for you is the one you enjoy the most and will continue to do. Few people are going to stick to a routine that is boring and dreaded.

Mindfully Moving

Yoga and other mindful movements continue to grow in popularity, especially among those with depression and other mental health concerns. These ancient disciplines unite the mind and body by combining physical postures, breathwork, and meditation, which offer the benefits of both exercise and mindfulness. Mindful movement brings gentleness and curiosity to the exercise world's mentality of "No pain, no gain" that many of us were taught or internalized growing up.

Did anyone else once suffer through Jane Fonda's exercise videos in the 1980s? I used to scream at her, usually internally, but sometimes out loud, every time she overly enthusiastically encouraged me to "Feel the burn!" Despite my groans, I religiously kept doing her routines, believing that the pain would lead to physical fitness gain.

It is no surprise I bought into this paradigm. I spent over twenty years taking dance classes, mostly ballet. My childhood dance teacher was a strict, classically trained dancer who kept a horse whip beside the record player in the corner of the studio. She would whack the whip against the floor beneath our feet to "encourage" us to jump higher. I will admit it was an effective technique, but not exactly the kindest. As I progressed in dance, adding more and more classes and hours of practice, I would bleed through my pointe shoes and keep dancing. I learned to power through pain. It never occurred to me to listen to my body and stop.

After college graduation, when I was no longer dancing daily, I was shocked at how quickly my body became tight and constricted, and how that affected not only my mood, but also how I felt about myself and my body. I discovered yoga as a way to keep the body supple, and was gratefully surprised to discover a radically different way of relating to my body than I had experienced in my ballet classes.

Pain is not a sign of "gain" but an indicator of pushing too far, too fast; a signal to pause, listen, and see what the body needs. Sometimes this means easing up, just long enough for the body to relax and deepen into a pose. Sometimes it means backing away to avoid getting hurt. We can only distinguish between the two by learning to listen and experiment. If we always back away from physical or emotional discomfort, we remain trapped in boxes of limitations that may not be real. Push too hard or too fast and we create more strain, tension, pain, and even damage. Like everything else in life, it is all about balance.

Yoga has taught me to tune in and listen to my body, not my ego, with kindness and acceptance. Some days I need a more vigorous workout to energize and empower my body. Much of the time my practice has become gentler. Sometimes I barely move, and just focus on the breath. Sometimes we need to lean into edges to recognize our own power and strength, or wake the body up if it has been too sedentary. At other times we may need to slow down and offer the body rest and reprieve.

Yoga, and other forms of mindful movement, also offers a way to release buried emotions and memories that can get locked in the body and nervous system from early traumas. Traditional psychotherapy involves talking through these experiences. Although this offers support and guidance that can be helpful and healing, a decade or even a lifetime of talk cannot rebalance and recalibrate a hypervigilant or shut-down nervous system, or release the trauma from the body. It cannot reach the preverbal limbic system of the brain, where remnants of trauma reside that cannot be expressed in words.

Working through traumas requires working with the body itself. In the last chapter, we learned a different way of being with and relating to the body by bringing awareness to its sensations. This is essential to healing, but our bodies also require movement. Yoga offers many physical and emotional benefits demonstrated in a growing body of scientific literature (though it should be noted that there are many disciplines of yoga, some of which are as aerobically intense as a Jane Fonda class; here, I am talking about restorative and mindful practices). Yoga allows emotions to move through and muscle tension to soften while toxins are released via the improved flow of lymphatic fluids. The flow of breath and blood oxygenate and energize the body. Yoga balances the autonomic nervous system, downregulates the HPA axis, modulates the stress response, and decreases inflammation. Beta and theta brain waves can increase by 40 percent after just one yoga class, allowing one to relax and turn inward, connecting with emotions, intuition, and creativity.

Yoga also reduces depressive symptoms and improves mood, well-being, and self-efficacy. It enhances connections in the brain, allowing the brain to function and regulate itself better, so that one is less easily hijacked by intense emotions and stress. One study found yoga to be as effective as medication in reducing depressive symptoms and rumination, although most of the literature has studied the use of yoga only as an adjunct to traditional medication and therapy. What psychiatrist wants to find out that yoga therapists can treat you as effectively as all of our fancy pharmacology?

Yoga also stimulates the release of oxytocin, the "love" hormone, encouraging us to connect with others, and perhaps even connect more kindly with our bodies and ourselves.

We have already looked at the benefits of breathing, mindfulness, and exercise, so you may wonder whether the effects of yoga might be attributed more to the physical postures or to the mindfulness. One interesting study examined this question by comparing a group of treatment-resistant patients assigned either to yoga postures, or a combination of yoga and meditation, for six weeks. Although both groups showed improvement, the yoga-only group experienced a 42 percent reduction in anxiety, while the yoga and meditation group improved by 72 percent. This certainly suggests that combining mindfulness with movement offers additive benefits.

Even the American Psychiatric Association has become interested in the use of yoga as a possible treatment option for depression and other mental illnesses—at least as an adjunct to medication!

It is clear from the research that exercise and movement are valuable and effective tools for managing mood, but the key to success is commitment to action. Just the act of setting an intention to move changes old fixed patterns and alters the signals sent to the brain. It offers possibility, motivation, and empowerment. It feeds the Wolf of Hope and puts you back in the driver's seat of your destiny. So grab your journal and let's take a few minutes to set an intention for yourself. Sure, your mind may be reminding you of a long list of other things you could or should do right now, but if pulling yourself out of your depressed state or preventing a relapse into another one is your hope and goal, then what better way to spend these next few moments?

WELLNESS RX: CREATE AN INTENTION TO MOVE

STEP 1: MOVING NOW   What can you do right now? If you are reading this, you have some free time available, if only for the next few minutes. If you wait to exercise until you get a gym membership, or a new pair of sneakers, you, like so many others before you, may lose your motivation, momentum, and window of opportunity. The Master Storyteller will spin tales about why moving is not possible or why now is not a good time: "I'll just do it later." Put the book down and use this time, this moment.

What if you just stood up and shook for a few minutes? What if you walked to the end of the street, or the end of the driveway? What if you turned on your favorite music and danced to just one song? Are you having fun? Play another song. Need to clean your house? Turn up the music and mindfully pay attention to your body sensations as you perform your chores. See if you can add some extra steps, dance moves, and movement to your chores. Do you need to go to the grocery store later? Instead of parking at the closest available spot, pick the one farthest away. Exercise does not have to be yet another thing on your to-do list. Find ways to creatively weave it into your day, beginning right now.

STEP 2: PLANNING AHEAD   Journal, draw, and brainstorm possible exercise ideas for the future. Which ones excite you, or at least feel less onerous than others? Make a list of ideas to consider over the next few weeks and a plan to put it in action. If you are stuck and cannot think of one thing you might possibly enjoy, consider that old stories and beliefs may be getting in the way here. Perhaps start with a commitment to shake for a couple of weeks and see if new possibilities emerge as fixed ideas and resistances get shaken lose. If you really dislike the shaking, commit to walking five minutes every day to get started. Keep reminding yourself of the benefits. Is turning on some music and dancing for a few minutes every day worth a bit more energy, motivation, and a brighter mood and outlook? Write down in your journal your specific goal: I will walk for ten minutes a day, three days a week.

STEP 3: CREATING AN INTENTION   Let's combine some mindfulness and imagination to shift the goal you have set, from act of willpower toward an intention. Find a comfortable position on a chair or the floor, closing your eyes and tuning into your breath for a few moments. Breathing in, fill your body with fresh oxygen and energy. Breathing out, release and let go of what is no longer serving you.

Bring to mind the goal you set in the last step. Imagine and feel yourself carrying out that goal as if it is happening now. Let's use walking as an example. Imagine yourself motivated and anticipating your walk. Imagine how that feels in your body. Sense the growing strength and ease as you follow through with your intention. Feel your energy and motivation. Feel a smile spread on your face. Sense the blood pumping through your body, invigorating you and your heart.

Allow an intention to form for yourself: "I feel motivated and energized to walk three times a week. My mood brightens, my body strengthens, and my sleep improves. I am healthy and well in every way." If you feel resistance to the words, you may try adding, "I release any and all blocks or resistances to moving and caring for my body." Find your own words and write the intention down in your journal. Take a few minutes every day to imagine and feel your body and senses carrying out this intention.

Making the Most of Your Time

Perhaps as you were considering the specifics of your intention, you wondered how little exercise you can get away with doing to benefit from your efforts. A recent research study demonstrates that exercise, if done for as little as one hour weekly, can reduce the risk of future depressive episodes by 44 percent. These findings are based on the largest, most comprehensive population-based study conducted on the benefits of exercise for depression. It involved nearly seventy-five thousand participants who were followed for nine to thirteen years in Norway. The results showed that if the entire population of Norway had been physically active for at least an hour a week, regardless of intensity of the exercise, 12 percent of depressive episodes could have been prevented. This does not even account for the additional physical benefits, including improved heart health, improved bone density and muscle strength, decreased risk of diabetes, and possibly even increased longevity and decreased risk of some cancers.

Let's think about the potential here. More than sixteen million Americans are affected by at least one major depressive episode every year. That means that one hour of exercise a week could potentially prevent nearly two million episodes of depression in this country annually. When I bring up exercise with my patients, I have those who are excited at the possibility that exercise alone could keep them off medication and immediately start taking a class or setting aside time for a daily walk. However, the more common response is feeling completely overwhelmed by one more thing they should be doing, but have no energy or motivation to pursue. The magnetic pull of that couch or reclining chair is a strong one.

Yet one hour a week breaks down into less than nine minutes a day. Unlike the many YouTube videos promising "abs of steel" in six minutes or less, this nine minutes has solid evidence behind it.

The intensity and type of movement do not seem to matter, just that you *are* moving, so pick activities you enjoy. You can walk, jog, bike, skate, swim, or run around and play with your kids (or someone else's kids). You can do strength training or aerobics or alternate between them. You can search You-Tube for a virtually endless list of possible short and long workouts including Zumba, reggae, hip hop, yoga, *qi qong,* or kickboxing. You can move indoors or outdoors, alone or with others. You can do high intensity or low intensity. You can exercise here or there, just nine minutes a day anywhere. The goal is simply to make movement a part of your daily life, and in the process improve your mood, health, and vitality. Can you think of one good reason not to try?

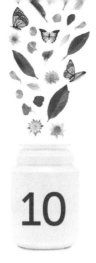

Nourishing the Body

Let food be thy medicine and medicine be thy food.

—HIPPOCRATES

The doctor of the future will no longer treat the human frame with drugs, but rather will cure and prevent disease with nutrition.

—THOMAS EDISON

Just as quickly as fashion shifts from miniskirts to bell-bottoms, stilettos to platform shoes, puffy sleeves to cold shoulder tops and back again, magazine and cable news headlines advocate the newest and latest fads in nutrition. The Atkins diet, the Zone diet, the Grapefruit diet, the Lemonade diet, the Paleo diet, the Ketone diet—all promise health, healing, and weight loss.

The latest research and advice changes and contradicts with an ever-evolving list of dos and don'ts, superfoods and super villains. Avoid fat. Eat carbs. Eat more fat. Don't eat carbs. Eat more meat. Eat less meat. Eat raw foods. Eat cooked foods. Eat fewer calories. It's not about the calories. Clearly, all this advice is not making us healthier or happier. What is one to do with all of this confusing information?

As I look back over my own life, I can see how my dietary patterns have shifted with these changing beliefs and fads. When I was a kid, my mom was never a big fan of cooking. For my mom, and millions of other women, the allure of cheaper and less time-consuming processed foods was magnetic, and they were, and still are, considered a godsend.

Our usual family meals were some form of meat and potatoes or pasta, with the occasional serving of defrosted peas or carrots in the winter, or corn on the cob in the summer. Dessert was never hard to come by in our house. My mother often served leftover cake for breakfast. Of course, that is not a whole lot different from the sugar-loaded cereals or Pop-Tarts marketed to kids today as a quick, "healthy" breakfast option. After school, we were often greeted with a bowl of raw cookie dough—my favorite!

At some point in high school, it occurred to me that my diet was not the healthiest. The news headlines spewed information about decreasing fat intake for health and weight control, so I turned to low-fat alternatives for everything—milk, cookies, cereal, peanut butter, and even white Wonder Bread.

One day, at my favorite after-school restaurant (you know, the one with the golden arches?), a Hindi friend of mine asked if I felt bad about eating my burger. "Because a cow is killed to make that burger," she explained. I suddenly felt sick and guilty as I bit into the burger, which right then looked and tasted revolting. In that moment I realized that meat came from somewhere—that it did not just magically appear in little patties ready to eat. I stopped eating beef and pork. With that, I was pretty convinced my diet was not only healthy, but humane.

Through the rest of high school, college, and graduate school, I basically subsisted on uncooked, processed, low-fat foods. I do not recall ever buying a vegetable or a can of beans for protein, or cooking. In fact, after living for almost a year in an apartment, I decided to prepare dinner one night, only to discover my stove did not work. I called the landlord, who came over to check on it. After turning the dials, he looked at me quizzically, and asked if I had ever used the stove before. I shook my head no. He explained that it was a gas stove, and I would need to contact the gas company to get my gas turned on in order to use it. I never did.

You might think (or hope) that medical school substantially shifted my relationship with nutrition and food, but you would be wrong. The only nutrition I learned about in four years of medical school were the biochemical pathways of the vitamins and the major diseases of gross deficiency like scurvy, if one is severely depleted of vitamin C, or rickets, if one is depleted in Vitamin D. Perhaps now you can understand why many physicians do not consider nutrition a viable option for improving health.

Fortunately, this is changing. Medical students at schools like Tulane University, George Washington University, and others now learn about nutrition, and even go into the kitchen and learn how to cook.

For me, like many others, change only began with a problem. In medical school, I started feeling incredibly fatigued, anxious, irritable, ravenously hungry, hot, and sweaty—so sweaty that I had to bring extra clothes on my rotations. I felt like I was going to pass out when forced to wear my white coat. My heart raced and my muscles felt heavy and weak. I dismissed all these symptoms as anxiety and mere hypochondriasis, a common problem among many medical students.

It turns out, however, that I had a different problem—one that took me two years of feeling lousy before finally turning to an endocrinologist for help. I was diagnosed with Graves's disease, an autoimmune disease of the thyroid. Instead of my metabolism being slowed down, like the more common Hashimoto's, mine was revved way up. I have no doubt now this was related to the stress of medical school, and the accumulated damage of years of processed sugary foods.

I was prescribed propylthiouracil, which made me nauseous, queasy, tired, and achy—so I stopped taking it. I was told my only other option was to get my thyroid ablated with radioactive iodine. That did not seem like a safe alternative, so I ignored the advice and tried to bandage the symptoms with a beta-blocker. This reduced some of the anxiety and sweating, but also made me feel weak and tired, like my brain was trapped in a thick, tangled cobweb.

Fortunately, a holistic physician with whom I had rotated suggested I come see her for an alternative approach. She treated me with a protocol involving a combination of kinesiology, homeopathy, and acupressure to balance my energies and desensitize my system. It may sound kooky, and I still cannot explain how it worked, but it did, and it has worked for many of my family members and patients as well.

Within two weeks, I was feeling like myself again. I will be forever grateful for Dr. Cheryl's intervention, since I now have a healthy thyroid to thank for it. This experience planted a seed in my brain about the relationship between food, food sensitivities, and health.

After resolving the hyperthyroid issues, I was left with mild Hashimoto's hypothyroidism, which was more easily treatable with thyroid medication. I continued to follow up with an endocrinologist, who remained puzzled as to how my Graves's had resolved itself, but he wrote it off to my thyroid finally burning itself out. I let him think what he wanted.

My diet and health remained relatively stable until after the birth of my second child, when my belly seemed to settle into a permanent bloated state that made me look three months pregnant. My brain and body felt trapped inside a heavy fog. Once again I dismissed these symptoms as just part of being an older, exhausted working mom with two small kids, limited sleep, and no time to myself. It would take another couple of years to finally see an integrative doctor who did lab work and determined I had a moderate gluten sensitivity.

Now, my diet changed radically. Good-bye cereal, bread, cakes, and cookies. I discovered that not only was my belly less distended, but I felt less fatigued and, miraculously, less irritable. Thanks to changes in my diet, daily meditation to reduce stress, and more sleep, my thyroid normalized over a three-year period, and I got off all medications.

The point of this story is to let you know that I totally get it. As you can see, like many of you, I grew up on the standard American (mostly processed) diet, appropriately called the SAD diet, and paid a steep price for it emotionally and physically. If I can learn to eat healthier and cook simple foods (I do mean simple; I am still a lousy cook), really, anyone can. If I, and many others, can overcome allegedly chronic and irreversible diseases with nutrition, it is possible for you too.

Since that discovery nearly eight years ago, I began to listen more closely to my patients' vague physical complaints about abdominal discomfort, bloating, fatigue, aches, and brain fog, which so often led to the prescription of an antidepressant in doctors' offices, and instead consider whether a food sensitivity, or just a mostly processed-food diet, may be at play.

This is not exactly new or radical. Hippocrates figured this out over two thousand years ago. Of course the food we put into our bodies affects how our bodies function and how we feel. Our bodies require nutrients to create the neurotransmitters in our brains, to balance the microbiomes of our guts, to support our immune systems, to provide energy and life itself to our minds and bodies.

In the name of efficiency, and the power of marketing and unproven nutritional advice, we have forsaken our bodies and our health by forgetting the very basic fact that what our bodies require is *real* food.

Eat Real Food

It sounds so simple, right? Eat real food. But what does this mean? In my search for answers, I read countless books and research articles on nutrition, with many more on my shelf still waiting their turns. If I was struggling to figure this out, how on earth could I help my patients to sort through this mass of information?

Fortunately, I discovered two very important books that simplified things for me. The first was Michael Pollan's book *In Defense of Food*. Pollan is a journalist, not a nutritionist, so he examined this crazy world of dietary contradictions with a fresh eye, free from school-taught dogmas. Pollan ultimately reduced his findings to the seemingly simple yet actually quite complex statement: "Eat food. Not too much. Mostly plants."

The key here is to learn to discriminate between processed food and "real" food. Pollan offers a few simple questions for clarification:

1. Would your great-grandmother recognize these foods?

2. Can you identify and pronounce all of the ingredients on the label?

3. Are there fewer than five ingredients?

If you answer yes to these three questions, you are probably eating real food. If not, it is likely processed.

WELLNESS RX: FOOD JOURNAL

For the next week, journal everything you eat to get a sense of your starting point. Notice how much of it is real food and how you feel after meals. Just the act of noticing your patterns with curiosity, not judgment, may start to subtly change these habits, just as focusing on the breath changes our breathing.

What did you discover? Perhaps you, like me, were surprised by how many unrecognizable and unpronounceable ingredients are listed in one simple loaf of "whole grain" bread. Sure, it may look like great-grandma's bread, but it is a cheaply processed approximation that can sit on store shelves for long periods of time without rotting or molding. Probably not real food!

You may wonder what all this talk about food has to do with healing depression. Remember that depression is a common symptom, like a fever, stemming from multiple roots, mainly stress and inflammation, that in turn, leads to many physiological issues unrelated to our brains. Part of the synergistic recipe for healing depressive symptoms almost always includes nutrition.

One of the few things not disputed in the world of nutritional research is that eating a SAD diet of processed, sugary foods increases the risk of chronic diseases, including type 2 diabetes, cardiovascular disease, stroke, and cancer. It is also associated with a 50 percent increased likelihood of depression. Conversely, those who eat healthier whole foods have a 30 percent decreased risk of developing depression. This applies to young and old, men and women. There is also emerging evidence that changing these dietary patterns can prevent and treat depression as well as other chronic diseases.

The recent Supporting the Modification of Lifestyle Interventions in Lowered Emotional States (SMILES) trial sought to discover whether teaching nutritional basics to depressed adults with highly processed diets might impact their health and emotional well-being. A nutritional education group was encouraged to mindfully eat a whole-foods Mediterranean-style diet with lots of vegetables, fruits, and legumes, along with whole grains, some dairy, lean meats, eggs, and olive oil. A control group received social support for the same amount of time. At the end of twelve weeks, researchers found that one-third of those in the nutritional education group remitted from depressive symptoms, compared to 8 percent in the social support group. They also discovered that those who changed their diets the most experienced the greatest improvement in mood.

I want to stay clear of declaring a super villain in the world of nutrition, but the data consistently suggests that higher consumption of sugary beverages, desserts and pastries, fried foods, and processed meats are all associated with increased risk of depression in longitudinal studies, while increased intake of vegetables, fruits, and fiber decreases risk. Sugar and processed foods become super villains when they dominate our dietary habits and we lose moderation and balance, which has happened to the majority of us in this country.

Wisdom of the Blue Zones

The data is overwhelmingly clear that we should not be eating diets full of processed foods. But the question remains, what foods *should* we be eating, when there is so much contradictory information? The 2012 Food and Health Survey found that a majority of Americans consider it easier to do income taxes than to figure out how to eat a healthy, nourishing diet.

To answer the question of what to eat, I turn to my second-favorite guide, *The Blue Zones Solution: Eating and Living like the World's Healthiest People,* by Dan Buettner. National Geographic paid Buettner to travel around the world to those places where people live the longest and healthiest lives in order to learn their secrets. Sounds like a fun job, doesn't it? Buettner discovered that although specific diets vary from region to region—with the people of Okinawa in Japan eating more sweet potatoes, tofu, and miso, and the people of Nicoya in Costa Rica eating mostly rice, beans, corn, and eggs—all consume real, whole foods local to their environment and free of pesticides, hormones, and antibiotics.

Here are the Top 10 pearls of wisdom gleaned from the healthy centenarians of the Blue Zones, backed up by Pollan's research:

1. Grandma was right: **Eat your vegetables, greens, and fruits.** The more colors and variety, the better. Spinach, watercress, beet greens, Swiss chard, lettuces, fresh herbs, peppers, pumpkin, cauliflower, broccoli, brussels sprouts, lemons, and strawberries are all foods particularly beneficial for depression. Mix in sweet potatoes, avocados, blueberries, and grapes. Yum!

2. **Eat your beans.** Eating at least half a cup a day of lentils, chickpeas, pinto, black, great northern, or cannellini beans is part of daily life in most of the Blue Zones.

3. **Eat whole grains** like oats, brown rice, barley, and non-GMO ground corn. Pass on the white Wonder Bread and other breads with long lists of unpronounceable ingredients. Minimize gluten. Avoid it if you have or suspect a sensitivity.

4. **Breakfast like a king, lunch like a prince, dinner like a pauper.** Breakfast really is the most important meal of the day. In this country, so many of us skip breakfast and eat heavy dinners. Intuitively this makes no sense, since a full stomach when we sleep does not serve us. Choose breakfast foods wisely, and do not forget to include mostly plants! How about a bowl of warm oatmeal mixed with flax, hemp, and chia seeds, honey, and fresh berries? It sets the stage for the rest of your day.

5. **Avoid processed foods** that great-grandma would not recognize, or that have more than five ingredients. This one bears repeating, since it is so fundamentally important.

6. **Save sugary treats for special occasions.** Savor them slowly. Satisfy your day-to-day sweet cravings with honey, fruit, or a piece of dark chocolate. Skip sugary beverages and stick to filtered water, organic teas, and coffees.

7. **Limit meat intake to the size of a deck of cards,** and eat it no more than two to three times a week. Pick high-quality lean, free-range meats without growth hormones and antibiotics. As Thomas Jefferson said,

eating meat should be a "condiment for the vegetable." If you do not eat meat, consider adding one tablespoon of spirulina daily, or taking a vitamin B complex to make sure you get enough B vitamins.

8. **Practice *hara hachi bu*.** This is a Japanese phrase that sets an intention before beginning a meal to stop eating when you feel 80 percent full. It takes our bodies 20 minutes to notice we are satiated, yet most of us have finished our plate long before that.

9. **Eat slowly and mindfully, ideally with family or friends.** This means turning off the TV and putting away your phones and devices. Commit to at least taking your first bite mindfully, free of all distractions. Practicing this one will help make number 8 easier to achieve.

10. **Keep healthy snacks of nuts, seeds, fruits, and vegetables readily available** so you do not grab the bag of chips or chocolate bar.

Just to keep things real, please know that these rules are difficult with children. My son's friends bring sugary, processed foods for him to eat at school since I do not pack them. Let go of what you cannot control. Model an alternative option that, hopefully, one day will resonate.

Since most of us do not live in Blue Zones, do the best you can, and do not beat yourself up for falling short of these ideals. Small changes add up, so consider what small changes you are willing to make. See if you can create a community of friends and family who support you. Consider sharing a Blue Zone potluck dinner monthly.

Vitamins, Minerals, and Supplements

Notice that the healthy Blue Zone centenarians are not obsessing over which specific vitamins and supplements they might need. Although nutritionists break food down into different components, food is more than the sum of its parts. Spinach is more than the vitamin K, vitamin A, vitamin B_2, vitamin B_6, folate, magnesium, iron, zinc, potassium, vitamin C, and fiber that are released into our body after we eat it. I once saw a patient who considered herself fit and healthy despite being emotionally anxious and depressed. As we discussed the specifics of her daily diet, she disclosed that she ate virtually no actual food, but instead devoured bottles and bottles of vitamins and supplements. She did not return after I suggested that real food nourished us physically, emotionally, and spiritually in a way that bottles of supplements cannot.

This is not to say there is not a place for supplements in our nutrient-depleted world, but food is our best source when possible. A 2018 article offered the first nutritional guidelines, based on the best available evidence, for prevention and treatment of depression. The researchers recommended traditional dietary habits like those consumed by Mediterranean, Norwegian, and Japanese cultures that focus on whole foods with lots of vegetables, fruits, legumes, whole grains, nuts, seeds, fiber, and fish. They also suggested a steady source of omega-3 polyunsaturated fatty acids, mostly through the consumption of fish, and a limited intake of processed and sugary foods.

Sound familiar? These dietary patterns offer the many vitamins and nutrients necessary for emotional and physical health, and have also been shown to increase brain-derived neurotrophic factor (BDNF), a peptide essential for the growth and survival of neurons and brain neuroplasticity. Conversely, studies have shown that a Western diet leads to shrinkage of the hippocampus, likely due to the reduction of BDNF.

Although following these traditional eating patterns would meet most of your nutritional needs, there may be times that a supplement could be helpful or necessary. Unfortunately, fewer than one in ten American adults eat enough vegetables or fruits daily, so the majority of us are deficient in many vitamins and minerals.

Folate (Vitamin B₉)

Folic acid, a synthetic form of folate, has been mandated by the FDA to be added to processed grain products like breads and cereals to prevent neural tube defects in newborns. Yet 75 percent of Americans remain deficient in folate. Low folate levels are associated with more severe and chronic depressive symptoms. Part of the reason for this may be that up to 40 percent of the U.S. population may have a genetic variation of the gene for methylenetetrahydrofolate reductase (MTHFR).

MTHFR is an enzyme required to convert the folate we consume from food sources, or the folic acid in supplements, into the active form, which is needed by the body to create new red blood cells, regulate neurotransmitters, detoxify the body, and protect our DNA. Those with MTHFR variations are less efficient in breaking down the synthetic folic acid. Methylfolate (5-MTHF) alterations are more common among those with treatment resistant depression than the general population. Multiple studies have shown that folate supplementation, along with B_{12}, improves depressive symptoms. For those with TRD, you may want to consider working with an integrative or functional medicine doctor who can help you start L-methylfolate, the active form of folate, and B_{12} supplementation. Meanwhile, try eating more leafy vegetables.

Vitamin D

Vitamin D is another vitamin (and hormone) that at times may need to be supplemented, especially for those of us lacking exposure to enough sunlight, which is our primary source of this vitamin. A 2007 review article in the *New England Journal of Medicine* estimates that over a billion people worldwide are deficient in vitamin D. Five to ten minutes of sunscreen-free exposure to sunlight offers about 3,000 IU of vitamin D_3, which is the active form of the vitamin. Few foods offer significant doses of this nutrient. Fresh wild salmon offers about 600 to 1000 IU of vitamin D_3, yet the more frequently eaten farm-raised salmon offers only 100 to 250 IU. Cod liver oil, if you have the stomach for it, has 400 to 1000 IU. Fortified milk, yogurts, or orange juices usually add about 100 IU.

Vitamin D is needed to maintain strong bones, absorb calcium, strengthen the immune system, and optimize nerve function and neurogenesis. It is also required for the synthesis of neurotransmitters. Again, low levels are associated with increased frequency of mood disorders, and likely play a role in seasonal affective disorder. Low levels are also associated with low energy, fatigue, insomnia, decreased immunity, and increased risk of many chronic diseases. A small study found that adults taking 400 to 800 IU of vitamin D for five days in winter showed an improvement in mood and positive affect.

Getting your levels checked by a physician is the best way to determine what dosage you may need, but 1,000 to 3,000 IU of vitamin D$_3$ is where I start if someone cannot afford the lab work, depending on level of sun exposure, time of year, and health status. Consider getting ten minutes of daily sun exposure on at least your arms and legs before putting on the sunscreen, so your body can synthesize and store this critical vitamin for free. A sunscreen with an SPF of 8 has been shown to reduce vitamin D synthesis by 92 to 99 percent.

Omega-3 Fatty Acids

Omega-3 fatty acids are essential for brain and neuron structure and function, regulating inflammation, modulating the HPA axis response, memory, and mood. Two-thirds of the brain is made up of lipids. Without fatty acids, the brain cannot function optimally. A study by researchers at UCLA found that those who consume inadequate omega-3s have lower brain volumes and cognitive impairment. Yet it is estimated that 90 percent of Americans are deficient in omega-3s, and 95 percent of women of childbearing age have this deficiency. This is alarming since low levels are associated with postpartum depression, and adequate levels are needed for brain development of offspring.

Low intake of fatty fish, along with dietary recommendations to drastically reduce intake of fats and exploding numbers of statin prescriptions, may have inadvertently played a role in rising rates of depression. On top of that, a huge shift in the ratio of anti-inflammatory omega-3 and pro-inflammatory omega-6 intakes has occurred over the past 150 years due to drastic dietary changes. In the past, the ratio between these forms of omega fatty acids was fairly equal, but with the advent of processed foods high in corn and soy oil, and high consumption of animal fats, Americans now consume nearly 20 times as many omega-6s, leading to chronic inflammation and disease. Studies show that those with depression and anxiety tend to have lower levels of omega-3 and higher levels of omega-6 in their blood and brain compared to a healthy population, and that this omega-3 to omega-6 ratio in the blood correlates with duration of depressive symptoms and degree of inflammation.

A growing body of data specifically links low levels of fatty acids with increased risk of suicide. One particularly disturbing study compared the omega-3 levels of eight hundred active-duty U.S. military personnel who died by suicide with eight hundred randomly selected controls. Researchers found that suicide risk was 62 percent greater among those with the lowest omega-3 levels. Adding two grams of omega-3 has been shown to reduce suicidal thinking, depressive symptoms, and perception of stress.

The three primary forms of omega-3 are alpha-linolenic acid (ALA), eicosapentaenoic acid (EPA), and docosahexaenoic acid (DHA). ALA comes from plants and vegetable oils like flaxseed, canola, soybean, and walnut oil. But only about 5 percent of ALA is converted in the body to the EPA and DHA fatty acids needed by the body and brain, so even in large quantities it has negligible effects. Studies show the best results for improving depression, anxiety, and PTSD use higher concentrations of EPA than DHA.

The best food sources of omega-3 come from fatty coldwater fish like mackerel, salmon, and sardines. Chia seeds, flax seeds, hemp seeds, soybeans, walnuts, and brussels sprouts are also good sources. If these foods are lacking in your diet, and you prefer supplementation, I recommend 1,000 to 2,000 mg of a fish oil, ideally with a higher ratio of EPA to DHA. For vegans, one tablespoon of flaxseed oil provides a whopping 7.5 grams of omega 3s. Those on anticoagulation medications should avoid taking more than 1,000 mg daily. Besides a fishy aftertaste, the only other side effects are loose stools.

Magnesium

Nearly 70 percent of Americans are deficient in magnesium. Studies associating low magnesium levels with depression date back nearly a hundred years. Magnesium is involved in hundreds of roles and reactions that include regulating the heart and blood pressure, producing proteins, cell growth and division, maintaining electrolyte balance, regulating blood sugar levels, and roles in sleep, cognition, and neuroplasticity. Common medications like protonpump inhibitors, antacids, blood pressure medications, stimulants, corticosteroids, oral contraceptives, some antibiotics, and many others may further deplete magnesium levels.

One small trial compared the effects of 2,000 mg of magnesium chloride to no treatment in a group of depressed adults. Within two weeks, the group on magnesium showed reduced depressive symptoms, along with increased energy and decreased headaches, constipation, muscle aches, and cramps. Fifty-eight percent of participants reported improved mood. One-fifth reported diarrhea, a common side effect of magnesium, usually resolvable by decreasing the dose. Although the magnesium was helpful while taking the supplement, within two weeks after discontinuation, depressive symptoms returned. If you are seeking a safe, quick, inexpensive, and easily available option for improving mood and sleep, it is certainly a supplement to consider.

Magnesium glutamate and aspartate should be avoided, as case studies suggest high doses of these can be toxic to the brain. The safest choices are magnesium glycinate, taurate, or citrate, at a starting dose of around 350 to 400 mg. Spinach, kale, avocados, bananas, raspberries, nuts and seeds, black beans, chickpeas, broccoli, green beans, and peas are all excellent sources.

Curcumin and Theanine

As I am writing this, I am sipping a cup of hot green tea mixed with turmeric and black pepper for warmth, comfort, and health. Turmeric, the golden spice, has been used for over four thousand years in India and China for flavor and healing. Its active ingredient, curcumin, has powerful antioxidant, anti-inflammatory, and neuroprotective properties. It promotes neurogenesis in the hippocampus and increases serotonin, dopamine, and norepinephrine levels. Better yet, turmeric is tasty and well tolerated with few side effects.

Recent trials have demonstrated curcumin's antidepressant properties. One study showed that it worked as effectively as fluoxetine but with fewer side effects. Try adding turmeric to your food or tea, ideally with a bit of black pepper, which increases curcumin's bioavailability. If you do not like the flavor, consider taking a 1,000-mg capsule for a safe, effective antidepressant.

My green tea also provides me with the amino acid L-theanine, which reduces stress and anxiety. Animal studies suggest theanine increases serotonin, dopamine, and gamma-aminobutyric acid (GABA). Human trials show that 50 mg of L-theanine increases alpha brain waves, which are associated with a relaxed, but alert and attentive, state of mind.

Another small but interesting placebo-controlled trial found that 200 mg of theanine worked as well as the benzodiazepine alprazolam (Xanax), but without the side effects and addictive potential. A 2018 Korean health and nutrition survey, including nearly ten thousand participants, found that consumers of green tea had a 21 percent lower prevalence of depression compared to nonusers. For the coffee lovers out there, the same study found a 24 percent lower depression rate for those who drink coffee (but adding sugar, cream, and chemical flavors likely cancels out any possible benefits). You can get your daily dose of theanine with green tea, or by taking a 200 to 400 mg chewable or capsule once to twice a day for anxiety and insomnia. Some people do report mild sedation and prefer to take it at night.

Healthy Gut, Healthy Brain

When we stop and reflect for a moment, it seems fairly obvious that our bodies require nutrition to feel and perform optimally, but it may be harder to understand why the sugary processed foods are so bad for us. As long as we get our nutrients, what does it matter what else is going down the tube? What most of us do not consider, when living a plant-depleted lifestyle, is that our food choices not only affect "us," but are also vitally important to the forty trillion bacteria, viruses, fungi, protozoa, and other microbes residing in and on our bodies.

According to the Human Microbiome Project, we are outnumbered ten to one by our microbial companions, although a recent study suggests that the real ratio is closer to one to one. Whether we are vastly outnumbered or equal cohabitants within this body of ours, we are most definitely not alone. Because of the vast ecosystem that considers our bodies "home," the journal *Nature* has advocated that a human should be referred to as "we" rather than "I." It appears that just as our rigid concepts of what defines gender and sexuality are challenged, so too must we reconsider our definition of ourselves as individual beings.

Although this may be fascinating to reflect on, you may wonder, yet again, what the gut has to do with depression. There is a good chance your psychiatrist did not suggest healing the gut as a way to heal your mood, yet an exploding body of research is revealing that the gut, not the head, may play the leading role in so-called "mental" illnesses. This complex ecosystem sharing our bodies influences every part of our growth and development, from conception to death. The microbiota regulates the metabolism and digestion of nutrients; the synthesis of vitamins, enzymes, and neurotransmitters; the development and regulation of the immune, nervous, respiratory, and endocrine system; and, yes, our moods and behaviors.

The balance and health of our inner flora largely depends on the food we eat. The gut and brain form a bidirectional network that continuously conveys information back and forth via the vagus nerve, neurotransmitters, hormones, and messengers of the immune system known as cytokines. Each mouthful of food shifts the balance of microbes in our guts. This information influences our moods and behaviors. In turn, our moods, stress, and behaviors send messages from the brain to the gut, shifting the microbial balance. What this means is that if our diet and gut are chronically out of balance, our emotional and neurological health will follow.

The research on all this is fascinating, but a bit overwhelming, so here is the oversimplified, cartoonish version of the story. Let's go back to our bus-driving analogy with the teenagers, only now you are on a bus with forty trillion microbes with competing agendas and desires competing for your attention and control of the bus. You have determined you want to make healthier food choices for the sake of your mood and well-being, but a group of angry, sugar-craving, beer-bellied microbes are demanding sugar—*now!*

The craving for sugar is overwhelming, overpowering your willpower to deny it. You grab a chocolate bar. You are rewarded with a pleasant dopamine rush to encourage you to continue this behavior. For a moment there is peace on the bus, until the potato chip–craving mob rushes in, demanding their turn at a fatty meal. You give in and feed them too. Meanwhile, the vegetable-loving populations are dwindling toward mass extinction. With each mouthful of sugary and fatty treats, the sugar- and fat-feeding microbes expand in size and power, like the Hulk. Eating vegetables tastes bland, because that population is now so weak after years of a SAD diet and accumulated stressors that they have no say in your taste preferences.

Meanwhile, the imbalance in the gut is triggering a chronic low-grade inflammatory response. This causes the one-cell-thin lining of the gut, designed to let nutrients through and keep pathogenic bacteria out, to become more permeable. This means bigger food molecules, bacteria, and toxins can now cross into the bloodstream. One of the nastiest offenders that crosses this barrier are the gram-negative bacteria, which have a lipopolysaccharide (LPS) outer membrane and are supposed to stay inside the gut. Even small amounts of these guys crossing sets off a full-blown inflammatory response, and increases activity of the amygdala fear center, leading to classic "sickness behaviors" like fatigue, avoidance behaviors, anxiety, depression, difficulty concentrating, increased pain, and GI symptoms.

Large food molecules start crossing over the gut lining as well, which the body perceives as yet another unidentifiable threat, triggering another red alert and more inflammation. That yummy bread, slice of cheese, or corn tortilla you devoured with relish, now in the belly of an overreactive immune system, becomes tagged as a threatening enemy to be attacked. You may experience an array of "unexplainable" symptoms like fatigue, joint pain, muscle tightness, bloating, and diarrhea or constipation. These are all symptoms of food sensitivities. All of this chaos in the gut is sending warnings to the brain, triggering neuroinflammation and leading to anxiety and depression.

Let's say, however, that you set an intention to ignore the cajoling, deceiving pleas of the expanding sugar and fatty microbial gangs, and for one week eat whole foods with lots of vegetables, fiber, fruits, and legumes. You will have to use all your willpower, maintain your position in the driver's seat, and stay on course. If you do, the fiber-, vegetable-, and fruit-loving populations will regain their power. These guys cringe at the idea of a fast-food meal or second helping of cake. The sugar and fatty microbes will shrink, no longer controlling your cravings and taste buds.

The happy, peaceful, anti-inflammatory, earth-loving microbes, who have coevolved with us humans for millions of years, reestablish control and balance over the microbial world. Peace reigns, at least temporarily. You no longer crave sugar and fat as strongly. Fake foods start to taste more like chemicals than actual food. Your mood improves. You feel more energized.

At this point, however, there is more unknown than known about our inner flora. The key, as always, to a healthy gut is balance and diversity. We all start off with unique flora based on what is passed down to us from our mother's flora; whether we were born vaginally or by C-section; whether we were breastfed or formula-fed; whether we were exposed to antibiotics or not; whether we were allowed to play in the dirt or constantly wiped down with

Purell; whether we ate a wide variety of foods or subsisted mostly on chicken nuggets, fries, and cookie dough. Childhood trauma and stress also shift the microbiome, which is yet another explanation for the strong link between adverse childhood events and future risk of chronic disease.

Although we cannot change our starting point, we do have control over how we nourish our microbes. The data is evident that as diets become more Westernized, the variety within the microbiome declines precipitously, leading to a state of chronic inflammation and chronic disease. The good news is that we can add back some variety, and increase the total population of microbes, by returning to real food, especially adding sources of fiber and reducing intake of sugar and fat.

Unfortunately, we are still a long way from fully understanding the best balance of different types of microorganisms, but we do know enough to begin to restore balance to our guts, bodies, and brains by providing the nutrients upon which our flora flourish. The most powerful intervention for improving our mood, vitality, and health is nourishing ourselves with healthy whole foods. Picture a lush green salad full of ripe tomatoes, your favorite nuts, broccoli, and green and red peppers, sprinkled with chia and hemp seeds. Perhaps you suddenly have a craving?

WELLNESS RX: TO EAT OR NOT TO EAT

This exercise takes only a few seconds, but it allows you to become more aware of triggers that may lead to sugary, processed food choices that may temporarily boost your mood or energy, but make you feel worse down the road.

Before eating, take a moment to pause and take a few deep breaths. During this pause, notice with curiosity the **thoughts** and stories circulating in your head around the subject of food and your body. Pay particular attention to judgments and criticisms, and offer yourself kindness.

Notice your **emotions.** If you are craving something sweet, salty, or fatty, check in and see what you may really need in that

---

moment. Perhaps you are tired or stressed and just need a few minutes of breathing to reset. Perhaps your body needs fresh air or movement. Listen. Perhaps you are feeling sad or angry and trying to numb your emotions with food to avoid fully feeling it.

Notice any **body sensations.** Are you actually hungry? Is your stomach gurgling? Or are you eating out of boredom, or to numb emotions or stress?

After making these observations, you may still choose to have the doughnut, cookie, or mocha Coffee Coolatta with cream, and that is fine, once in a while. But if these choices are made daily, your mood and health pay a price. Offering kindness instead of criticism, and awareness instead of reactivity, begins to gently change our responses. By bringing awareness to the patterns, thoughts, emotions, and sensations behind cravings, this offers a space to choose what is in your highest good.

As always, be sure to write down your observations. Do you notice any patterns among your moods, behaviors, and energy and certain food choices? Do you notice certain triggers, like being tired or stressed, that lead you to crave certain foods? Do certain thoughts or feelings change your eating patterns? Do certain foods change your thoughts and feelings?

How We Eat

Using this variation of the Breathing Space activity offers an opportunity to pause and reflect on what we actually need in any given moment. It keeps us in the driver's seat, rather than reflexively reacting to thoughts, emotions, and the urges of our microbial companions. The Blue Zone elders teach us not only the importance of whole-food traditional diets but also that *how* we eat may be as important as *what* we eat.

In the Blue Zones, food is primarily consumed during meals, usually at home with family and friends. Here in the United States, 62 percent of us snack throughout the day; 52 percent work and eat at the same time; 31 percent eat while in the car; 57 percent while watching TV; and 37 percent while on the phone. A whopping 60 percent of our meals are eaten alone. It is difficult to mindfully eat while working, driving a car, watching TV, or talking on the phone.

In the Blue Zones, people are not stressing about eating the right foods, or worrying about their waistlines. When they eat dessert, they savor it. When they eat a meal, they are not counting calories. When the Okinawans start a meal, they pause to murmur *"hara hachi bu,"* to set the intention to pause when they are 80 percent full. Others offer a simple thank-you in gratitude. Briefly pausing our busy lives and reincorporating some simple eating rituals can help return sacred nourishment to our bodies.

WELLNESS RX: MINDFUL EATING

Begin by feeling your body seated at the table. Feel your feet planted on the ground. Straighten your back to allow a fuller breath and better digestion. Take a few belly breaths. Notice your body and areas of tightness or restriction. Notice the thoughts in your mind. Notice your emotions.

Offer a simple thank-you, or a prayer of thanks, for your food. Gratefulness diminishes the stress response and activates the parasympathetic nervous system, which is in charge of digestion. Just thinking about food activates the release of enzymes required to break down our food. Stress influences the speed at which food travels through the body and the absorption of nutrients. Being mindful allows our food to be better digested and absorbed.

Now, bring your focus to the food on your plate. Notice the colors of the food in front of you. Notice the smell. Observe your own anticipation. Notice the movement of your arm as it travels toward the plate and lifts some of the food onto a utensil. As you bring the food closer to your face, again, notice the smell. Perhaps you can feel the heat of the food. Putting the food in your mouth, notice the first burst of flavor and the texture in your mouth as you take a bite. Chew slowly and observe the movement of your jaw. Notice how the flavor of the food changes as you chew. Notice the urge to swallow and then the sensation of swallowing.

After your meal, record your experience in your journal. Set an intention to add this practice for at least the first bite or two of each meal. Notice how it influences your relationship with the food on your plate, and even your digestion. Notice too, without judgment, how easy it is to forget to take this mindful pause.

Small Changes, Big Effects

Changing what we eat and how we relate with food can drastically alter our mood and well-being. Molly is the perfect example. I happened to meet her for the first time the day after she was diagnosed with diabetes by her primary care physician. She blamed herself for being so "stupid" for "letting this happen." She was understandably devastated to be told she had a chronic irreversible disease requiring medications for life. Sounds like the same soul-crushing verdict psychiatrists routinely cast on those with depression, does it not?

In her case, Molly had suffered from depression as long as she could remember. Research shows that depression is two to three times more common in those with diabetes, which is not surprising since stress and inflammation play a role in both. Molly had experienced a sad, lonely childhood. Molly learned at an early age to turn to food for the comfort and nurturance she was not getting at home.

I assured Molly that recent research suggests that neither diabetes nor depression are irreversible, and that both stem from stress, inflammation, and imbalanced food choices. I taught her the breathing exercises you learned in chapter 5. Then we explored her dietary patterns and lack of exercise. She started taking turmeric, omega-3 fatty acids, vitamin D_3, and a multivitamin with L-methylfolate, since we discovered she had an MTHFR variation. She committed to going on at least one hike and cooking three whole-food meals a week. Her new diagnosis gave her an incentive and motivation to implement these lifestyle changes. Molly was excited about the possibility of having the power to make changes in her life and not be a passive victim to her body and emotions.

Molly started hiking with her husband, and felt joy for the first time in decades as they explored new parks and trails. She eliminated processed, sugary foods and was exploring new food possibilities and ways to cook real, whole foods. Within a couple of months, she was free of depressive symptoms for the first time in her teenage and adult life. She was standing up for herself and setting limits at work, no longer willing to work extra hours for no pay at the cost of her health and well-being. She stopped smoking. Her relationship strengthened with her husband as they hiked and played together. On top of all that, Molly's blood glucose levels dropped to normal levels. Her primary-care physician attributed the improvement to her medications. She proved him wrong when she stopped the medications and her numbers continued to improve.

This is the power of food, exercise, and breathing. Everything is intercon-nected. Although research is helpful in understanding parts and pieces, healing is a product of multiple changes within a complex system, each creating a ripple effect that leads to other changes. Sometimes it requires a crisis to wake us up and call us to action, as it did for Molly and me.

Perhaps it is time to consider what small nutritional changes you could make, starting today, to help improve your mood and health. Commit to one small step that feels doable and not overwhelming to you. Decide to try one new vegetable weekly. Replace one processed food with a whole-food option. Begin to notice how certain foods make you feel. If you feel tired, cranky, or bloated after a meal, try eliminating a potential culprit for a couple of weeks and see how you feel. Add it back in after two weeks and notice how that feels. Record your findings so you do not forget. If you notice a difference, that is probably a food for you to avoid, not because it is "bad," but because it is not healthy for you and your body. There is no one perfect diet for everyone. We are all biochemically unique.

Maybe it is time we stop heeding the advice of "experts" and diet books, and return to the wisdom of our ancestors, the healthy centenarians living in the Blue

Zones, and our own bodies. If you are feeling chronically tired and depressed, or want to avoid feeling tired and depressed in the future, food choices cannot be ignored. The good news is that even small adjustments can lead to rapid and significant changes in your microbiome and, in turn, your health.

Set the intention to follow through as best you can. Be kind to yourself, especially in those moments when the microbes, and old reflexive habits, take over the bus. If you temporarily lose control, it is no different from getting lost in thoughts while meditating. It is expected. You notice you have strayed from your intended focus, and you start over. Just as each breath is a chance to start again, each meal is a chance to begin again as well.

It is unhelpful to add stress about food choices and eating to your list of stressors. This is not a win-or-lose game with superfoods and super villains, but one of balance. The centenarians do not deprive themselves of sugars and sweets. They savor these treats in moderation. It is hard in our world to entirely avoid processed foods, but we can choose them mindfully. When you cannot decide what to eat, remember the brilliantly straightforward advice of Michael Pollan: "Eat food. Not too much. Mostly plants." Once again, it really can be that simple.

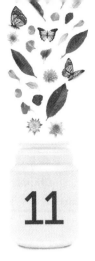

Restoring the Body with Sleep

Sleep is that golden chain that ties health and our bodies together.

—THOMAS DEKKER

While our microbiome reminds us of our interdependence with the complex ecosystem residing within and on our bodies, sleep reminds us of our connection to the natural rhythms of the world around us. The mystery of sleep also connects us with our ancestors who, like us, have pondered for millennia why we need to sleep.

Ancient civilizations believed sleep offers us access to messages of the gods. The Egyptians and Greeks traveled to dream temples to sleep on special "dream beds" to seek divine wisdom and healing. In the Book of Genesis, the pharaoh called upon Joseph to interpret a dream that nobody else could understand. By wisely predicting seven years of bounty, followed by seven years of famine, Joseph not only spared the people from starvation, but also earned himself a position of power and prestige.

Six thousand years later, Sigmund Freud turned to the dream world for buried clues to the psyche and healing, although he placed dreams within the confines of the brain and psychology rather than within the realm of gods.

In our modern industrialized world, many dismiss sleep and dreams as an unproductive nuisance. Thomas Edison famously declared that "sleep is a criminal waste of time and a heritage from our cave days." Yet, the fact that nearly all living organisms require periods of sleep implies that sleep must somehow be essential to living. Some creatures and humans require lots of sleep, and some far less, but we all need sleep to function. The brown bat sleeps away most of the day and night, totaling about twenty hours of rest. Opossums, armadillos, and pythons sleep around eighteen hours. The tall, lanky giraffe sleeps while standing for five-minute "giraffe naps" totaling about thirty minutes a day.

Dolphins, whales, and birds rest one-half of their brain at a time, so that the other half can remain alert for dangers and keep them afloat or flying. More astonishingly, even primitive worms and one-celled organisms, like bacteria, plankton, and yeast, display fluctuating periods of rest and activity that correspond with the cycles of light and dark.

In Greek mythology, Hypnos, the god of sleep, and his twin brother, Thanatos, the god of death, resided in neighboring caves in the underworld through which Lethe, the River of Forgetfulness, flowed. Although the deep stages of sleep resemble "mini deaths," research is revealing that the restorative powers of sleep keep us away from Thanatos's side of the cave for a longer period of time. Clearly, we living beings require rest, relaxation, and reprieves from the demands of living.

Although the function of dreams remains mystifying, we can no longer dismiss the importance of sleep for restoration and physical and emotional well-being. Sleep deprivation, defined as less than six hours of sleep a night for adults, leads to chronic inflammation and increased risk for dementia, strokes, heart disease, obesity, cancer, psychosis, depression, and, death. Yet according to the CDC, eighty million American adults are sleep deprived and relying on caffeine and other stimulants to get through the day. Our busy lifestyle with bright lights, TVs, tablets, and smartphones has disconnected us from the natural rhythms of day and night, light and dark, sun and moon.

Adults and youth are paying a price for this lack of balance. Kids require sleep for growth and development, yet they are suffering from even greater sleep deprivation than adults. A 2017 study found that children who do not get enough sleep in early childhood exhibit issues with attention, memory, problem solving, and increased impulsivity at age seven. Yet over a quarter of children fail to get the recommended nine to eleven hours of sleep each night.

The problem of not enough sleep only grows as kids get older. A 2006 Sleep in America poll found that 87 percent of high school students in the United States get far less than the recommended eight to ten hours of sleep. Yet, in a strange disconnect, 78 percent of parents believe their children are getting sufficient sleep. Unfortunately, sleep-deficient kids are more likely to suffer from anxiety, depression, suicidality, difficulty concentrating, and poor grades. They are at increased risk of alcohol and drug addictions. Over time, the poor sleeping patterns of adolescents and teens become a dangerous norm, leading to chronic inflammation and a host of chronic illnesses, including increased risk of depression, anxiety, and addiction.

We have all experienced the immediate effects of a poor night of sleep. We feel moodier, more irritable, and short-tempered. We suffer from poorer judgment and increased impulsivity. We crave sugar and caffeine to counteract the lack of energy and motivation. We find it harder to focus and remember. Our reflexes slow.

Imaging studies reveal that a night without sleep heightens amygdala reactivity by a whopping 60 percent. Just like trauma and stress, sleep deprivation activates the amygdala and hijacks the frontal lobe. A full night of quality sleep keeps the amygdala and frontal lobe connected. These findings explain the strong associations between sleep deprivation and increased impulsivity, suicidality, and aggression.

Severe lack of sleep affects us so deeply, in fact, that the United Nations torture report declared sleep deprivation to be a form of torture. In response to the United States' use of sleep deprivation to break the will of prisoners at Guantánamo Bay, the Supreme Court ruled that depriving prisoners of sleep for more than thirty-six hours violates due process. In 1944 Supreme Court Justice Black wrote, "It has been known since 1500 at least that deprivation of sleep is the most effective torture and certain to produce any confession desired."

The deleterious effects of sleep deprivation on our ability to think and respond can be deadly: it actually leads to more car crashes than alcohol and drugs combined. One study found that "after being awake for nineteen hours, people who were sleep deprived were as cognitively impaired as those who were legally drunk." If a person sleeps less than five hours, the risk of a car crash increases threefold. If you sleep less than four hours, the risk of an accident rises nearly twelvefold.

In my psychiatry residency class, every one of us was involved in at least one motor vehicle accident after a night on call, which at that time meant staying up for a thirty-hour shift. Fortunately, nobody was seriously harmed, but that is an eye-opening example of how dangerous lack of sleep can be, and how cavalier many of us, especially physicians, can be in denying the issue. This may be attributed to the fact that, like being drunk, the more sleep deprived we are, the less aware we are of our deficits. Clearly, our bodies desperately require sleep for optimal and safe functioning.

Unfortunately, medications are usually the first-line strategy for most patients encountering difficulty with sleep, often without taking the time to seek underlying causes. Sound familiar? Combining sleep deprivation with sleep medications, like Ambien, Restoril, trazodone, or benzodiazepines, only creates a deadlier cocktail and a more massive public health concern. The risk of crashing while on these medications is similar to the risk of crashing while driving drunk.

The medicalization of insomnia, like depression, has changed a nearly ubiquitous human experience into a pathology, overtreated with harmful pharmaceuticals. Between 1993 and 2007, the diagnosis of insomnia increased sevenfold. Over this same fourteen-year period, prescriptions for sleeping pills, or "Z-drugs," increased thirtyfold from 540,000 to 16.2 million. Not only do these medications fail to resolve the problems causing a lack of sleep—most frequently stress and poor sleep habits—but they are dangerous and extremely difficult to discontinue. They also lead to side effects that include sleep driving and increased car accidents, sleep eating and weight gain, sleepwalking, short-term amnesia, daytime sedation, cognitive impairment, dementia, dependence, cancer, and a threefold increased risk of premature mortality.

Given the dangerous and potentially deadly side effects of these medications, one would hope that they are at least effective. But sadly, this is not the case. A review of sixty-five trials, involving over four thousand people from different countries, found that the difference in extra sleep time between placebo and any of the sleep medications amounted to about twenty minutes. This is an extraordinarily small benefit in relation to the profound risks.

A disturbing study examined the risk of psychiatric disorders over a six-year period for those on sedative medications. The trial compared those with insomnia who were prescribed hypnotics, those with insomnia who were not prescribed hypnotics, and those without insomnia or medications. The data showed that those prescribed benzodiazepines or hypnotic drugs were at increased risk of developing depression, anxiety, and bipolar disorder. More alarmingly, a 2017 study, published in the *American Journal of Psychiatry,* concluded that these medications can not only worsen depression but increase suicidality. For an extra twenty minutes of sleep, does this make any sense?

Once again, it is clear that our treatments are causing more harm than good. As the data becomes more difficult to refute, physicians are being encouraged to de-prescribe, but are offered no tools to help patients do that. I have recently seen far too many patients who have been abruptly discontinued from these medications, or even "fired" as patients and left to fend for themselves, primarily because many physicians simply do not know how to solve the problem they created.

Impaired sleep certainly carries its own risks, including tripling to quadrupling the risk of a future depressive episode. Three-quarters of depressed patients experience difficulties falling asleep or staying asleep. The best way to exacerbate a sleep issue, however, is to add a sleeping pill, as we just saw in the data above and, worse, to add fear and helplessness to the mix. The fear of not being able to function the next day and the frustration at not being able to sleep is precisely what fuels so much of modern-day insomnia. "That which we resist persists" most certainly applies to sleep. The first place to begin to address sleep issues is not to pop a pill, but to examine sleep habits and establish a sleep routine.

WELLNESS RX: ESTABLISHING A SLEEP ROUTINE

When it comes to sleep, our brains are wired for routine and consistency to set the sleep cycle into action. Here are some simple guidelines to consider for setting a sleep routine. Keep a sleep diary (you can find one at the National Sleep Foundation website, https://tinyurl.com/yy5x4f26) to help you to gain clearer insight into your sleep patterns.

1. Go to bed at the same time every night, as often as possible. Our dog, Bean, will encourage us to all go upstairs at 8:30 p.m., which is the kids' bedtime on school nights. Sometimes Bean will wait for us, but often he will give up and go upstairs on his own. Eventually, we will come to our senses and join him. Our brains, like Bean's, function best when we stick to the routine.

2. Avoid caffeine and stimulants after noon. If sleep is not an issue for you, avoiding caffeine after 1 p.m. is best. Caffeine has a five- to seven-hour half-life, which means that the latte you had at 3 p.m. to get over the mid-afternoon hump will slowly dwindle to half the original concentration over the next five to seven hours. This means that between 8 p.m. and 10 p.m., depending on your metabolism, you still have 50 percent of the original concentration of caffeine in your body, masking your fatigue and preventing you from falling asleep as easily.

3. Avoid eating a large meal three hours prior to sleeping. The body cannot rest if it is busy digesting.

4. Create a bedtime ritual beginning thirty minutes to one hour before bedtime. Sleep requires consistent cues and conditions that let the body know that sleep time is approaching. For example:

   • Dim the lights an hour before bed. Fading light stimulates the production of melatonin, which cues the body to prepare for sleep. Keep the bedroom dark.

   • Turn off the TV, or at least watch something soothing.

   • Turn off the electronic devices, and keep them outside the bedroom. The blue light can decrease the rise of melatonin by 23 percent, and decrease REM sleep.

   • Read or listen to calming music.

- Have a cup of hot chamomile or lavender tea (only if it will not wake you up in the middle of the night with a full bladder).

- Take a hot bath with a drop or two of organic lavender oil.

- Meditate or do some gentle yoga or stretching.

5. Turn down the thermostat. Darkness and a drop in body temperature by two to three degrees Fahrenheit are required to initiate sleep. As a bonus, you can save some money on your heating bill.

6. Keep a separate "gratitude journal" by your bed and write down three things for which you are grateful. We will discuss this further in chapter 15.

7. Keep another notepad by your bed to write down any thoughts bouncing around in your head, or items to be added to tomorrow's to-do list, so that you can let them go and clear space for sleep.

8. Use the bed only for sleep. Watching TV or checking your phone sends mixed messages to your body. If sleep is not an issue, and reading with a dim light is part of your routine (I can't fall asleep if I don't read for at least a few minutes), that is fine, but if sleep is an issue, then read the book somewhere else until it gets regulated. Sex is the one exception to this rule.

9. Surrender. If you cannot fall asleep, stop trying to force it. If you haven't fallen asleep within 20 minutes, get up and do something relaxing. No, this does not mean playing a quick game of Candy Crush or Mortal Kombat on your phone. Try focusing on belly breathing or left nostril breathing (chapter 7), the Body Scan (chapter 9), or imagining yourself in a peaceful place with a friend, beloved pet, spirit guide, or other supportive resource beside you (chapter 6). Notice your frustration and see if you can find

---

where you are holding the tension in your body. Observe your thoughts about how you should be asleep, and your subsequent frustration that things are not going your way. Tend to the upset inner child with tenderness, rather than a critical rebuke. What if you shifted your perspective about being up in the middle of the night from being a problem to an opportunity to practice the skills you have been learning during the day?

10. Get up at the same time every morning and avoid napping. Yes, especially if you had a lousy night of sleep. Sleeping in or napping will only perpetuate the cycle. The goal here is to create a new pattern so you can sleep. Once that is accomplished, if you want to sleep in once in a while, or feel the need for a nap, go for it.

11. Get outside in natural light. If your job prevents this during the winter months when daylight is scarce, consider a light box or dawn simulator light.

Options for Sleepless Nights

Cognitive Behavioral Therapy for Insomnia

Poor sleep hygiene is the most frequent cause of sleep disruption. If poor sleep is a problem for you, hopefully some of the suggestions above provide relief. If not, consider taking a class on cognitive behavioral therapy for insomnia (CBTi). Despite its infrequent recommendation by physicians, the National Institutes of Health Consensus Statement recommends it as the first-line treatment for insomnia. CBTi offers a combination of sleep education, relaxation techniques, and sleep hygiene. Most importantly, it teaches cognitive restructuring to shift self-defeating, anxiety-producing stories and beliefs about sleep. This option has been found to be more effective than medications, without the life-threatening risks, and offers a lifetime of tools and strategies to incorporate if or when insomnia strikes again, which it does from time to time for most of us. CBTi is equally as effective whether taken online or in person, which makes it a much more affordable and accessible option. As a bonus, it has also been shown to improve depression, anxiety, bipolar disorder, and even suicidality.

Herbs and Supplements

Calming teas, tinctures, and oils may also help lure you into a peaceful slumber. **Chamomile** has been recommended since 1550 BCE as a medicinal tea to quiet the mind and induce calm. Try drinking a cup of tea near bedtime or taking a 3 to 5 ml tincture. It is also helpful for bloating and indigestion. I usually drink a cup of tea after dinner for its digestive and calming benefits.

Lavender is a safe, gentle herb used for insomnia, anxiety, and depression for over 2,500 years. Today, Silexan, a patented capsule form of lavender oil marketed in Europe, has been shown to benefit sleep and anxiety as effectively as lorazepam, a commonly prescribed benzodiazepine—without any of the side effects. Try diffusing some organic oil in your bedroom, sipping a cup of tea, or placing a drop of oil on your pillow. Sweet dreams!

Valerian and **hops** have been used for centuries all around the world for their anxiety-relieving and sleep-inducing properties. Valerian works as well as the benzodiazepines, which replaced the use of the herb in the United States thanks to effective marketing. A review of data consistently suggests that this combo is effective for falling asleep more quickly, and improving quality and quantity of sleep. Research suggests valerian's benefits increase over a period of two weeks, so do not give up on it if you do not notice an immediate effect. Try a tincture of 5 to 10 ml a half hour to an hour before bed, or a capsule of about 200 mg of valerian and 40 to 60 mg of hops. Although side effects are rare with this combo, a small subset of people does feel restless, so be sure to start at a low dose.

The supplement I am most frequently asked about in my practice is the use of **melatonin.** Over three million Americans take this supplement in hopes of getting a good night's sleep. Although melatonin is quite effective for jet lag and shift work, for other forms of insomnia it increases time to fall asleep by about seven minutes, and total sleep time by about eight minutes. The most common side effects for melatonin are grogginess, impaired balance, headache, dizziness, or nausea—a much safer profile than possible dementia and death with sleeping pills! Melatonin, however, is a hormone, and the consequences of long-term nightly use are unknown.

As we have seen with antidepressants, messing with the body's balance may have unintended consequences. A small study in Great Britain showed that melatonin increases the risk of fractures, as it may interfere with the normal cycle of bone formation. If you choose to try it, experiment with when you take it. Some find better results when taken closer to dusk, rather than just before bed. This allows melatonin to set the timing in place for sleep later in the evening.

Magnesium and **L-theanine,** both discussed in the last chapter, are also helpful options to consider. While all of these supplements are fairly safe and may improve your slumber, remember that sleep hygiene and CBTi should always be the first choice, as these will help resolve, rather than just cover up, the problem.

WELLNESS RX: YOGA FOR RESTFUL SLUMBER

A national survey found that over 55 percent of people slept better after some relaxing yoga. How about giving it a try? Viparita Karani, the Legs Up the Wall Pose, is a great resource for settling the body for sleep.

If you have a yoga mat or blanket, place it perpendicularly against the wall. Scoot your bottom close to the wall. Lie back on the mat, blanket, or carpet, and extend your legs up the wall, scooting in a little closer, so that the backs of your legs rest comfortably against the wall. Allow your arms to relax by your sides with palms up, or gently joining the tips of the ring finger with the thumb in the Surya Mudra, the sun gesture. If it is difficult to get your legs up the wall, lie on your back and rest your calves over a blanket on a chair instead. You will want your thighs to be at a 90-degree angle to the shins.

Feel your body on the ground. Notice the breath in your belly. With each exhalation, invite your body to sink deeper into the ground, releasing and letting go. Notice areas of tension in your body and breathe into them with curiosity and kindness. Feel the weight of your legs against the wall. Stay here for five to ten minutes, focusing on the breath and the body.

For additional calming, you could try adding a couple of minutes of left nostril breathing (chapter 7).

Plenty of videos are available online with various yoga routines designed for sleep. Try some and see what works for you. As always, jot down your observations, but be sure to do so in the morning after you wake up from a good night of sleep!

Light Up Your Life

You may notice that issues with sleep and mood are acutely affected by the shorter days and longer nights of winter, when our bodies receive the signal for sleep earlier and earlier, making some of us long to curl up under a warm blanket in cozy jammies until spring brings light and thaws the snow. It is estimated that 1.6 million people around the world are affected by seasonal depressive symptoms. During the fall transition from daylight saving time to standard time, there is an 11 percent increase in depressive disorders. This can last for up to ten weeks, until the body starts to adjust or, perhaps, the increase in daylight and the hope it brings dissipates the symptoms.

For those of us especially sensitive to reduced exposure to the sun and abrupt desynchronization with our circadian rhythms, we can begin with honoring our bodies' desire to slow down. Unfortunately, this is difficult, since the shortest days of the year coincide with holidays and some of the busiest days of activity and socializing. But sometimes just saying "no thank-you," or at least leaving early from yet another holiday gathering, is the biggest gift we can offer ourselves this time of year. To better align ourselves with nature's rhythms, it is even more important to dim evening lights, even though we may want to do just the opposite.

Other tools that can help us more smoothly navigate the transition to standard time and the shortening days of winter are bright-light boxes or a dawn simulator device. These devices changed my formerly adversarial relationship with Ohio's long dreary winters. I used to blast winter blues away with the 10,000 lux of light emitted by my light box. I sat in front of it for twenty minutes in the early morning while I meditated.

A 2015 study in *JAMA Psychiatry* compared the effects of light boxes with placebo and an antidepressant in patients with nonseasonal depression. It turns out the light box outperformed the medication and the placebo. Ironically, the placebo outperformed the antidepressant.

These days, I rarely use the light box as I am now a big fan of my light dawn simulator. It requires less work. I do not even need to turn it on. This device acts as a gentle alarm clock that gradually increases the intensity of light over a half-hour period before my alarm is set to go off, just as if the sun were actually rising outside my window on a sunny summer day. Studies have generally shown that these two devices work equally well in helping to improve fatigue, cognition, and mood, although, like everything else in life, some people may respond better to one than the other.

As you move toward the winter solstice, consider dimming the lights, pausing, and enjoying the darkness. An evening walk can be the perfect way to end the day, allowing the darkness to attune your body's natural rhythms. Remember to notice and honor your body's own unique rhythms and its connections with the rhythms of the world around you.

Why We Sleep and Dream

So far, we have explored some of the ways to create or enhance our sleep routine, and the consequences of becoming disconnected from the natural rhythm of sleep. But we have not yet answered the age-old question of why we sleep and dream. To better understand some of the research, it would be helpful to have a basic understanding of the stages of sleep, as each has a unique role.

Sleep Cycle

Our bodies alternate between NREM (non–rapid eye movement) sleep and REM (rapid eye movement) sleep in four stages, which repeat themselves in roughly ninety-minute cycles. NREM sleep dominates during the first half of the night, while REM sleep rules in the second half. If we go to bed late, we miss out on the NREM, and when we wake up early, we get less REM.

Like everything else in the body, and in life, it is all about balance. NREM sleep prunes unnecessary neural connections in the short-term storage area of the hippocampus to clear space for new information. REM sleep links new information, experiences, and skills from the day with relevant older memories, consolidating the synthesized information in the cortex for long-term storage. It is an amazingly wise process that balances the forgetting and letting go of what we no longer need so that we can make space for remembrance of new ideas, skills, and behaviors. The functioning of this complex system depends on our circadian rhythms, time spent awake, exposure to light and darkness, movement of the body, and sleep habits.

Stage 1: This stage of light sleep only lasts about five minutes. Our heart rate, breathing, and brain waves begin to slow down, creating space for a deeper sleep. Our eyeballs move from side to side beneath our eyelids. At this stage, we are easily awoken by outside sounds or disturbances. We may drift in and out of this stage without even realizing it.

Stage 2: As we drop into stage 2 sleep, brain activity continues to slow down, but now with occasional half-second sparks of activity, referred to as spindles. The breath and heart rate slow further, muscles relax more deeply, our eyes stop moving, and our body temperature drops.

Stages 3 and 4: As we fall deeper into sleep, the tempo of the brain waves slows down, becoming more synchronized and harmonious. We are now in slow-wave sleep in which the slow, rolling delta waves first appear. In stage 3, the delta waves are present less than 50 percent of the time, while in stage 4 they predominate. The body becomes immobile and pain-free, and the brain activity resembles that of a brain death or coma. Here we can see why the ancient Greeks personified sleep and death as twins. Yet it is during this stage that the body works to restore and rebuild the muscles, bones, organs, and brain from the stresses of the day so that we may continue to grow and thrive. Much of this work is supported by the secretion of growth hormone by the pituitary gland, which promotes neurogenesis, increased protein synthesis, and stimulation of the immune system.

In this deep sleep, glial cells that surround and support the neurons deflate by 60 percent, creating space for the toxins that accumulated during the day to be washed away by the cerebral spinal fluid. Without sufficient deep-wave sleep, beta-amyloid peptides and tau proteins cannot be purged from the brain and accumulate, becoming entangled and toxic. This leads to impaired communication among neurons and increased risk for Alzheimer's and other neurodegenerative diseases. Although the body requires this essential stage for health and vitality, the body does not want to dwell in the underground realm for more than about thirty minutes before we shift into REM sleep.

REM Sleep: This stage is often referred to as "paradoxical sleep," since the brain is awake but the body is asleep. Unlike the slow rolling deltas of deep-wave sleep, brain scans for this stage resemble the waking brain, with super-fast and chaotic brain waves. MRI scans show that parts of the brain during REM sleep are 30 percent more active than when we are awake.

"Perchance to Dream"

The oldest known book of dreams, written on papyrus, dates to 1275 BCE. This ancient document, now kept in the British Museum in London, includes 108 dreams divided into those that were auspicious and inauspicious. "Good" dreams included seeing oneself eating crocodile meat, seeing the moon shine, slaying a hippopotamus, or plunging into a river. "Bad" dreams included being bitten by a dog, seeing oneself in a mirror, looking like an ostrich, or feeding cattle. Clearly, cultural context plays a role in the images we see while asleep. But what benefits, if any, do these hallucinations of the night bestow upon us?

Although plenty of mysteries remain, neuroscience has begun to reveal some of the amazing treasures offered to us by the dreaming state. For these answers, I turned to the intriguing book *Why We Sleep: Unlocking the Power of Sleep and Dreams*, in which neuroscientist Dr. Matthew Walker unlocks some of the amazing treasures offered to us by the dreaming state. During REM sleep, the activity in the prefrontal cortex—our logical, rational part of the brain that is front and center during our waking hours—slows down. Meanwhile, the areas of the brain responsible for visual imagery, motor activity, emotions, and autobiographical memory increase in activity. The amygdala becomes 30 percent more active than while awake.

Amazingly, research has revealed that dreams act as a form of free "overnight therapy." The emotional themes from the day emerge in our dreams at night. While we work through the emotional residue of the day, the stress hormone epinephrine gets turned off, essentially creating a safe, stress-free space for processing our emotional discharge. At the same time, softened, processed memories are amalgamated into our memory banks. In essence, REM sleep balances the act of forgetting that which we no longer need, and remembering that which we do.

To figure this out, Walker conducted a clever experiment. While inside an MRI scanner, two groups of participants viewed emotionally charged images and were assessed for emotional reactivity. Twelve hours later, they were all once again presented with the same images. The key difference was that one group viewed the images in the morning and later that evening, while the other group viewed the images in the evening and again in the morning, after a night of sleep. Those who did not sleep between the two viewings displayed the same degree of emotional reactivity at each session. For those who slept, however, the emotions had softened, and the amygdala was less reactive.

Sleep researcher Rosalind Cartwright has spent the past half century studying the role of sleep and dreams in our lives, particularly the relationship between REM sleep and depression. She has found that those with more severe depression spend more time in REM sleep and less time in restorative deep sleep. It is as if those with depression are stuck repeating their dreams of the night until they can finally work through their emotional turmoil and find resolution. Cartwright proposes that the purpose of dreaming may be to diffuse emotional experiences by merging memories from the past and present into a new cohesive story line in the brain, which over time may offer new perspective and insight.

To test her theory, Cartwright followed a group of depressed individuals undergoing divorces for a period of one year, witnessing how dreams and sleep influenced their moods during this emotionally turbulent time. She discovered that those who dreamed about their spouse and painful experiences successfully resolved their depressive symptoms, while those who avoided the pain, even in their dreams, got stuck in their despair. It sounds a lot like the principles of mindfulness, does it not?

By leaning in and fully feeling our emotions, we allow them to move through and release. Avoiding or resisting discomfort keeps us trapped in its unrelenting grasp. This makes me wonder if learning to lean into emotional discomfort during our waking hours offers us better access to the pain in our dreams, so that it may be diffused and set free. I do not think this question has yet been researched.

Walker's research not only shows that dreams can soothe our emotions, but also gift us with the ability to accurately read facial expressions and body language while awake. Being social creatures, detecting the emotions of others is an essential skill to navigating our world. Walker describes REM sleep as the "master piano tuner, that adjusts the brain's emotional instrumentation at night to pitch-perfect precision, so that when you wake up the next morning, you can discern overt and subtle covert microexpressions with exactitude." He discovered that sleep-deprived brains lose the ability to discern a friendly expression from a threatening one. The world appears more hostile, uncertain, and fearful. This perception of the world further amplifies the amygdala reactivity, making it more difficult to sleep, depriving us of more REM, and entangling us in a vicious spiral of anxiety, fear, and depression.

Dreams free us from the confines of our logical and rational selves, offering us access to our imaginative, colorful, creative, insightful, and intuitive aspects. In the process of synthesizing old and new memories, dreams create opportunities to arrive at new possibilities and perspectives. Connecting with those aspects of ourselves has been used for healing purposes for thousands of years.

Wouldn't it be interesting to see what wisdom you might discover by starting a dream journal and writing down even just a few sentences about your dreams when you wake up? If you do not remember them, that is OK, but keep a pen and paper by your bed for what tiny remnants you may recall, even if it is only a feeling, color, or word. Like the activities in chapter 6, this may access insights that are not available to the overly rational parts of the brain.

Sometimes just posing a question before you go to sleep, or taking a few moments to acknowledge emotional difficulties, may direct your brain to work on some decision you are trying to resolve, or emotional pain that needs healing. Writing the dreams down offers yet another means of processing and releasing remaining emotional charge. If you have frequent nightmares, it may be best to see a therapist to help you work through these. Nightmares are less scary once exposed to the light of a caring supporter.

What we have learned from the neuroscience of dreams is that we dream not to escape reality, not to hide repressed emotions and desires, as Freud suggested, but to face them head on, so the pain may be acknowledged and dissipated. We travel down the River of Forgetfulness to release what no longer serves us, but then return to the Shores of Remembrance to assimilate and consolidate memories. Remembering too much, we become overwhelmed by the excess clutter preventing us from accessing pertinent information, like unmanaged emails. Forgetting too much, the information we receive falls through our grasp like a sieve, unable to be utilized.

We must remember and forget in order to learn, grow, and transform. We must face our distress so that it may soften and release. When we do not sleep, or worse, when we sedate ourselves into medicated slumber, we may lose our way on the River of Forgetfulness as brain connections unravel. We risk floating perilously close to the shores of Thanatos sooner than we had hoped. In order to spend adequate rejuvenating time each night in the cave of Hypnos, we must reconnect with the rhythms of our bodies and the world around us. By doing so, restorative sleep balances the time spent in NREM and REM sleep, in forgetfulness and remembrance, so that we may remain resilient, healthy, and well.

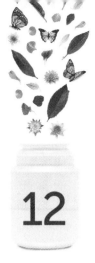

Environment as Sustenance or Poison

Everybody needs beauty as well as bread, places to play in and pray in,
where nature may heal and give strength to body and soul.

—JOHN MUIR

"Are you feeling tired, irritable, or stressed out?" asks a good-looking bearded man sitting on a rock, beneath a shady tree, beside a peaceful lake. "Well, you might consider Nature." We hear the caw of a crow in the background of this YouTube video, as the logo pops up for the new and approved prescription-strength Nature Rx, "a nonharmful medication shown to relieve the crippling symptoms of modern life."

The scene shifts, and we see the bearded man walking on a wooded trail with a couple of friends and the requisite cute fluffy dog. While his friends explore a rocky creek, the man looks into the camera: "Nature is recommended for humans of all ages, and is great for pets too." An adorable blond-haired pony-tailed girl appears out of nowhere to offer the man a yellow daisy. The man looks into the camera again as he cuddles his pooch, who has her hair pulled back with a barrette, accentuating the perky puppy eyes and snout. The voice of a narrator lists the benefits of the prescription: "Nature can reduce cynicism, meaninglessness, anal retentiveness, and murderous rage."

Near the end of this parody the man warns, "Caution: Nature may cause you to slow down, quit your job, or consider what the f— you are doing with your life." As we watch the man paddling away in a canoe at sunset, the narrator notes, "If you are overly jaded, cynical, or numb, you may need to increase your dosage." The scene shifts to the quintessential cheery scene of a good-looking, smiling circle of friends gathered around a campfire. A written disclaimer appears in the lower right corner: "Nature doesn't solve everything. It just may help."

Although the *Nature Rx* video is a clever spoof on pharmaceutical commercials, research is proving that nature is indeed an amazingly effective healing balm. It has been prescribed for centuries to soothe the body and soul. Cyrus the Great, founder of the Persian Empire, created gardens for rest and relaxation 2,500 years ago. Hippocrates described nature as "the physician of diseases." In the late 1800s, sanatoriums were established in the pine forests of Germany, Switzerland, West Wales, and the Adirondacks of New York to treat tuberculosis with the "exhalations of turpentine" from the trees.

In 1865 the landscape architect Frederick Law Olmsted, who not only created New York City's Central Park but also played a key role in the development of the national park system, wrote that immersing oneself in nature "reduces mental and nervous excitability, moroseness, melancholy, or irascibility." At an American Medical Association meeting in 1898, Dr. Frederic Thomas presciently linked the increasing rates of mental illness to noise, smoke, and pollution of industrialized cities.

Physicians all around the world are once again turning to the healing properties of nature. In Great Britain, physicians prescribe green gyms, where patients improve their communities by helping plant trees, sow meadows, and establish wildlife ponds instead of doing push-ups and leg lifts. Dr. Robert Zarr of Washington, D.C., founded *Park Rx America*, whose mission is to "decrease the burden of chronic disease, increase health and happiness, and foster environmental stewardship by virtue of prescribing Nature during the routine delivery of health care." The U.S. National Park Service created *Healthy Parks, Healthy People*, which partners with medical schools, health care leaders, businesses, and scientists to use public park lands to reconnect Americans to nature for "mental, physical, and spiritual health, and social well-being and sustainability of the planet."

My absolute favorite program is sponsored by the national health board in the Shetlands, which encourages physicians to prescribe mindful activities in nature to counteract depression, anxiety, stress, diabetes, and other chronic health conditions. This program includes a beautiful online nature prescriptions calendar that offers stunning photographs and a list of monthly ideas to mindfully connect with nature and wildlife.

In January, the brochure suggests readers step outside and "be still for three minutes and listen," or use a magnifying glass to "really look at lichen." A suggestion for April is to "Find a bud on a tree ... feel the texture." In May, it suggests, "Bury your face in the grass," or "Make a daisy chain."

You may roll your eyes at how this could possibly help resolve depression, but a growing body of evidence suggests that these are not just the whimsical ideas of tree huggers. Studies from around the world demonstrate that those living more than half a mile from green space are more likely to report higher stress, anxiety, and depression, and an overall increase in diseases of all kinds. Conversely, those living closer to parks report decreased stress, depression, and anxiety as well as a decreased risk of cancer, stroke, and death.

A study at the University of Essex tracked households over a three-year period, comparing those that moved from rural areas to cities and vice versa. Researchers found that those who moved to greener areas experienced less depression and improved mental well-being, while those moving into urban areas had an increased risk of depression. You may be thinking, places with more greenery may just be more economically advantaged communities, and the benefits may have nothing to do with nature. To rule out that possibility, another study examined comparable inner city neighborhoods, differing only in the amount of green space. This study arrived at the same conclusions: the presence of green spaces decreases the risk for stress, depression, and disease.

Although getting outside and interacting with nature is ideal, research suggests that just views of nature soothe our bodies and emotions. Studies have found that postsurgical hospital patients with rooms viewing nature recover more quickly and have fewer complications and a decreased need for pain medications than their unfortunate controls with views of buildings or brick walls. Prisoners with a view require fewer visits for medical care. Elementary school children with views of nature perform better in school. Office workers are more productive at work.

MRI scans show that viewing nature increases activity in the hippocampus, particularly an area dense with opioid receptors, increasing positive thoughts and affect and decreasing the perception of stress. Views of nature also decrease the firing of the amygdala, and increase activity in areas of the brain associated with empathy and altruism. Imagine the effect on our society if we all added a bit more nature to our daily lives!

In contrast, those who viewed urban scenes showed increased activity in the amygdala, leading to increased feelings of stress, fear, and anxiety. Other studies suggest urban views even shift value systems from altruistic desires for helping others to more self-centered pursuits of money, fame, and power. Clearly, we as individuals and as a society are suffering more than we know from our disconnection from nature.

For those city dwellers without access to a view or a nearby park, do not despair. It seems that even pictures of nature offer some reprieve from stress and sullen moods. One study had a group of students, fresh from college exams, view a series of pictures. Half of the students viewed nature scenes, while the other half viewed urban buildings. Those who viewed the scenes from nature reported feeling calmer and happier, while those viewing the urban scenes felt sadder.

Brain scans and labs confirmed this finding. Those viewing nature displayed more alpha waves, indicative of a calm, attentive state, as well as lower cortisol levels and heart rate, and increased serotonin levels.

Why not take advantage of your body's response to nature and tape a picture of a beautiful calming scene next to your computer, and look at it every hour or so, while taking a few deep breaths? Better yet, buy a plant. The presence of plants at work can decrease anger, anxiety, depression, and fatigue by 40 percent, and decrease stress by 50 percent.

As I am typing this, my cat, Moonshadow, who has been sitting in front of my computer screen for the past hour, turns to look at me, and offers an insistent meow. Pictures of animals or beloved pets offer a nature reprieve as well. In fact, one study on watching cat videos online suggests that those who watch these videos report feeling more energized and positive, with decreases in anxiety, irritability, and sadness. Even better, studies suggest pet owners may experience decreased stress and anxiety, improved mood, lower blood pressure and heart rate, less loneliness, fewer health problems, and even a longer life. In exchange for food, water, and shelter, these companions, with whom we have cohabitated over the past fourteen thousand years, offer unconditional love and acceptance, wet sloppy kisses when we are sad, and a reason to get up off the couch and go for a walk on even the dreariest and coldest of days.

Forest Bathing

Much of the research on the healing benefits of nature has come from Japan, where two-thirds of the country is filled with forests, and there is a deep spiritual attachment to the wonders of the natural world. In 1982, Japan instituted a national program for *shinrin-yoku,* or forest bathing. The first of over 60 forest therapy bases was created within the Akasawa Forest. There, one could receive a medical consultation amongst the trees, and hike trails designed to offer physical, emotional, and spiritual benefits. At the time, these benefits were based on nothing more than intuition and ancestral wisdom.

Beginning in 2004, a new field of study was initiated to seek evidence for this ancient hunch. The research reveals that time spent in nature decreases stress, anxiety, depression, and anger. It increases energy and vitality and improves sleep. It boosts the immune system, not just while you are in the woods, but for up to a month afterward. Labs show that forest bathing decreases cortisol levels, blood pressure, and blood sugar. It balances the autonomic nervous system, breaking the stress-induced sympathetic response, and activating the parasympathetic nervous system to allow for rest, relaxation, and rejuvenation.

Better yet, we do not have to escape to the forest for extended periods of time to benefit. A study conducted by Dr. Qing Li, one of the world's leading experts on forest bathing, found that a two-hour hike offered roughly the same benefits as a long weekend in the woods. Everyone returned to the city feeling happier, calmer, and more energized. Why not find a park near you and see for yourself? This prescription offers lots of benefits without any side effects, at least if you stay out of the poison ivy, and do not offer your finger to local wildlife as a chew toy!

WELLNESS RX: SENSING NATURE

For this exercise, return to a favorite trail or, if you are feeling more adventurous, pick a new park to explore. Take a few moments before beginning your stroll to notice your breath, thoughts, body sensations, and emotions. As you walk toward the trailhead, take a few breaths to clear out old worries and stress, and create space for a new experience.

Feel the movement of your body. Feel the connection of your feet with the ground.

Tune in and use all your senses. **See** the colors of the sky, the trees, the grass, the flora. Notice the light as it passes through the leaves or across the ripples of a lake or stream. Look for signs of wildlife.

Listen to the sounds around you: the wind in the trees, the rustle of flora as a small critter scurries by; the songs of birds; the sound of your own footsteps, breath, and heart.

Smell the air, the trees, the flowers, the dirt.

Touch the texture of a leaf or lean against a large tree and feel the bark. Sense the energy of the tree. Feel the air, the sun, the wind on your face and skin.

Experience nature for at least 20 minutes. Walk, sit, run, stand, lie on the ground, whatever feels right. Notice how your breath, thoughts, body, and emotions may shift as you engage with all your senses to the world around you. Notice whatever arises, and then find a quiet spot to write or draw to record your experiences.

Did you notice your body relaxing? Perhaps your mind quieted? Maybe there was even a moment of awe that caught you by surprise, or a sense of deep familiarity and knowing, like seeing your best friend from childhood after decades apart? Americans now spend 93 percent of their days inside the walls of homes, office buildings, and cars, and ten hours a day tethered to technology. Fewer than 10 percent of teenagers spend time outside daily! We have truly become disconnected from our very roots.

Like the research on viewing urban scenes versus natural ones, multiple studies around the world have examined our different responses to walking through an urban area versus a park setting. Whether in Ann Arbor, Michigan, South Korea, or Palo Alto, California, participants who walk in nature show additional benefits above and beyond the exercise. By hiking through parks, individuals saw improved mood and cognition, increased capacity for memory recall, and decreased rumination and negative affect.

Other research has compared exercising indoors versus outdoors. Those who exercised outside felt greater energy, vitality, and enthusiasm. They reported enjoying it more, and being more likely to do it again.

Healing Power of Nature
Smelling

Why does being in contact with nature dramatically improve our well-being on so many levels? Nature appeals to all of our senses, especially smell. Have you ever walked through a pine forest and felt calmed, energized, and centered by the smell of pine? Ever wondered why pine scents are used in so many cleaning products and candles?

Modern research shows that the "exhalations of turpentine," first described back in the 1800s as a treatment for tuberculosis, are natural oils produced by the trees, known as phytoncides. These natural aromatic chemicals are released into the air to protect the tree from bacteria, insects, and fungi, and to communicate with other trees. Each tree sprays its own unique scent, composed of various terpenes, such as D-limonene, which unsurprisingly smells lemony; alpha-pinene, which smells, yep, piney; beta-pinene, which has a more herby smell; and camphene, which smells like turpentine.

Dr. Li conducted a study in which he diffused Japanese cypress oil into the hotel rooms of participants who slept in the room at night, but went to work as usual by day. Even without being in the woods, the aroma of trees improved sleep and energy, increased pain tolerance and immunity, and decreased stress, anxiety, and cortisol.

This is the powerful basis of aromatherapy. We can bring the forest into our homes with a simple diffuser. An earlier study on the diffusion of D-limonene to depressed inpatients showed that this approach was more effective than antidepressants at improving mood. We have much to learn from the natural world.

Seeing

We have already seen that simply viewing images of nature can offer physical and emotional benefits, but it is more than just the beauty. Research suggests that viewing the patterns of nature—the branching of trees; ferns and butterfly wings; the spirals of shells, roses, and pineapples; a moth drawn to light; the scales of a pine cone; the ripples in water and sand; or the cracks in dry earth or shattered ice—can decrease stress by as much as 60 percent.

Take a moment to look out your window or walk into your backyard, or if you are at work, search for a picture of a flower and spend a few moments just noticing the patterns of color and structure, while breathing deeply into the belly. Notice any shifts in your body or emotions. On your next walk in the woods, consider gathering pine cones, twigs, rocks, and grasses to create a nature mandala on your table, or a larger-scale one in your yard or a park. My kids love to build rock sculptures in creek beds in the summer. Bring your journal on your next hike and draw some of the patterns you see.

Hearing

We all know how it feels when we are surrounded by loud, artificial sounds. I used to dread the birthday parties of my kids' friends that were held at places like Chuck E. Cheese. My shoulders and neck tightened, my jaw clenched, and I would feel an incredible urge to escape the clangs, pings, chimes, rings, whirls, and shooting sounds of the video games, coin machines, and loud, excited, sometimes irritable and angry children all confined in a relatively tight space. I usually left my husband in charge of those events. Contrary to the stress-inducing sounds of the modern world, the sounds of nature calm us.

Nature's sounds quiet the sympathetic nervous system and amplify the parasympathetic nervous system. Unlike artificial sounds, which turn our focus myopically inward, the sounds of nature direct us outward, to something beyond ourselves. Better yet, these sounds provide the most benefit to those who are the most stressed.

Most humans gravitate to the sounds of a babbling brook, waves lapping against a shore, rain falling on the rooftop or on a canopy of trees, and the song birds chirping.

Gordon Hempton, an acoustic ecologist, said that with all the noises created by the modern world, silence, or the absence of human-made sounds, is becoming an endangered species "on the verge of extinction." Hempton has traveled the globe recording and preserving the sounds of the natural world, including thunder in the desert, sunrise on the shores of Cape Cod, babbling brooks in Belize, evening mist in Sri Lanka, the inside of a Sitka spruce, and the sound of silence within a volcano in Hawaii.

During his travels, Hempton created a list of the world's "Last Great Quiet Spaces." He has found only twelve silent sanctuaries in the United States where one can go without hearing the noises of the modern world. He chooses to keep most of these secret so that the spaces remain quiet. If you are interested, he has created over fifty soundscape albums you can download or stream to reconnect you with the natural world outside your office or home.

Touching

A powerful tool of healing, largely unrecognized and barely noticed, is the earth beneath our feet. Our synthetic and rubber-soled shoes have separated us from the energy of the earth. I understand this may sound kooky, but there is evidence to back me up. Before I explain it, though, try connecting with the earth for yourself.

WELLNESS RX: GROUNDING

If the weather allows, take off your socks and shoes and stand in the grass or dirt. Feel the contact of your feet with the earth. Notice any sensations in your toes and feet. Scan your body for other shifts in sensation as you stand there. As you continue to

---

notice body sensations, take a few deep relaxing breaths. Stay here, paying attention to the connection of your feet with the earth and notice any shifts in energy or mood that may occur.

You may want to experiment further and lie down in the grass, allowing the whole back side of your body to be supported by the ground. Notice where the body is making contact with the ground. Feel the body sinking into the ground, allowing the earth to support you. Imagine releasing emotions, thoughts, or even uncomfortable sensations into the ground. Notice any shifts in the breath, emotions, thoughts, and body as you lie there. Write your observations in your journal. The point, as always, is to be open and curious.

Although the earth, throughout history, has been honored as a sacred source of sustenance and life, the evidence for its healing potential is fairly recent—and astonishing! Clinton Ober, an electrical engineer, has pioneered research in this area, which he details in his book *Earthing: The Most Important Health Discovery Ever?* He describes the planet as a "six sextillion metric ton battery that is continually being replenished by solar radiation, lightning, and heat from its deep-down molten core."

This battery offers an endless supply of negatively charged electrons. This matters because our bodies are flowing with an excess of positively charged free radicals, which play a critical role in our immune system. These free radicals are incessantly in search of negatively charged electrons to pair with for stability. In cases of acute inflammation, the free radicals will pair with electrons from pathogens and damaged tissue, which effectively kills the pathogens and cleans up tissue debris.

Unfortunately, in states of chronic inflammation, the overabundant radicals go rogue and start killing healthy cells. Contact with the flow of electrons from the earth neutralizes the body's positive charge and this inflammatory response, freely offering the most potent anti-inflammatory in existence.

It appears that our bodies require connection with the earth to synchronize our circadian and biological rhythms. A series of studies was conducted at the Max Planck Institute involving hundreds of volunteers who were isolated in underground rooms shielded from the earth's electrical field. All the participants developed sleep and hormonal disturbances. These disturbances were normalized when electrical rhythms similar to those of the earth's were pulsed into the rooms, showing that our body's biological rhythms require calibration by the rhythm of the earth for optimal functioning.

Subsequent research has shown that grounding with the earth, by reducing inflammation and coordinating our biological rhythms, increases sleep and energy; decreases stress, anxiety, irritability, and depression; and improves a range of physical symptoms that include gastrointestinal issues and hormonal imbalances.

It is not only the earth's electrical power we require for health, but the sustenance of her soil for food—and microbes! Our bodies need dirt and germs to develop a strong immune system.

The Cebu Longitudinal Health and Nutrition Survey has followed a group of over three thousand pregnant women and their children from a variety of urban and rural neighborhoods in the Philippines since 1983. The study reveals that early and chronic exposure to harmless microbes is critical to immune development and future health. Our overly sanitized society is disabling our immune systems and leading to chronic diseases.

The good news is that by making our lives simpler, we build a more resilient immune system for ourselves and our kids. Forget daily baths. Forget throwing away food that falls on the ground. Definitely ditch your Purell. Make some mud cakes. Garden. Play in your pesticide-free yard and get dirty! In the summer, my kids are lucky to get a bath every week. Their hands and feet are coated in dirt. This is one of my small contributions toward more time for play now, and less inflammation, depression, and disease when my kids are older.

Toxins and Poisons

Despite the warnings of the Lorax, who spoke "for the trees," and ecologist and author Rachel Carson, who alerted us that chemical pesticides were poisoning the environment, nearly two thousand new, untested chemicals enter the marketplace each year in the United States.

These chemicals wind up in our shampoos, detergents, hand lotions, beauty creams, deodorants, toothpastes, sunscreens, household cleaners, clothing, carpets, paints, and plastics. They are in the air we breathe, the water we drink, and the food we eat. Stop and look around for a moment. Consider how many products within view are made of these cheap, ubiquitous, untested toxins. We put chemicals on our skin, sinks, toilets, countertops, yards, and food, naively assuming they have been tested and found safe. They have not.

Until 2016, when President Barack Obama instituted reforms, the 1976 Toxic Substances Control Act prevented the U.S. Environmental Protection Agency (EPA) from examining the safety of chemicals unless there was evidence of harm. Doesn't that make you feel safe and protected?

Unfortunately, the 2016 reforms, which granted the EPA the right to review and regulate new products and theoretically prevent companies from withholding "trade secrets," have already been weakened and undermined by the Trump administration.

BPA and Endocrine-Disruptors

Even with regulations in place, with so many chemicals being created annually, it is a Sisyphean task to research and regulate them. Consequently, we have all become part of a massive, unintended, unmonitored science experiment—and we are the guinea pigs. Until enough of us squeal—or die, like the Truffula Trees and Bar-ba-loots in *The Lorax*—our safety will remain largely unaddressed.

One of the most ubiquitous chemicals in our environment is bisphenol A (BPA), a component of plastic and epoxy resins first invented over a hundred years ago. The CDC found BPA is in the urine of more than 90 percent of Americans, and in the umbilical cords of nine out of ten infants.

The first evidence of BPA's toxicity dates to the 1930s, when scientists discovered it acts as a synthetic estrogen, similar to diethylstilbestrol (DES), a chemical prescribed to pregnant women between 1940 and 1971 to prevent miscarriages. By the 1950s, it was clear that DES did not reduce pregnancy complications, although the medication continued to be prescribed. DES was finally banned in 1971, after it became undeniably clear that the medication increased the risk of reproductive cancers, some by as much as fortyfold, as well as the risk of breast cancers, premature births, fertility issues, and even depression among the unfortunate daughters exposed to this chemical in utero. Unfortunately, it took thirty years for these risks to come to light. We keep forgetting to learn from our mistakes.

Despite evidence of toxicity, and similarities in properties and structure, BPA continued to be used in common household products, including plastic water bottles, baby bottles, sippy cups, dental sealants, and the lining of canned foods, including baby formula. By the late 1990s, studies indicated BPA increases breast and prostate damage, and leads to early puberty and neurobehavioral issues, yet the FDA continued to insist the product was safe for consumer use.

In 2003, the NIH recommended a full evaluation of BPA, but hired industry contractors to do the assessment, which, of course, declared BPA "safe." Meanwhile, accumulating evidence documented that BPA was leaking into baby formula at dangerously high levels, sparking multiple congressional hearings and investigations.

The determination that BPA poses a risk to humans led to restrictions in 2012 in canned infant formula and baby bottles, yet billions of pounds continue to be produced annually.

A 2008 study suggests higher BPA levels in the body are associated with increased likelihood of obesity, coronary artery disease, diabetes, asthma, liver toxicity, and immune and reproductive dysfunction. Exposure in the womb has been shown to increase the risk of anxiety and depression in children, especially boys, ten to twelve years later. A Harvard study found that college students drinking from BPA-containing sports bottles for one week increased their urinary BPA concentrations by 70 percent. A 2014 study found that even one exposure to a plastic bottle raises blood pressure within a few hours. The FDA's assurance that BPA is "safe" does not seem to match the accumulating data indicating otherwise.

Largely due to media coverage of the potential health risks from BPA, and subsequent public concern, many products now carry the label "BPA-free." This may seem assuring, but all this means is that the BPA has been replaced with yet another untested chemical, likely with similar properties and consequences.

The point of this story is simply to point out that our wisest course of action, in a world filled with untested and unregulated toxic chemicals, is not to be consumed by fear but to be aware and make simple choices that can reduce our contact. Ditch the plastic bottles and use glass or stainless steel. Avoid canned foods and foods covered in plastic or lots of packaging. Read labels. If there are a ton of unrecognizable long words, reconsider whether you really want to be a lab rat for the untested chemicals.

Cosmetic and Beauty Products

I suppose I could just say "ditto" to the advice above for plastics, but since the average American woman uses twelve personal care products daily, exposing herself to around 170 untested chemicals, and teens are using seventeen products a day, exposing themselves to even more toxins, I think it is important to comment on these toxins specifically.

You may want to start reading the labels of the products you use on your body. You may think it is "just your skin," but once products get absorbed into your skin, they travel into your bloodstream and lymphatic system. The best rule of thumb is, if you would not eat your hand lotion, makeup, deodorant, bug spray, or sunscreen, you should not be putting it on your skin either.

Not only are these products contaminated with untested chemicals, but many also contain heavy metals. When Environmental Defence tested forty-nine beauty products, including foundations, powders, mascara, and lipsticks, nearly all of them contained beryllium as well as lead and other heavy metals, including arsenic.

To find safer alternatives, go to the Environmental Working Group (EWG) Skin Deep cosmetics database (www.ewg.org/skindeep). The site also offers a user-friendly app for your phone so that you can check out products in the store before you buy them. Flooding our bodies with fewer toxins reduces stress on our bodies, allowing us to prevent disease and heal rather than remain constantly in crisis mode.

Antimicrobial Soaps and Products

Triclosan and triclocarban are broad-spectrum antimicrobial agents used, for the past twenty years, in over two thousand products, including soaps, hand lotions, household cleaners, toothpastes, deodorants, acne products, toys, pencils, scissors, and clothes, in our fear-based desire to destroy germs and microbes. Unfortunately, these so-called "protective" products—which many moms carry in their purses at all times, and schools encourage kids to use routinely—are endocrine disruptors, which bioaccumulate and break down into carcinogenic compounds that are found in lakes, rivers, and streams, as well as human blood and breast milk.

Triclosan is found in the urine of three-quarters of people tested. At even low levels, broad-spectrum antimicrobial agents have been shown to disrupt thyroid function, reproduction, and embryonic development. Neither the CDC nor the FDA has found any evidence that the use of these chemicals "improves consumer or patient health or prevents disease" or offers any advantage over nonantimicrobial soap and water.

Due to growing health concerns, the FDA banned the use of these chemicals in soaps in 2017, yet they still appear in hand sanitizers, wipes, lotions, and even some toothpastes. Since hormonal disruption can lead to all kinds of physical and emotional dysfunction, it is best to avoid these products and use good old-fashioned soap and water to wash your hands. Avoid any products labeled "antibacterial," "odor fighting," or "keeps food fresh longer," as these are all code phrases for the presence of antimicrobial agents.

A revealing NIH-funded study involving over eight hundred children found that higher levels of triclosan in the urine directly correlated with food and environmental allergy risk, especially for boys. This may explain why it has become "normal" to have a separate lunch table at school for those with allergies. These chemicals are disrupting the body's microbial balance, dysregulating the immune system, and leading to chronic allergies and illness.

Shortcuts in the forms of pills, powders, and sanitizers lead to unintended consequences, especially when poorly researched and regulated. Just like with emotions and body sensations, that which we fear and avoid gains power. In our attempts to protect our children and ourselves from feared microbes, we have become further disconnected from the natural world in which we coevolved. Just as we need our emotions and body sensations to guide us, we need exposure to bacteria and viruses for our immune systems to thrive.

Pesticides

We talked earlier about the therapeutic value of grounding your feet and body in the earth. Yet, one hundred million pounds of herbicides, fungicides, and insecticides are sprayed by homeowners annually in the name of maintaining a perfectly manicured yet entirely unnatural lawn. According to Congress, 90 percent of these pesticides lack health and safety testing, yet they continue to be sprayed on parks, playgrounds, school grounds, and our food, all with the assumption they are safe.

These chemicals get tracked into our homes with shoes, furry paws, and the air we breathe. In a CDC study, 100 percent of participants tested positive for the presence of pesticides in their blood. Children's levels are ten times higher than those of the original application, which may explain why children growing up in or near homes with pesticide-treated lawns have a significantly increased risk of leukemia, brain tumors, asthma, and behavioral issues. For adults, exposure to these chemicals has been shown to increase the risk for brain, prostate, kidney, breast, and pancreatic cancers, as well as non-Hodgkin's lymphoma. It seems like an unnecessarily scary risk for the sake of the perfect yard.

If you want to see how poorly these chemicals are being regulated today, check out the EPA's 2017 annual cancer report to find a long list of chemicals used in pesticides. As you scan through the list, the chemicals are categorized as "not classifiable," "data inadequate for assessment," "suggestive evidence for carcinogenicity," "possible carcinogen," "likely to be carcinogenic," and, the only slightly more reassuring "not likely to be carcinogenic." Your lawn care service may assure you that their products are safe, but it is not based on research and data, only hopeful assumptions and marketing propaganda—including from agencies who are supposed to be protecting us and the environment.

My husband and I were recently sent letters by our homeowners association requesting that we treat our yard in the name of maintaining the "health, safety, and general welfare" of the residents in the neighborhood. I replied that we do use a fertilizer, an organic one, which keeps our yard, kids, and pets healthy. Yes, we have more dandelions and clover than our neighbors, yet I would argue that the increased risks for cancer, birth defects, reproductive issues, liver and kidney damage, and disruption of the endocrine system outweigh the need for a picture-perfect weedless yard. Maybe it is time to establish a new "ideal" yard with a rich microbiome that nourishes ourselves, our children, our pets, and the wildlife around us.

The safety of Monsanto's pesticides sprayed on our food is another area of controversy. Despite a recent court decision ordering Monsanto to pay $289 million to Dewayne Johnson, a school groundskeeper, who attributed his non-Hodgkin's lymphoma to the toxic effects of the Roundup he sprayed on school grounds, and other evidence suggesting increased risks of cancer, gluten intolerance, irritable bowel disease, celiac disease, diabetes, thyroid disease, and dementia, most of our food supply is being sprayed with these potential toxins.

In 2015, the World Health Organization classified the active ingredient in the herbicide—glyphosate—as a probable carcinogen. Residue from this chemical is found in our food, soil, air, and water. EWG recently examined twenty-eight cereal and breakfast products. All but two had levels of glyphosate higher than recommended for safety. Research has shown that this chemical disrupts the gut microbiome and increases anxiety and depression-like behaviors in mice.

Human studies of pesticide sprayers, farmers, and their spouses found an 80 percent increased risk of depression and suicidality. What kind of doses lead to these significantly increased risks remains unclear, but once again, do we really want to wait a few more decades to find out?

Our safest play for now is to avoid these chemicals when we can, both in our yards and our food. A 2018 study in *JAMA* confirmed the benefit of eating organic foods free of these toxins. Those who primarily eat organic foods have a reduced risk for cancers.

Unfortunately, this can get costly. Check out the EWG's list of the foods with the highest levels of pesticides on them, the "Dirty Dozen," and the foods with the least pesticides, the "Clean Fifteen," to determine how best to spend money on organic produce. The "Dirty Dozen" list currently includes strawberries, spinach, nectarines, apples, grapes, peaches, cherries, pears, tomatoes, celery, potatoes, and bell peppers. To give you a sense of the range of pesticides on various produce, 99 percent of conventional strawberries sampled tested positive for at least one pesticide, and some had over twenty different pesticides.

On the safer side, fewer than 1 percent of the nonorganic avocados tested positive for pesticides. The 2018 "Clean Fifteen" list of produce that has low levels of pesticides includes avocados, sweet corn, pineapples, cabbage, onions, frozen sweet peas, papayas, asparagus, mangoes, eggplant, honeydew, kiwi, cantaloupe, cauliflower, and broccoli. These resources can help you limit your exposure to untested toxins to reduce the total burden of these unavoidable chemicals on our bodies.

Medications as Toxins

These days, for American adults, taking prescription medications is as common as plastic water bottles, chemically treated lawns, and antibacterial hand sanitizers. According to a 2018 survey published in *JAMA,* more than a third of adults in the United States are taking at least one of two hundred prescription medications that increase their risk of depression or suicide. Those on three or more of these depression-inducing medications triple their risk of a depressive episode. Some of these commonly prescribed drugs include statins, proton-pump inhibitors, beta-blockers, hormonal contraceptives, and antibiotics.

Statins

Half of Americans over the age of sixty-five are prescribed statins, and probably far more have been encouraged to take them and refused. Every time my father goes to see his primary-care physician, he is reflexively prescribed one, even though he has no history of cardiovascular disease. Every time he follows his doctor's orders and takes the pill, his cognition suffers, and I try to convince him to stop.

I cannot begin to count the number of patients I have seen who suffer from memory issues and muscle weakness that magically clear, or at least improve, after stopping this class of medication. Accumulated data suggests that statins reduce the chance of a heart attack from 2 percent to 1 percent, which is indeed a 50 percent decreased risk, which is why your physician likely recommends it. Put another way, if 100 patients are treated with a statin, one patient will have one less heart attack in a given year. This might be fine if the medication is safe, yet there are over three hundred documented side effects of statins. Twenty percent of those taking it discontinue the medication due to intolerable side effects. Many more continue the medication oblivious to the potential harm, which includes increased risk of muscle weakness, cognitive impairment, hormonal disruption, heart disease, depression, and diabetes. In fact, the risk for diabetes increases up to 46 percent, especially in postmenopausal women.

Although the reasons for all these risks remain unclear, a big piece of the puzzle is simple: we need cholesterol. As discussed in chapter 11, cholesterol is needed for the structure and integrity of all cell membranes and the coatings around neurons. Our brain is 60 percent fat and requires cholesterol to function efficiently. Low levels of cholesterol are associated with depression, violence, and suicide. The chance of dying by suicide or violence is double for those on statins as compared to those not on them.

Ironically, research also suggests that as we age and start these medications, lower cholesterol levels are associated with increased mortality. It seems, once again, that our quest for "health"—as in ever-lower cholesterol levels—may cause more harm than good.

It may take another decade before prescribing patterns reflect the evidence. Meanwhile, I am not suggesting you stop your medication, but I do strongly recommend consulting with your physician to see if statins really are the best choice for you. Other options include exercise, relaxation, sleep, and avoiding processed, fatty foods. These steps will not only improve your cardiovascular health but also your mood, overall health, and well-being.

Proton-Pump Inhibitors

Proton-pump inhibitors (PPIs) are one of the top-ten most widely used medications in the world. They are deemed so safe that you can run to your local pharmacy and pick one up over the counter for your heartburn after eating too much at Thanksgiving dinner. For infrequent use, PPIs are probably safe, but chronic use can lead to a host of other problems. Even the FDA advises that PPIs should only be used for four to eight weeks, yet millions of Americans take these for years or decades.

Long-term use inhibits absorption of critical vitamins and nutrients, including calcium, iron, magnesium, and vitamin B_{12}, and leads to increased risk of hip fractures, gastrointestinal infections, kidney disease, pneumonia, stroke, depression, and death. Studies examining stool samples of those taking PPIs have discovered a significant disruption of the microbiome, with decreases in beneficial bacteria and diversity, and increases of potentially pathogenic species.

A healthy whole-food diet and good stress management are the two most important strategies to avoid the need for PPIs. Eating smaller meals more mindfully several hours before bedtime as well as avoiding spicy or fatty foods will help. After eating, relax and have a cup of chamomile or ginger tea with honey. Although I could not find any research to back me up on this one, chamomile is where I turn for digestive discomfort; it has been used, as has ginger, for thousands of years for digestive issues.

Hormonal Contraception

The discovery of the modern-day birth control pill was lauded as one of the "Seven Wonders of the Modern World" by the *Economist* in 1994, and listed as an "essential medicine" by the World Health Organization. Today, over one hundred million women worldwide use "the pill" as a means to assert some control over their own bodies and reproduction. Yet research on the pill's potential side effects has been contested since its first trials on psychotic inpatients and later on Puerto Ricans in the 1950s.

Women who expressed concerns at that time about side effects such as nausea, headaches, breast tenderness, and mood swings were dismissed as mere hypochondriacs—a historically familiar refrain when women speak up and complain. Since then, the pill has been modified, and various formulations approved, yet one of the most common reasons for discontinuation remains depression and mood liability.

In 2016, a nationwide prospective study was published in *JAMA Psychiatry* that followed over one million girls and women ages fifteen to thirty-four over a period of fourteen years. They found that the use of all hormonal contraception options was associated with a 20 to 30 percent increased risk for depression. Fifteen- to nineteen-year-old girls showed the greatest risk, especially during the first year of use. For this already high-risk group, the use of combined oral contraceptives, with estrogen and progestin, increased the risk of depression by 80 percent compared to the risk for those not on the medication. Those using progestin-only pills doubled their risk of depression, while those on the patch or vaginal ring had triple the risk compared to nonusers.

A follow-up to this study, published in the *American Journal of Psychiatry*, used the same extensive Danish database to assess the risk of suicide attempts in users of hormonal contraception compared to nonusers. Shockingly, the users of hormonal contraception showed double the risk of a suicide attempt and triple the risk of a completed suicide. This risk rose rapidly within the first month after starting contraception and remained doubled for the first year. After that, the risk remained about 30 percent higher for users than for nonusers.

In this study, all of the oral products showed the same increased risk. The risk of the patch, however, was more than tripled, and the users of the depot injection showed a 6.5-fold increased risk. Once again, those at highest risk were the adolescents. It is unclear whether aging and time decreases the risk, or if those most at risk have already discontinued use due to significant mood issues.

So, what is one to do with this information? Like most things in life, we do not have a tidy, one-size-fits-all answer. What the data from these studies suggests to me is not that we should panic and never prescribe or use hormonal contraception again. Pregnancy obviously carries even more risks, especially unplanned ones. But it is critical for physicians and patients to take the time to have a conversation and carefully assess the individual risk factors against potential benefits.

I have seen way too many teenagers in my office—and worse, adult women who have been on antidepressants since they started birth control decades ago—who complain of depression after starting the pill to manage acne, irregular bleeding, or painful periods. From my perspective, the potential benefits of prescribing a pill to alleviate these symptoms to a non–sexually active adolescent are difficult to rationalize against the possible risk of depression or suicide. There are many other options for those issues, including dietary changes, exercise, supplements, and stress management, that will help with minimal to no risk.

For sexually active adolescents and adults, the calculations become more difficult, and each woman's particular life circumstances must be evaluated. It would be helpful to know if your mother or other female relatives had issues with the pill, since research shows that women with certain genetic predispositions are at increased risk. Another group at higher risk of side effects is those with a history of childhood trauma. In fact, research published in *Nature* suggests that many of the long-term physiological consequences of taking the pill resemble chronic stress, which at least partially explains the increased risk for depression.

Obviously, health risks like smoking and obesity must be considered, as these factors combined with the pill further increase the risks for blood clots, strokes, and cervical and breast cancer. These risks must be weighed against the possible reduction in risks for ovarian and endometrial cancer among pill users.

If you choose to go the route of hormonal contraception, the data suggests oral forms appear to be significantly safer, with fewer side effects than the patch or injection. Most importantly, during the first few months on the pill, be mindful of any mood changes. If your mood darkens, do not let your doctor tell you it is "all in your head," or "Let's just try another brand," or add an antidepressant. Recognize that it is likely the medication, and other nonhormonal options like condoms, cervical caps, or the diaphragm may be better alternatives for you.

Antibiotics

Although Alexander Fleming's discovery of penicillin in 1928 has saved countless lives, the careless overprescribing of antibiotics is causing harm that we are only beginning to comprehend. In 2015, there were 269 million antibiotics prescribed. The CDC estimates that at least 47 million of these were for viral colds, sore throats, and bronchitis that would not respond to the medications, and thus were completely unwarranted.

The average American child receives seventeen prescriptions for antibiotics by her eighteenth birthday, more often to relieve concerned parents than to cure the kids. Exposure to unnecessary antibiotics increases the resistance of the bacteria that the medicines are attempting to destroy, which is dangerous for all of us. Taking antibiotics strengthens the pathological microbes, while simultaneously destroying the beneficial ones needed to maintain our immunity against future invaders, which is harmful to individuals.

Not only does overuse of these medications place us all at risk of bacterial resistance, but even a single treatment of antibiotics is associated with an increased risk of depression and anxiety, with the risk increasing with recurrent exposures. Hundreds of reports document their potential neurotoxicity, ranging from milder irritability, insomnia, and depression to more severe mania and psychosis. This makes sense given what we have already learned about the link between the gut and the brain, and the importance of a balanced gut microbiome to physical and emotional health.

Studies have shown that "even short antibiotic exposures disrupt the gut microbiome for up to a year or more," decreasing the flora by about a third, and significantly reducing the diversity and richness of the microbiome. When you consider this possibility, maybe prevention and natural antimicrobials are a better bet for most ailments.

Boost your immune system with curcumin, vitamin D_3, a multivitamin, and some elderberry, especially in the winter, along with plenty of sleep, exercise, and whole foods. For an extra boost, add garlic to your food. Your breath may stink, but garlic has natural antibacterial, antifungal, and antiviral properties.

How about some echinacea tea with honey? Both have been used for hundreds of years throughout the world for their taste and antimicrobial benefits. Manuka honey has even been shown to be effective for wounds infected with methicillin-resistant *Staphylococcus aureus* (MRSA). The world would be safer for all of us if we first turned to the remedies of our ancestors, saving antibiotics for times when they're truly needed.

WELLNESS RX: REDUCING TOXIN EXPOSURES

1. Eat organic when possible, especially when choosing produce in the "Dirty Dozen."

2. Avoid plastic. It is bad for you and the environment. Choose glass, ceramic, or stainless steel.

3. Avoid antibacterial products for your body or your house. Use plain soap and water.

4. Avoid chemical air fresheners. Use a diffuser with organic essential oils. Try pine oil and add the beneficial aroma of the forest to your home or office.

5. Check EWG's Skin Deep cosmetics database (www.cosmeticsdatabase.com) before buying products for your skin. If you would not eat it, do not put it on your skin.

6. Make your own cleaning products. All you need is two cups of vinegar, two cups of water, and ten to twenty drops of organic orange or lemon essential oils for natural fragrance for a basic cleaner. Check out Women's Voices for the Earth (https://tinyurl.com/y62z9zrl) for other suggestions. If you prefer to buy cleaning products, check the EWG website (www.ewg.org/guides/cleaners) for recommendations.

7. Avoid pesticides, especially if you have kids or pets.

8. Use iron or stainless-steel pans for cooking instead of non-stick cookware, which is coated with untested chemicals that will seep into your food.

9. Exercise to release toxins.

10. Sleep so that toxins in your brain can be washed away.

11. Check with an integrative physician or provider to see if you really need all the medications you may be on, or if there are safer alternatives.

12. Reduce stress, using all the skills you have already learned.

This list may seem overwhelming. Honestly, it overwhelms me as I consider how many toxins are still lurking in my drawers and cabinets. Remember, it is a process. Take it in baby steps, and transition slowly. As old products run out, seek new ones on the EWG website. Approach the detox of your environment with curiosity and a sense of exploration as you seek new, safer products. Do not add this to a long list of fears, but rather make it an opportunity to cleanse your life and your home.

Reconnecting with Our Environment

Clearly, it is time to heed the warnings of Rachel Carson and the Lorax. Just as Mohini the tiger confined herself within the imaginary boundaries of her enclosure at the National Zoo, we trap ourselves not only within the stories in our heads but also within the confines of our offices, houses, and cars. We have lost connection with the beauty of the world around us, losing our wildness and aliveness. Being disconnected from the natural world, we fail to see the harm we bestow within us, and around us, with the toxins we add to our inner and outer environments.

This week, set aside time to begin to remove some of the toxins in your home and yard. Regardless of the weather, take time to reconnect with the natural world around you. Find a new park or return to one of your favorite spots. Why not seek guidance from the physicians in the Shetlands, and "turn o'er a rock and see what's there," "follow a bumblebee," "make a meal of dandelions" from your pesticide-free yard, or, if it is cold, "feel the exhilaration of wind and rain or snow on your face"?

Imagine if your physician offered you a prescription for a daily dose of nature, instead of one that would add toxins and side effects. If you seek "spontaneous euphoria, taking yourself less seriously, and being in a good mood for no apparent reason," connect with nature today, and every day. Kick off your shoes, stand in the grass, and breathe in the smells, sounds, and feel of the world outside your home, office, and car doors. Nature is the free and ultimate antidepressant.

In the words of my favorite poet, Mary Oliver, "The world offers itself to your imagination, calls to you like the wild geese, harsh and exciting—over and over announcing your place in the family of things." Listen to the call.

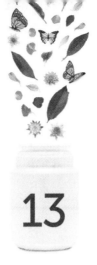

Heart, Energy, and Soul as Conductors and Synthesizers

People often ask me what the most effective technique is for transforming their life. It is a little embarrassing that after years and years of research and experimentation, I have to say that the best answer is—just to be a little kinder.

—ALDOUS HUXLEY

Without thinking, point to yourself. It may seem silly, but just take a second and point to You. Pause. Notice where you pointed. If you are like most people, you pointed not at your head, but toward your heart. Throughout history, people and religions have recognized the heart as the core of our being, the source of our intuition, wisdom, and spirit. Only in fairly recent history in the Western world has the logical, rational, thinking mind taken center stage.

So far in this book, we have focused on the roles of the breath, mind, body, and environment for emotional and physical healing and well-being. Now we turn to the inseparable heart, energy, and soul.

In Carl Jung's book *Memories, Dreams, Reflections,* he describes a visit to the pueblos of Taos, New Mexico, where he talked with the Hopi chief Mountain

Lake. As they sat on a rooftop watching the sun rise, the chief described his confusion about and distrust of Caucasians. "The whites always want something; they are always uneasy and restless. We do not know what they want. We do not understand them. We think they are mad."

Jung asked why he thought this. The chief replied, "They say they think with their heads." Jung was puzzled and asked, "Where else would one think?" Mountain Lake pointed to his heart and answered, "We think here."

After a moment of reflection, Jung realized the Native chief "had struck our vulnerable spot, unveiled a truth to which we are blind." As he looked over the "rolling plateau of Taos," he realized the limitations of the thinking mind. "Knowledge does not enrich us; it removes us more and more from the mythic world in which we were at home by right of birth."

This is not to say we should throw out books, stop taking classes, and ignore the vast wealth of information we store in the mind; instead, to heal and access our wholeness, we must relearn how to listen to the intelligence of the heart.

In school, we learn about the stunning capacity of the heart to beat a hundred thousand times a day, and distribute two thousand gallons of blood daily through sixty thousand miles of blood vessels, providing life-sustaining nourishment to every cell in the body and carrying away its waste. This is awe-inspiring, but we never learn about the heart's even more fantastic role as conductor and synthesizer of our body's symphony, which it broadcasts to the world around us.

The heart's electromagnetic field is five thousand times more powerful than the brain. Its electrical energy can be measured up to several feet away from the body. As we interact with others, and the environment around us, the heart senses information and conveys it to the brain and body via forty thousand sensory neurons, hormones, pulse waves, electrical and electromagnetic fields, and the rhythm of its beats. Despite our reverence for the brain, far more information moves from the heart to the head than the other way around. Although the brain cannot function without a pumping heart, the heart can function independent of the brain. In fact, if you removed the heart from the body, the heart would continue to pump at its own intrinsic rhythm established by internal pacemaker cells for up to an hour.

Just like poetry, art, and music, the heart speaks the language of emotions, translating its energetic messages to the body via changing rhythms. The heart both responds to our emotions and has the capacity to transform them. It is the conductor of our unique emotional symphony. When we are trapped in fear or frustration, the heart becomes so focused on maintaining its own beat that it loses control of the orchestra. Readings of HRV form jagged and chaotic, angry, sharp-toothed waves spreading a message of alarm and disharmony.

In contrast, shifting our focus to gratitude, acceptance, and compassion, the heart confidently returns to the conductor podium to coordinate the players into a synchronized, harmonious melody. This shifts the HRV into a powerful, smooth wave and rhythm that sends a message of safety throughout the body, aligning the systems to the heart's unified beat.

Because of the heart's powerful electromagnetic energy, once in a state of coherence, the heart pulls respiration, blood pressure, brain waves, hormones, digestion, and immunity into a synchronized harmony of balance and order. In this state, we not only feel calmer and think more clearly, but our body has time and space to stop focusing on putting out the real, and imagined, small fires of daily life. Instead, our body can focus on healing and restoring balance.

HRV provides a window through which we can assess the state of our heart and emotional resilience. As we discussed in chapter 7, HRV measures the beat-to-beat variation between heartbeats. A healthy heart, like a flexible body, is responsive and adaptable to change. Research has shown that increased rigidity and loss of flexibility is a marker of depression, anxiety, PTSD, and other chronic diseases—all states associated with a decreased ability to adapt to stressors and change. More severe symptoms are associated with worsening HRV. Some research suggests that antidepressants may actually decrease HRV further, potentiating the imbalance of the autonomic nervous system that lies at the core of the problem.

The good news is that the heart, like the brain, is incredibly malleable. By learning how to create a state of coherence within our own hearts, we can foster greater emotional stability and resilience, regardless of age and life circumstances. This helps balance the autonomic nervous system. Rather than perpetually fueling an overactive sympathetic system, we can amp up the parasympathetic system, creating a calmer and more stable brain and body.

Many tools you have already learned increase our HRV, including deep breathing, meditation, yoga, exercise, sleep, and connecting with nature. Even omega-3 fish oil and theanine have been shown to increase HRV. Let's add one more powerful technique, a heart-centered meditation, to your heart coherence tool box. This increases our capacity for compassion, offering us a way to connect more deeply with ourselves and others.

WELLNESS RX: HEART-CENTERED MEDITATION

Begin by sitting tall and taking a few deep breaths into the belly. Breathing in, fill the body with fresh oxygen and energy. Breathing out, release and let go.

Bring your focus to the area around your heart. Imagine breathing in and out of the heart center. Feel the sensations around the heart with each inhalation and exhalation. Notice any tightness or restriction, and breathe into it. You may begin to notice the rhythm of your heartbeat.

Now, tune into a feeling of gratitude, appreciation, or love. To generate these feelings, you may bring to mind something or someone for whom you feel appreciation or love. It could be the memory of a beautiful sunset; the love for a pet or child; the sound of the waves on a beach—anything that stirs warm feelings of benevolence. The key is to tune in with the feelings in the heart center, not thoughts about the memories or scenes. If that is happening, recognize that you are lost in thoughts and return to the feelings themselves, all while continuing to breathe in and out of the heart.

Imagine sending this heart energy first toward someone you love, then someone you struggle to understand. Next, send that same love and compassion to yourself. Finally, send it out to all beings everywhere. Notice how this feels in your body, and take a moment to journal about your experience.

Thank-you to HeartMath for this simple but effective technique.

For many people, especially those with depression, the idea of offering oneself kindness may be met with a critical inner voice and resistance. That is perfectly OK. The idea is not to judge or avoid that inner critic, but to simply acknowledge that voice, that hurt part of yourself, with kindness, compassion, and breath. You may try gently placing your hand over your heart to offer yourself touch and warmth. While doing this, like all forms of meditation, painful emotions may be stirred. Do not try to use the meditation to push these away, but to offer the same compassion and kindness toward yourself that you would offer to a loved one.

Self-compassion is a concept foreign to many of us raised in a culture that reveres willpower, where we are taught to strive harder, do better, and be better. We are taught to distrust forgiveness of our flaws and mistakes, with the mistaken belief we may "slack off" and repeat them. Instead of offering acceptance and kindness, we offer judgment and condemnation. Instead of recognizing failure as an inevitable part of growth and learning in this human experience, we label it a personal flaw.

In many ways, lack of self-compassion is at the very heart of depression. So many describe themselves as "broken," "nonfunctioning," "not normal," "incapable," "weak"—basically "less than" in so many ways. These are not words we would use to describe our friends, yet they are words we toss around mercilessly to describe ourselves. Being stamped with a pathological label and handed a prescription only reinforces the low perception of one's abilities, resilience, and possibility for healing.

Our bodies are starving for self-compassion. Fortunately, compassion for ourselves and others is a skill we can practice and learn. One study found that just seven minutes devoted to the practice of "loving-kindness" meditation can improve mood, self-acceptance, and a sense of social connection. Feeling more deeply connected to others decreases the risk of depression and improves overall health. It also increases altruism, trust, and cooperation, which all lead to increased feelings of connection. It creates a path out of the downward spiral of sadness and despair.

Another study found that after eight hours of training, the brain scans of meditation "novices" resemble the brain patterns of experienced meditators. The data suggests that compassion changes the brain more quickly than other forms of meditation. In the words of Daniel Goleman and Richard Davidson in their book, *Altered Traits,* "the brain seems primed for love."

Perhaps this should not be surprising. According to Karen Armstrong, who has spent her life studying and writing about religion, despite different rituals, beliefs, and teachings, the common thread in all religions is the practice of compassion, not just in words, but in action.

Every religion teaches some variation of the Golden Rule, written in the Christian Bible as "Do unto others as you would have them do to you." In the Hindi Hitopadesa, dating to 3200 BCE, it is declared: "One should always treat others as they themselves wish to be treated." The Buddhist Udanavarga, around 560 BCE, states, "Hurt not others with what pains yourself." Taoism, Jainism, Islam, and Judaism all point us in this same direction, suggesting that compassion is the way out of our misery, out of our overidentification with ourselves and our own suffering. It offers a template for healing ourselves, our spirits, each other, and our communities. It offers us a pathway out of fear and disconnection—the sources of much of our pain.

Practicing this skill increases our capacity to navigate the daily stressors of life so that we are less easily hijacked by events around us. Tuning in regularly with the heart helps us to recognize the different vocabularies of the heart and the brain so we are less likely to get duped by the urgency of the thoughts in our heads. While the brain speaks insistently, incessantly, and often judgmentally, the heart's voice feels more like a whisper and deep knowing. The brain often sounds like a whiny two-year-old who sees herself as the center of the universe, while the heart sounds like the wise, intuitive grandmother who wraps you in her arms without questions or advice, just unconditional love and support. As we let go of the brain's thoughts and checklists, blames and judgments, we arrive at a quiet intuitive place of knowing.

Practicing compassion also increases our capacity to empathize with the suffering of others. One study found that just six hours of at-home online training in compassion meditation activated the empathy circuits in the brain. Empathy enables us to sense the feelings of others. It is all too easy to turn away from the pain of others to avoid our own discomfort. Neurobiology teaches us that the witnessing of the suffering of another activates the same circuits in ourselves activated in the other. When your amygdala fires, so does mine. This may sound like an unnecessary drain on our resources—and it is—unless we add compassion to the mix.

Compassion activates circuits associated with concern and love. While empathy viscerally connects us with the suffering of others, compassion allows us to feel another's suffering and induces us to act on their behalf. Compassion is the antidote to the unavoidable empathic response triggered when we watch the nightly news or witness the suffering of others. Compassion is the remedy for our stressed-out, burned-out, fear-based lives.

Counterintuitively, despite leaning in and feeling more pain, studies find helping others activates the pleasure center of the brain, and we feel happier. We are wired to follow the Golden Rule and help others as we would want to be helped. The script for happiness has been buried inside religious teachings and texts for centuries. Unfortunately, the fear part of the brain keeps attempting to divide us into different groups. If you believe this, you are one of us, and therefore right; if you believe something else, you are one of them, and therefore wrong.

Tuning into empathy and compassion, and sensing the suffering of others, grants us a wider perspective of our own suffering. It connects us with others by reminding us we are not alone. So many of my patients come up with endless reasons to wait before volunteering or reaching out to help others. They insist they must wait until they are "fixed," "healed," or "feeling better," yet they fail to recognize that it is the act of helping others that gets us out of our own way so that we can heal.

Depression creates myopic blinders that draw us inward, so we only see our own pain and suffering. We fail to see or we disconnect from the suffering of others, perhaps feeling that it is too much pain to bear. Yet as we connect with the pain of others, we recognize we are not alone and that we can help each other. Reaching out to others helps the other and yourself at the same time. We heal each other. This is the power of compassion.

Another desirable individual and societal outcome of the practice of compassion is the decrease in implicit biases. These are our unconscious prejudices that influence our perceptions of others without our conscious awareness. A 2013 study at Yale measured implicit biases of students before and after six weeks of practicing loving-kindness meditation. These students were compared with a group taught about meditation in a similar setting, but without learning the practice. The group that practiced the compassion meditation for twenty minutes daily at home, and participated in a one-hour class weekly, showed reductions in unconscious prejudices against stigmatized groups.

Imagine if we all began learning this skill at a young age in schools, churches, synagogues, and mosques. What if this was required training and encouraged practice for police forces, first responders, physicians, politicians, and, dare I say, presidents? What if instead of required professional ethics classes, which have little evidence-based value, we all sat and practiced compassion meditation together? We could create a more loving, caring world for all of us. Based on existing research, I would be willing to bet rates of depression and other chronic diseases would plummet, as would violence and fear.

Don't just imagine the possibilities wistfully; begin your own practice. Set aside seven minutes of your time. You will strengthen the muscles of compassion in yourself and others. If your brain argues that you do not have the time, or that you won't make much of a difference, check in with the wisdom of your heart.

Cultivating Gratitude

While appreciation powers the synchronicity of the heart, many of us may find difficulty harnessing these feelings, especially during periods of sadness or despair. The practice of gratitude can increase our ability to connect with appreciation. One of the simplest ways to add gratitude to your life is to create a gratitude journal.

WELLNESS RX: GRATITUDE JOURNAL

The idea here is simple and will take only a few minutes nightly. Keep a special journal by your bed reserved for listing at least three things for which you are grateful. This gives you a chance to focus for a few moments on your day, and recall small moments of grace, beauty, and synchronicity, or things that went smoothly.

This shifts you out of the mind's natural tendency to replay over and over all that is wrong.

Try to look for unique moments of gratefulness in each and every day. These can be small or large: the words of a favorite song that popped in your head just when you needed it; the smile from the cashier at the grocery store; a hug from a loved one; a cuddle with your dog or cat; the warmth of the sun; finishing an amazing book; sipping a cup of warm tea while watching the sunset; a funny moment on a TV show; the first buds of spring; a letter from an old friend.... The list of possibilities is endless, even if you do not leave the house today.

In the words of Ralph Waldo Emerson, "What we seek we shall find." If we seek moments of beauty, grace, and kindness each day, we will undoubtedly find it. A gratitude journal can capture these moments, and at least for a few minutes, shift our focus toward appreciation. It can also serve as an anchor when we are lost in despairing thoughts and feelings, a resource we can pull from to generate memories to focus on while breathing in and out of the heart.

I know this is not always easy. The pull of negativity and wallowing in our own pain can be alluring, like the call of the Sirens luring sailors to shipwreck with their enchanting voices. We know it will not end well if we go there, but the pull feels so overwhelmingly powerful, it seems we cannot resist. Often, patients feel indignant at the suggestion that turning away from the downward spiral is a choice. To be clear, this is not to deny one's sadness or suffering. These feelings need to be acknowledged with tenderness. But getting stuck in the story line about everything that has gone wrong, and how it is impossible to fix, keeps us stranded there unnecessarily.

It's like getting a boot stuck in the mud. Jerk out too quickly and you will likely pull your foot out minus a boot. But staying too long just sinks you and the boot deeper in the mud. Noticing you are stuck, and then slowly easing out, keeps the boot on your foot and freed from the muck.

In the *Odyssey,* the sailors plugged their ears to avoid hearing the Sirens' call, and Odysseus had his men tie him to the ship's mast. In this same way, a daily practice of gratitude, as well as breathing, meditation, and the other skills you have learned, can keep you grounded, so you are less likely to be stuck in the mud or shipwrecked.

Research comparing those keeping gratitude journals to those just writing about the hassles of daily life shows that gratitude journaling decreases physical complaints and depressive symptoms while increasing optimism, mood, gratefulness, and altruism. These improvements are not only subjectively experienced by the participants but validated by observable changes in the brain, with increases in neural activity in areas associated with gratefulness and altruism. Altruism, or selflessly acting on behalf of others, has been shown to reduce the likelihood of depression by half and lead to greater health, decrease inflammation, and improve immunity.

Remedy for Loneliness

Clearly, building the muscles of gratitude and compassion benefits all of us. Although most of us cognitively recognize the importance of kindness and compassion toward ourselves and others, this does not always translate into action in our busy lives. Embodying these qualities is a lifelong practice, and one at which we will fail many times. This is not to be judged negatively. Rather, it offers us yet another opportunity to practice self-compassion and forgiveness for our mistakes and, like the breath, begin again.

An intriguing study was conducted at the Yale Divinity School. A group of students were told they were to be evaluated on a presentation. Half the students were assigned to speak on future job opportunities for seminary students, while the other half were asked to speak on the parable of the Good Samaritan. In that story, a man traveling from Jerusalem to Jericho was beaten by robbers and left for dead at the side of the road. A priest and another religious man of the church passed by this man without stopping to help. Only a good Samaritan paused to bind the man's wounds and take him to an inn for further care.

After the students were assigned their brief presentations, they were asked, in various degrees of haste, to go one by one to another building to give their presentations. All passed by an actor, hunched over in pain, moaning and coughing. The question was who would stop to help? It turned out that whether a student stopped or not depended not on their religiosity or on the presentation they were about to give, but on their sense of hurry and pressure to be on time. Sixty-three percent of those with more time stopped to help, while only 45 percent of those feeling more hurried, and a scant 10 percent of those urgently rushed, stopped, even if they were on their way to speak about the Good Samaritan.

When we become overly busy and rushed, and myopically focused on ourselves and our own needs, we fail to notice those around us. I once was rushing out of a bookstore with two sleepy, crabby kids, desperately trying to get them to the car before they exploded. A kind tall man held the door for us. I thanked him but never looked up. Only after getting to the car did my husband, who had been trailing behind after paying for some books, inform me that the man holding the door had been a former preceptor at the hospital at which I had trained. I had seen only a shirt. Of course, when you walk through life at five feet tall, that is often what you see unless you intentionally take time to scan upward. But the point is that in our busy lives, we have habitually become more disconnected and less likely to pause and notice others, let alone help those in need.

According to former Surgeon General Vivek Murthy, this growing disconnection has led to epidemic levels of loneliness. Nearly half of Americans report feeling lonely as we go about our lives glued to our computers and phones, working more and socializing less. Yet research has shown that loneliness is more detrimental to our health than obesity and smoking. It amps up cortisol levels and increases the risk for depression, anxiety, dementia, heart disease, and stroke.

A fascinating study involving Stanford undergraduate students offers insight into how profoundly a sense of loneliness impacts our emotional well-being. Twenty-two undergraduate students were divided into two groups, both of whom were hypnotized. One group, while under hypnosis, recalled an experience where they felt isolated and lonely, while the other recalled a period in which they felt connected and had a sense of belonging. Both groups filled out depression, anxiety, self-esteem, and loneliness scales before and after the hypnosis.

The moods and self-esteem of those who recalled feelings of isolation plummeted, while those who recalled moments of connection revealed improved moods and self-esteem with lower fear and anxiety. This was just one session. Imagine replaying scenes of disconnection and loneliness over and over in our minds day after day, week after week. How would this not radically increase the risk of depression?

To combat the growing epidemic of loneliness, the British and Canadian governments are advocating the "social prescribing" of hobbies, sports, and art groups. Instead of pills, physicians in Great Britain are being encouraged to offer sources of connection through prescriptions of dance, cooking, improvisational comedy, singing and art classes, and volunteering opportunities, while doctors in Canada are prescribing free visits to art museums. These are not frivolous suggestions but preventive strategies that not only connect people socially but also have been validated by research to improve emotional and physical health.

One trip to a museum has been shown to increase serotonin levels and decrease cortisol as much as exercise. A study including fifty thousand participants in Norway found that participation in cultural activities is associated with better health and less anxiety and depression for adults and adolescents. Music has been used as medicine throughout human history. Modern technology proves that music causes the brain to release dopamine, inducing pleasure while calming the nervous system and reducing stress and anxiety. Group drumming has been shown to improve the immune system. Joy and creativity feed the Wolf of Hope, calming sympathetic, fear-based responses and activating the restorative parasympathetic response.

What have you done recently that brings you joy? Our tendency when we feel down is to avoid doing the very things that make us feel good and can pull us out of the downward spiral of isolation and avoidance.

WELLNESS RX: TAKE AN INVENTORY OF YOUR DAY

For this exercise, grab your journal and a pen. Divide a page into two columns. On the left side make a list of everything you do on a typical day. Wake up, brush teeth, take a shower, eat breakfast, and so on. After completing your list, in the second column note after each entry whether that activity replenishes or depletes your energy. Next to those activities that energize you, add a plus mark. After those that fatigue you, add a minus mark. If an activity sometimes does one and sometimes does another, you can put plus and minus there, but consider first whether it predominantly adds or subtracts energy and mark accordingly.

When you have completed this, scan over your second column and see what you notice. Are there more negatives or more positives? I am going to guess that if you are feeling depressed or have a history of depression, there is likely a predominance of negative energy-depleting activities. The point here, as always, is not to judge, but simply to notice the pattern of your days.

Now, consider if there are any ways to balance your energy ledger. Are there negatives that could be eliminated? If not, is there another way of looking at or going about the activity so that it is less draining and more enjoyable? Might there be ways to add more fun, nourishing activities to your day, even if for only a few minutes? Reflect on these possibilities in your journal.

Thanks to MBCT training for this useful exercise.

I used to dread cleaning dishes. Yet I found that if I slowed down and stepped out of the story line about how I have so much to do and so little time (that is my brain's number-one favorite story line that inevitably creates unnecessary tension), I can enjoy the feel of the water on my hands as I clean the dishes and place them in the dishwasher. Just about any task, if approached mindfully, instead of from a place of "not another f— plate," can become a relaxing and calming experience.

Are there ways to add more moments of replenishment and joy to your day? Your first thought may be, "I don't have any more time." Fine, but do you have a few seconds or minutes in your day that could be devoted to something meaningful and enjoyable? What about listening to your favorite tunes while doing your least favorite chore? What about treating yourself to a few minutes of reading a book you love before bed? Do you have a half hour once a week to go somewhere or do something you have been wanting to do for some time, but keep finding reasons why you cannot?

Sing, draw, listen to music, visit a museum, learn a new instrument (you can do this on YouTube these days; you do not have to pay for or commit to a class). Even adding in a few minutes for breathing exercises can help your mood shift. Notice how quickly your brain may try to find excuses, but realize these excuses are just more stories keeping you from happiness. We are rarely as stuck as we feel, no matter how loudly our brains scream otherwise. So, with an open mind, look at your list of daily activities again and see if there isn't somewhere you can tweak to add a little more joy and a few less shoulds to the list. Remember, any committed step, however small, creates a ripple effect that leads to more steps, which can lead to big changes, especially when approached with compassion.

I cannot tell you how many people, especially moms, I see in my practice who have an entire list of depleting activities and not one item for self-nourishment and fun. How could you expect to feel anything but depressed? I get it. When my kids were little, I was one of those moms too. Although I also meditated, I felt a twinge of guilt for taking any other time for me. Everything, every moment was about them. There are still days like that, but even then, is there a way to change the story line even if you cannot yet change the list?

Practicing compassion not only leads us to greater internal coherence and sense of connection, but actually creates a state of heart coherence between us and others—another antidote to loneliness. Loneliness is defined as the "subjective, unwelcome feeling of lack or loss of companionship" that occurs when there is a "mismatch between social relationships that we have and those that we want." Notice that by definition, loneliness is the perception, not reality, of disconnection and aloneness. This story of the mind leads to distrust and withdrawal, which leads to an ever-increasing sense of isolation.

When we feel alone, we tend to get self-absorbed and think that we are the only ones experiencing this. This makes it even more difficult to connect, creating a downward spiral and self-fulfilling prophecy. Although this feeling can be powerful and feel like truth, science informs us that in truth, we are all deeply and energetically connected in ways we cannot even imagine.

One interesting study had pairs of participants, who were previously complete strangers, meditate together for twenty minutes, which has been shown to harmonize brain activity. They were then separated and placed in Faraday chambers, basically a small cage or human-size safe, which prevented the possibility of any sensory or electromagnetic communication between the two partners. They were instructed to maintain a sense of their partner. One was exposed to a hundred random flashes of light while an electroencephalogram (EEG) recorded the brain waves of both participants. The brain recordings revealed that both brains responded in a similar pattern to the stimuli, despite the separation and the fact that only one experienced the flashes. Just twenty minutes of meditation created a state of harmonic entanglement and connection.

Group coherence amplifies this effect. Shared group intentions create coherent energy fields even when separated by distance. For the past year, I have met online weekly with eight others in different parts of the country in a Power of Eight group established by Lynne McTaggart's work on focused intentions. When we meet, we set intentions for each other and others. We have witnessed some amazing shifts. Two days after my group intended for me to find a publisher for this book, I was offered a contract. Another woman intended for a reasonably priced and safe used vehicle, and a few weeks later, she and her dogs were happily riding around in a reliable van. Another woman sought more clients for her therapy practice, which has been flourishing in some unexpected ways, including a growing online following. Another woman found the courage and trust to leave a living situation no longer working for her. This is the power of heartfelt intentions and connections. If this is possible, imagine the limitless possibilities.

We are connected in more ways than we can fathom. The act of choosing to focus on positive thoughts and actions has implications beyond our own lives. Dr. Masaru Emoto spent his career studying the effect of human thought on water molecules. He found that sending positive thoughts of love, gratitude, appreciation, and joy to water changed the molecules into beautifully symmetrical shapes. Thoughts of anger and fear led to messy, asymmetrical shapes.

If you consider that humans are 70 percent water, consider for a moment the immense implications this may have, not only on our own physiology and health but on living creatures and the world around us. More amazingly, these thoughts are not limited by time or space.

In one study, two thousand people in Tokyo directed positive thoughts toward water samples inside an electromagnetically shielded room in Petaluma, California. Control water samples were stored in a shielded room in a different location. One hundred independent judges viewed photographs of these water crystals and concluded that those "treated" with the heartfelt intentions were more symmetrical and beautiful.

In fact, we each have our own energetic imprint. A study at the Institute of Aerospace Thermodynamics in Stuttgart, Germany, found that our unique energy influences the pattern of water. Students were asked to fill a syringe with water and squeeze a drop onto a slide, which was then photographed under a microscope. The photos revealed that each individual's water drops were consistently unique, different from all the others, once again showing that our energetic fields change matter and the world around us.

Given this information, the power of our thoughts to influence not only our emotions, health, and perception of the world around us, but also the physical reality of our world, becomes apparent. With this in mind, finding moments throughout the day to check in with the thoughts, body, emotions, and energy becomes more essential for healing than previously imagined. Before drinking your next cup of water, tea, or coffee, you may consider holding the cup to your heart and offering a quick, simple thank-you or blessing.

Clearly, all of this evidence suggests that we are far more than just our body or mind. We radiate emotion and thoughts out in the universal field. We all benefit from offering more mindful attention to what we are broadcasting. Your health and well-being depend on it, as does mine, and everyone else's. Sometimes, when we cannot motivate ourselves to do the things we need to do to heal, taking action for the sake of those we most cherish may be a helpful place to begin. Focusing on another broadens our perspective. McTaggart's work suggests that intending for others has a boomerang effect that generates positive benefits in our own lives.

Energy and Healing

Energy has been harnessed for healing for thousands of years; this is hardly a new or radical concept. Ancient Egyptians used electric eels to generate powerful shocks to alleviate pain and improve blood circulation. Jesus and early Christians laid hands on the ill for healing. The practices of *qi gong*, tai chi, and yoga are designed to move energy. According to Nobel Prize–winning scientist Albert Szent-Györgyi, "In every culture and in every medical tradition before ours, healing was accomplished by moving energy." It is yet one more piece of wisdom we lost or dismissed, but are now rediscovering.

Ultimately, of course, everything is energy—every breath, thought, emotion, body sensation, and movement. Every cell in the body emits particles of light as part of intercellular communication. Energy is required for every function of the body. We are beings of energy and light.

Although conventional medicine remains skeptical of energy medicine and psychology, the modern medical world relies daily on energy and electrical fields for diagnosis and treatment. Instead of electric eels, we now use electric stimulation in the form of transcutaneous electrical nerve stimulation (TENS) units and other devices to speed healing and alleviate pain. Defibrillators shock the heart to reestablish its rhythm after a cardiac arrest. Electrocardiograms (EKGs) and EEGs read the electrical fields of the heart and brain.

In psychiatry, electroconvulsive therapy and now transcranial electromagnetic stimulation are accepted practices. One of the oldest recordings of energy healing techniques can be found in an ancient Chinese medical text called *The Yellow Emperor's Classic of Internal Medicine,* written in 2600 BCE. In this book, energy channels and hundreds of acupressure points that could be used to balance the flow of energy within the body were identified and recorded. This book is still in print.

Today, the use of a galvanometer can identity these acupressure points, which have two thousand times less electrical resistance than the surrounding skin. This enables more electrical charge to pass through with greater ease. Modern technology is now elucidating the effects of these specific points on the brain and body. Acupuncture has been shown to calm the limbic system and balance the sympathetic and parasympathetic nervous system as well as neurotransmitters.

Based on its effects on the brain, acupuncture would appear to be a good option for dealing with depression as well. Although there is still limited evidence with regard to its efficacy in depression, the studies that have been conducted suggest it might be a useful alternative, and certainly one worth researching further. One study in Great Britain compared acupuncture to counseling and found them equally effective. A similar study followed patients experiencing both pain and depression. For that population, the acupuncture group experienced the greatest reduction in both pain and depression.

Although I highly recommend acupuncture as part of treatment plans for anxiety, depression, insomnia, and medication withdrawal, another use of these acupressure points are self-healing techniques that fall under the umbrella heading of "energy psychology." The most popular of these is the Emotional Freedom Technique (EFT). This simple yet powerful tool incorporates the tapping of acupressure points with your fingertips while focusing on distressing thoughts, emotions, or events.

I will be the first to admit: it looks strange. When my patients and I do it together, I sometimes feel like a monkey playing Simon Says, but it works. Over one hundred randomized controlled trials and review articles published in peer-reviewed papers have demonstrated EFT's safety and effectiveness, and I am continually amazed by the results. Although it used to be considered a strange, fringe therapy, today it is recognized by the American Psychological Association as an evidence-based practice and is used by a growing number of therapists and millions of people around the world.

Sadly, EFT is still fringe in the world of psychiatry, even though data consistently demonstrates that it has a much greater effect size than any medications or talk therapy. A triple blind randomized controlled study that directly compared EFT to traditional talk therapy and a control group found that symptoms of depression and anxiety of those in the EFT group decreased by more than twice those in talk therapy. The EFT group also experienced a drop in cortisol levels nearly double that in the other groups.

Functional MRI studies show that, like acupuncture, EFT calms the limbic system and balances the nervous system. One study examining EFT's effect on gene expression found that a single one-hour session influenced the expression of seventy-two genes involved in decreasing inflammation, increasing immunity, and increasing synaptic connections in the brain. What a powerful use of one hour of your time, don't you think?

I teach this to most of my patients to help with reducing anxiety, ruminating or obsessive thoughts, phobias, pain, insomnia, and really, just about anything that disturbs them. Although EFT does not instantly eliminate all problems, it reliably reduces distress to a manageable level. There are many free online videos, which I have listed on my website (www.jodieskillicorn.com) that can teach you this tool better than I can here in words. I highly recommend setting aside some time to learn the basic technique so you can see how simple it is, and start using it in your life. Trust me, you will be grateful you did.

Another energy technique I use on a daily basis in my practice is eye movement desensitization and reprocessing (EMDR). This was originally developed by Francine Shapiro serendipitously in the late 1980s to alleviate the distress associated with traumatic memories. As Shapiro tells the story, she was walking through a park one day, reflecting on a distressing memory, when she noticed her eyes were rapidly moving back and forth, and she suddenly felt tremendous relief and release. Thus, EMDR was born.

When Shapiro first created the therapy, she would direct patients to move their eyes back and forth while focusing on a specific moment from a trauma, hence the awkward and off-putting name of the technique. The eye movements created are much like those in REM sleep, when the brain processes and integrates events from the day and acts as our nighttime therapist. The literature suggests, however, that any kind of bilateral stimulation works.

My preference is a small handheld device that vibrates back and forth, activating and connecting the right and left hemispheres of the brain. This is important because when we are highly stressed or traumatized, our frontal lobe is hijacked, as we have learned, and information is not getting connected throughout the brain. The memory gets stuck in time, never being connected, processed, or resolved. This technique connects the fragmented, frozen memories into a coherent narrative, while informing the body that the incident is in the past and the body is safe now.

Remembering the events activates the limbic system, and the bilateral stimulation simultaneously calms the system, rewiring the memory of the event, so that the memory no longer triggers a strong emotional reaction. The event becomes a memory of an event that happened in the past but is now over.

What I most love about this technique is how it combines everything we have discussed so far in this book. It combines mindful awareness of the breath, thoughts, emotions, and body as one leans into discomfort and distress, trusting that the body and mind can reassemble and synthesize the picture into a coherent, balanced whole. This shifts one's perceptions and cognitions about the event and often allows one to find a deeper meaning and understanding.

Although we may not fully understand how the technique works, the research has consistently found it to be a highly effective technique for PTSD, anxiety, phobias, and depression. Most of the research has been centered on PTSD, but let's remember the direct correlation between early adverse childhood events and mental illness. Processing these early childhood traumas and losses can shift limiting beliefs and perspectives, enhancing mood and well-being.

One study compared EMDR to Prozac and placebo. All three treatment groups improved. Ironically, but consistent with prior research, there was no statistical difference between those on medication versus those on placebo. After twelve weeks, the EMDR and medication groups showed equal reductions in symptoms, but at the six-month follow-up, 58 percent of those who received EMDR had completely recovered compared with none in the medication group.

Those in the EMDR group also had a greater reduction in depressive symptoms, which continued to improve over time while those on antidepressants leveled off. This once again suggests that although medications may numb symptoms, they are not getting at the core of the problem, and are often no more effective than placebo. It is also a reminder of just how powerful the placebo effect can be, especially in the context of a supportive relationship with a provider.

A 2018 study compared EMDR with CBT, which has long been considered the "gold standard" for therapeutic intervention. The trial randomized sixty-six patients to either EMDR or CBT. Both were found to be equally effective at reducing symptoms of depression, anxiety, and PTSD at the end of the twelve-week trial. However, at the follow-up six months later, 71 percent of those in the EMDR group fully recovered as compared to only 49 percent in the CBT group.

Another interesting finding was that those in the EMDR group continued to improve over time, while those in the CBT group leveled off.

What I find in practice is that EMDR speeds up healing and more effectively gets to the roots of the problem. This makes sense if you consider that talk therapy is primarily accessing the literal, logical left side of the brain, which is the side we use to verbalize and communicate. It is also the side that traps us in the endless whys for which there is often not a clear-cut answer, no matter how many hours and how many sessions we spend talking about it.

Yet, it is the right side of the brain where the remnants and emotions of trauma and losses get buried. In order for the two hemispheres to connect and integrate, we must access both sides of the brain, collecting all the fragmented pieces in their different forms. More importantly, talk therapy cannot access preverbal memories of the young nonverbal child. These are aspects of healing where EFT, EMDR, and hypnotherapy excel over traditional talk therapies.

Comprehending this process is like cognitively trying to understand swimming while sitting at the edge of a pool, but let's dive into one example to give you a sense of how this can work. A couple of weeks ago, Cynthia, a twenty-three-year-old who suffers from depression, anxiety, and panic disorder, returned to see me after a several-month hiatus. When I had first seen her a year earlier, she had not been out of the house alone in months. In fear of having a panic attack, she avoided just about everything. Cynthia deeply believed she was broken and unfixable. She had not driven alone in months and could not even get through a grocery store without panicking. She desperately wanted to at least be able to go to the store, so we started EMDR with that experience.

While she held the tappers, Cynthia imagined walking through the store. She could feel her body panic and freeze when nearing the back of the store, farthest from the door. She breathed through it while imagining a loving supportive light surrounding and protecting her. After the session, she had her mom take her to the grocery store, and she made it all the way to the checkout line before panicking.

On her next visit to my office, we "returned" to the scene, once again breathing into all the alarming sensations in her body, noticing all the catastrophizing thoughts in her mind, leaning into and feeling her fear. Cynthia's fears subsided as she breathed and imagined the light surrounding and protecting her while she walked through the checkout line with confidence and ease. That night she successfully made it through the grocery store line without panic. We built from there. Within a few months, Cynthia was driving again and hanging out with friends. She got a job and was enjoying life for the first time in years.

Over the holidays, though, her anxiety, panic, and depression reappeared. She was barely leaving the house again. Even in my office, where Cynthia normally felt calm and secure, she started to panic. She desperately wanted to escape the confining space of the room, and the intensity of distressing body sensations and emotions. I encouraged her to stay and lean into the fears so she could work through them.

We combined EFT and EMDR as she restlessly paced around the office, unable to sit down or settle. I encouraged Cynthia to reflect back on the first time she had felt this sense of being trapped and panicked. This immediately brought back a memory of her as a six-year-old girl waking up in her bunk bed in the middle of the night to see her older brother seizing on their bedroom floor. She remembered going to get her parents but then coming back in the room, where the memory was frozen with her watching in terror and helplessness as her parents tended to her brother and rushed to get him to the hospital. That terrified six-year-old girl was still trapped in that dark room.

Both the adult and child Cynthia wanted out of the confined space, so we put on our coats and sat outside on a stoop while she wrapped herself in a hug and tapped her right and left shoulders back and forth, back and forth. As she did this, she imagined her older sister taking the six-year-old Cynthia outside to play in the sunlight, while lovingly reassuring her that she was safe. They were OK. Their brother would be OK. A gentle smile replaced the tears as the little girl played outside, finally free of the dark, scary room. She was no longer trapped and helpless. She could now replay the original scary scene without fear and panic.

For homework, I encouraged Cynthia to keep connecting with the little girl, to reassure her and let her know she is safe. Now, instead of criticism and blame for the helpless scared little girl, who she saw as "weak, frail, and broken," Cynthia feels compassion for the six-year-old, who was just scared like any "normal" child would be in that situation.

The memory had become fragmented from the full story, which includes the fact that she grew up and survived, and so did her brother. By going back, processing and integrating the pieces, the adult Cynthia can offer kindness and compassion to the little Cynthia. A new story line emerges of empowerment and resilience. It is often through the hardest experiences that we find our meaning and purpose. This is not to say Cynthia will not experience that fear again, but by shifting this experience it enables her to meet future experiences with more compassion, tenderness, and confidence that she can manage and get through them.

What is more amazing is that as Cynthia leans in and works through her fear, this not only shifts and rewires her nervous system, changes her perceptions of herself and the world around her, and softens and opens her heart, but these changes will reverberate to those around her. Emotions are contagious. They influence not just water, but people around us.

As part of the Framingham Heart Study, a group of participants were followed for over twenty years to explore how their changing happiness levels influenced those around them. The researchers found that one person's happiness boosts the odds that those close to them will also be happy by 34 percent. More astonishingly, just living within a mile of a friend who has become happier increases your chance of happiness by 25 percent. Even having a friend's friend's friend become happier increases your odds of happiness by 15 percent.

Think about the implications of this. We are inextricably connected and influencing each other in ways we cannot even imagine. My happiness depends on yours, and yours on mine and those around you. Although negative emotions are also contagious, fortunately their influence is not as strong. Still, imagine what happens if we shun our neighbors, or build walls to artificially separate and divide us. The ripple effects of living from a place of compassion or fear influence us all, for better or worse.

These complex social networks through which we are all connected influence our moods and behaviors. A fascinating social experiment that nobody signed up for included 689,003 Facebook users. The study incorporated an automated system that changed the emotional content of a user's "news feed." Researchers found that people posted more negative posts in response to the appearance of more negative posts in their feed and, likewise, posted more positive content when exposed to more positive information.

We are unconsciously influenced by and influencing those around us all the time. Social media posts reflect not only our interests and beliefs, but also our moods. Those with depressed moods tend to post photos with darker tones, while happier folks post photos with warmer and brighter hues. In fact, just looking at the color tones in an individual's posts, a computer could accurately diagnose depression with 70 percent accuracy. By comparison, studies suggest that primary care physicians accurately diagnose depression 42 percent of the time! We truly are, in the words of Lynne McTaggart, "leaky buckets" broadcasting our thoughts and emotions not only into cyberspace but also out to the world around us all the time.

It benefits all of us to become more aware of what we are sending out into the world. Research suggests the gifts of the heart proliferate, as does the mongering of fear. By increasing our own heart coherence, we boost the coherence of our family, friends, pets, and even the environment around us.

In one study, a group of participants were trained in a heart-based meditation designed to create HRV coherence. Trained participants then sat at tables with untrained volunteers and were asked to either quietly relax, focus on raising their own HRV, or create their own state of coherence while directing compassion toward the untrained volunteer. The latter group was told to do this with the intention of facilitating a state of coherence in the person seated at their table.

The trial found that untrained participants entered a state of heart coherence 80 percent of the time just by being in the presence of someone in coherence. Intentionally attempting to facilitate coherence in the other actually decreased effectiveness. Perhaps our greatest offering to others is to be present and coherent ourselves.

Accumulating evidence demonstrates that as more members of a group achieve coherence—whether it is a large corporation, a police force, a health care organization, or a school—everyone benefits. The U.S. Department of Education funded a study involving one thousand tenth-grade students. Half of the students were taught to simply breathe in and out of the heart center while focusing on the feeling of appreciation, as you learned in the earlier exercise.

The results revealed that not only did the group that learned this quick simple technique improve their ability to self-regulate their emotions and improve HRV, but they also found a 75 percent reduction in test anxiety, improved moods, and significant improvement academically. On top of that, the students showed greater empathy in their social interactions with others. I hope for the day when these skills will be taught at all schools, as it will not only benefit the kids throughout their lives, but create a better society for all of us in ways we cannot yet fathom.

It appears that our hearts not only pick up emotionally laden information from the environment around us, but research suggests the heart picks up this information before we are consciously aware of the information. In a fascinating study conducted by Dean Radin at the Institute of Noetic Sciences, a group of participants' physiological measures were monitored while they watched a series of randomly selected photos on a computer screen. The photos, some calming images of nature and others emotionally charged, were designed to elicit different physiological responses. Amazingly, the body responded to the content of the photos before they appeared on the screen.

The HeartMath Institute later followed up on this experiment, to carefully monitor the signals of the brain and heart to see how each responded to the images and in what order. The researchers discovered that the heart responded to the randomly selected photos 6 seconds before the image appeared on the screen, and 4.8 seconds before the computer even chose the image! The heart sent the message to the brain, which received the info 1.5 seconds later, still prior to the event actually happening. Those who had engaged in a heart-centered meditation prior to the experiment sent a signal to the brain with a stronger effect on the activity of the brain, suggesting heightened attunement and intuition.

Dubious? This study was later repeated in another country, with different researchers and participants, and arrived at the same shocking conclusion. This experiment added a small additional twist by conducting part of the experiment in pairs. Researchers found that the presence of another participant amplified the effects seen in the earlier experiments. This suggests that our hearts are exquisitely designed to sense the emotional environment around us before the brain and sometimes, at least, before the event even occurs. Getting lost in our heads disconnects us from the inner intuitive knowing of the heart and disconnects us from each other.

As more of us take time to shift our coherence to improve our own mood, health, and well-being, we have the power to shift the coherence of society and the planet. Random number generator machines have been scattered in locations around the planet. As the name implies, they generate random numbers that are stored in databases. Researchers noticed that at times of massive emotional upheaval, the numbers appeared less random.

One notable example of such a shift was at 9 a.m. on September 11, 2001, just after the first of two hijacked planes flew into the World Trade Center. At that time, all the random number generator machines deviated dramatically. At this very same time, a spike appeared in the global network of ultrasensitive magnetometers, which measure the earth's geomagnetic field.

The data suggests that our emotions influence not only each other, but when experienced in mass, disrupt randomness and shift the earth's magnetic fields. If this is true, our individual and collective thoughts, prayers, and intentions matter immensely. If most of us are projecting fear into the environment, that influences all of us. Conversely, if we project love, appreciation, and gratitude, this raises our global coherence. We are interconnected. Your healing matters, as does mine.

Although these ideas may be unsettling, they are also freeing and empowering, because what is certain is that the truth of who we are is bigger and more complex than the stories in our heads that keep us trapped and small. We must each take responsibility for our energies and what we broadcast within our own bodies and out into the universe. Looking at it this way, my individual healing is imperative for the healing of the planet, and so is yours. This may sound heady and kumbaya-ish, but data supports the common threads of compassion taught in all religions. Your actions toward others influence not only your own well-being but all of ours. We are in this together. When we feel and perceive ourselves as alone, it is simply not possible.

Like Odysseus, we must bind ourselves to our masts through our practices of breath, mindfulness, healthy eating, exercise, and compassionate connection with ourselves, others, and the world around us. Odysseus could not do it alone, and neither can we. We must join together from the heart so that we are not lured by the call of negativity that leaves us wallowing on the shores of despair. Learning to listen to the language of the heart is essential to counteracting the fear-based thoughts in our heads.

Committing to seven minutes of a heart-centered meditation can change your health, mood, and well-being, and the rest of ours too. Better yet, meditate with others, in person or online, to amplify the effects of your meditations, prayers, and intentions for a more stable, balanced, and compassionate world. As Coretta Scott King said, "The greatness of a community is most accurately measured by the compassionate actions of its members." The compassion and vitality of your heart, energy, and soul matter to all of us.

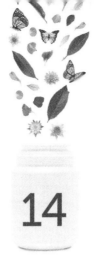

14

Connecting the Pieces

Wholeness is never lost, it is only forgotten.

—RACHEL NAOMI REMEN

Unlike lovable, furry Grover, who was terrified of getting to the last page of his book for fear of finding a monster lurking there, I hope that you have arrived at this last chapter with less fear and more hope than when you started. Hopefully you have learned that many of the monsters we most fear exist only in our storytelling minds. Rest assured, depression is not a monster forever lurking behind you, waiting to jump out and spook you when you least expect it.

Depression is a symptom of distress, imbalance, and disconnection, often created by our fears and our attempts to avoid and resist them. Instead of solving the problem, many of our "treatment" strategies only create more fear and stress. The disproven but widely propagated belief that depression is a chronic, incurable disease caused by faulty genes and neurochemistry, from which we can never escape, makes us powerless to manifest change. Conventional psychiatry is based on outdated notions about a static brain that once diminished in serotonin, norepinephrine, or dopamine is forever depleted without pharmacological intervention—once broken, forever broken.

The concept of neuroplasticity refutes this disempowering notion of the brain. You are not the same person you were when you started this book. You are not even the same person you were a minute or a second ago. Our brain and body are constantly regenerating and reorganizing based on our thoughts, actions, and experiences. In the time it took you to read the last sentence, your body replaced over eight hundred thousand cells, including at least one neuron. Today, your body will create over one trillion new red blood cells. In the time it took you to arrive at this final chapter, the lining of your stomach, small intestine, and colon was replaced, at least once, depending on how fast you read.

The only way your so-called "broken" brain will remain so is if you continue to input the same data or stop trying because you do not believe it will make a difference. Healing depression lies not in a magical pill, but in rebalancing your life and reconnecting the pieces severed by stressors, losses, toxins, and trauma.

It is not your fault for believing your brain cannot heal without pharmaceutical intervention. That is what we've been taught by doctors, TV commercials, ghost-written research papers, and news articles. Imagine if a child learning to walk was repeatedly told, "You can't do it. You will fall. You will hurt yourself. You will fail." When the child tries to walk and does fall, she is told, "See, I told you that you would fall. You can't do it on your own."

This is what doctors do to patients by authoritatively informing them they cannot survive without their medications. But just as the child will most certainly fall while learning to walk, we will all fail, we will all feel sad, anxious, and angry—this is a part of the human experience. This is neither failure nor dysfunction; it is part of learning, growing, and transforming. We must learn to listen to and manage our emotions so we can become stronger and more resilient.

Cutting ourselves off from our emotions disconnects us from our inner guidance, our bodies, from our own lives and the lives of others, and from the communities in which we live, work, and play. Is that not the deepest depression possible? With or without medications, sadness will inevitably appear. We must learn to acknowledge and listen to these feelings with curiosity rather than back away in fear and avoidance. The preponderance of evidence (at least unbiased evidence not marketed by pharmaceutical companies) suggests a radically different, far more hopeful story. Our bodies are designed to heal if given the chance.

Our bodies cannot heal, however, if we continue to breathe, think, act, eat, move, and interact in the same ways that we always have. We cannot heal if we numb ourselves and disconnect from the messages of the emotions and body, to avoid having to make difficult but necessary changes. This will invariably lead to the same results, over and over and over again, causing us to mistakenly believe change is not possible.

But change is possible. We are not powerless victims of our physiology and genes. Yes, of course, we have certain genetic predispositions, but our input and interaction with the environment play a much larger role than most of us were ever taught to believe or imagined possible.

To reiterate, I am not saying medications should never be used. Nor am I saying that if you are already on a medication or medications, you should just stop them. There are times someone may need medications, at least temporarily. But medication should be the last resort, not the first; the exception, not the norm.

My recommendation is always to first learn some of the basic breathing and mindfulness skills in this book, and create a regular practice of these so that you can build confidence in their power.

By not tending to the roots of depression, they will only rot and fester. The problem is rarely a brain malfunction, but rather a life that has become disconnected and out of balance. This is not to cast judgment on one's character or ability to cope. If anything, it is an indictment of our societal values and global disconnection from those things that sustain and nourish us. We learn what we are taught. As a society, we prize our minds and ignore our bodies. We value thinking over feeling, productivity and busyness over stillness and quiet, rationality over the imagination, fast processed foods over natural whole produce, watching TV over exercising, indoor spaces over the wilds of nature, sanitizers over dirt, money and power over meaning and purpose, and connecting with social media over intimate connections. We all pay the price.

Perhaps those grieving the disconnection and most sensitive to the imbalance are the sanest among us. Perhaps depression is the canary in the coal mine screaming for all of us to change: a messenger begging us to wake up, pay attention, and restore balance.

Having said this, it will not serve us to blame society, or our pasts, and abscond responsibility. We are the drivers of our own bus—and we do not travel alone. Not only are we accompanied by the millions of bacteria and microorganisms that ride along, on and within our bodies, but we are energetically linked to those traveling beside and around us. We are also intimately linked with the environment around us: the earth, trees, animals, water, microorganisms, and even the electromagnetic field surrounding our planet.

Our degree of balance and coherence, or imbalance and discordance, will influence how others respond to us, and how we respond to others and the world. When we are more balanced and coherent, we help others shift in that direction, so that it is a smoother and more enjoyable ride for all of us. If enough of us shift our priorities and values toward those that nourish and sustain, rather than toxify and deplete, we shift the cultural narrative. But we each have to do our own work, and find our own path and purpose on this road trip of life.

As I neared the end of writing this book, I discovered Johann Hari's thought-provoking *Lost Connections: Uncovering the Real Causes of Depression—and the Unexpected Solutions.* In the book, Hari traveled around the world talking to some of the top researchers to better understand the roots of depression. Perhaps like you, he had been diagnosed with depression at an early age and started on antidepressants. Yet he wrote, "no matter how high a dose I jacked up my antidepressants to, the sadness would always outrun it." He wanted to understand how he could still be depressed despite taking antidepressants and doing everything "right."

On his journey around the globe, Hari discovered, as you have here, that the answers lie not in neurochemistry and faulty brains in need of a lifetime of pharmaceuticals, but in imbalanced lives in a disconnected world. Hari offers much wisdom and insight, but one story I particularly loved exemplifies the different forms an "antidepressant" can take.

This is the story of a farmer and a healing cow. The farmer had lost his left leg to a land mine in the fields of Cambodia. Although he was fitted with a new limb, he remained profoundly depressed and anxious. The local doctor and villagers talked with the man to assess what he needed to lift his depressed state. He expressed hopelessness about the difficulties and pain caused by working in the rice paddies—the only life he had ever known. Believing there was no way out of the situation was a sure-fire recipe for despair and depression—for him, and for all of us.

But the community did not label his pain or despair as a pathology requiring a medication to fix. Instead, together, they brainstormed a creative solution to rebalance and restore his life. They bought him a cow, figuring that the life of a dairy farmer would cause less pain and distress than working in the rice paddies. They were right. The farmer's despondency lifted. His depression was not faulty brain neurochemistry, but rather a life disrupted and in need of change. The answer was not a pill, but reconnecting with a new purpose and meaning, while being encouraged in the process by a supportive community.

We can all get stuck in our stories at times, believing, like the tiger Mohini, that we are trapped. The story is told that the great magician Houdini was unable to escape only once. Frustrated and bewildered by his inability to free himself from a jail cell after two hours of failed attempts, he asked the jailor who had locked him in what he had done. The guard embarrassedly admitted that he had forgotten to turn the lock. Assuming he was trapped, Houdini failed to consider the possibility that he was already free. All he had to do was push the door open.

We all do this to ourselves far too often. The stories in our mind assume we are trapped by some circumstance, some pathology, some diagnosis, without realizing the only thing trapping us is our own beliefs and stories. If we can anchor ourselves with the breath, and mindfully step back and see our story from a different perspective, we are likely to find we are not as trapped as we believe. Even if we are, a solution may appear that was covered by the clouds of doubt, fear, and frustration.

I once heard a story on a podcast that stuck with me. A dog fell through the ice on a pond in a park. His owner ran out to save him, only to fall in himself. Terrified, he flailed frantically, unable to get a grasp on the slippery ice, until he finally heard his wife screaming. "Just stand up!" she repeated over and over until he finally heard her cries. In his fear and terror, he failed to realize the water was only waist deep. He was cold, but never in danger of drowning or being trapped. He could just stand up and get out.

This is what happens when fear hijacks our brains. Our limbic system takes over and we are at the mercy of fear. We lose the ability to think rationally. We lose the ability to find a way out. This ancient limbic system can save us in an actual emergency, but far too often it gets activated by the catastrophizing narratives of the Master Storyteller. We can get our feet back on the ground, by stepping out of the stories of the mind and focusing instead on slow, deep breaths to the belly, and noticing with curiosity the sensations of the body experienced as fear. Like the man in the pond, we will not remember these skills in an emergency if they are not practiced regularly. With practice, we rewire and restructure the brain so that we are less likely to get hijacked, less likely to forget to put our feet on the ground, and even if we do, we are able to pull ourselves out much more quickly. We can learn to recognize our fear-based stories as stories, and not spend as much time trapped there.

Ram Dass, a Harvard psychologist who traveled to India and brought back many of the ancient spiritual teachings of the East to the Western world, was once asked what he has learned from a lifetime immersed in meditation. He replied that before meditation he was full of fear, judgment, anger, anxiety, and impatience. After decades of practicing meditation, he said he was still all of those things, but now, instead of dragons, they were merely shmoos. They were still present, but no longer causing suffering.

Fear, anxiety, sadness, frustration, anger—these are all unavoidable parts of this human experience, yet we are only trapped by them if we believe that life should be some other way. We can resist these emotions, scream at or run from them, but, like the covered pot of water, they will only grow in intensity and boil over uncontrollably.

Ultimately, of course, no matter how fast or how far we go, it is impossible to outrun or avoid ourselves. Another option is to lean in with kindness and curiosity, and listen to the messages of our emotions, which guide us toward our destination and alert us to disruptions and imbalance. They are the roadmap on our journey. They alert us when we are short on gas, and we need to stop for rest and refueling. Perhaps we need higher-grade fuel, or food, for better performance. Maybe there is a tire blowout and we need to stop and get a new tire, new relationship, new job, or new perspective.

We can run away, or shoot the messenger for bringing news we do not want to face, or we can pause and listen, so that the whisper does not become a raging scream. We can listen to ourselves and our emotional "warnings" so that we do not find ourselves alone in the middle of the night without a phone, on a dark isolated road with a broken-down car. Even then, of course, we can walk for help and recover, but wouldn't it be easier to notice and tend to the signs of wear and tear, rust, deflated tires, and depleted fuel and oil before we get stranded?

Just as our bus needs to be driven, or will need a jump start to get back in action, we too must move our bodies on a daily basis to strengthen our immune system, balance the nervous system, and prevent and heal depression and anxiety. Getting outside in nature to do this is ideal. Our bodies thrive when exposed to the natural world of which we are a part. Pause and see the colors of grass, trees, sky, and birds. Listen to the sounds around you. Notice how the beating of your heart, the sound of your breath, the rush of the leaves and the wind, the song of the phoebe, the whoosh of a car passing by in the distance all join together in life's orchestra. Feel the ground beneath your feet, the movement of your body, the warmth of the sun or the tingle from the cold on your exposed skin.

The physicist Carlo Rovelli describes human beings as "a net of interactions." Our existence is based on our connection and relationship with others and the world around us. In depression, our interactions with the body, self, heart, family, friends, community, nature, meaning, and spirit become disconnected, or at least, perceived as such. To heal, we must figure out what pieces need to be reconnected and rebalanced.

We may never know the why, and often we do not need to in order to begin the journey of self-healing, one step at a time. The "whys" often lead us to an inescapable maze of the mind, trapping us with endless pondering and questioning, waiting for some clear-cut answer that may never come before taking action. What is clear is that we cannot heal soul wounds with biochemical solutions. They are only tourniquets that prevent you from bleeding on the white carpet, but do nothing to abate the internal hemorrhaging.

As we have learned, even the early formulators of the neurochemical imbalance theory understood that attributing depression to the levels of one of a few neurochemicals is preposterously simplistic and absurd. Yet pharmaceutical companies and modern medicine have convinced us otherwise in the name of money, power, prestige, simplicity, and comfort. It spares the physician the uncomfortable messiness of not knowing, not having an answer or cure, and feeling utterly helpless in the presence of another's pain and despair. It is just so much simpler to believe a pill can resolve everything, even life's pain and suffering.

Yet just as listening and acknowledging our own pain is a powerful tool in healing, so too is listening and acknowledging the pain of another without feeling compelled to take action to do anything about it. Sometimes it is enough just to be heard, acknowledged, and supported. That is perhaps the most powerful, most ancient, and most forgotten tool in the healing arsenal.

Listening, not just with our heads but with our hearts, helps guide us toward finding tools to reconnect and rebalance the pieces so we can see the whole puzzle and access the whole being. Most likely, a cow is not the answer to your depression. There is no one answer. Depression is a wake-up call, a compass pointing you in a different direction—your direction, not the farmer's or mine or anyone else's. It points you back to your center, back to balance, back to the breath, the body, back to movement, nature, community, purpose, and spirit. There is no end point.

Healing requires reconnecting the assorted pieces of the puzzle, shuffled and shaken by life's disruptions. The tools and skills you have learned in this book can help you do that. You can reconnect the puzzle pieces of your own life to enhance the quality of your experience and your time on this planet. To achieve this, you can:

- reconnect the parts of the brain with tools like imagery, breathing, meditation, EMDR, EFT, and REM sleep.

- reconnect the mind and the body with breathing, body awareness, exercise, nutrition, movement, and nature.

- reconnect the mind and gut by consuming healthy, whole foods and by mindful eating.

- reconnect the fragmented pieces of the self through imagery, breathing, meditation, journaling, EFT, and EMDR therapy.

- reconnect with family, friends, and community through art, dance, or singing classes, trips to the museum, volunteering, or heart-centered meditations.

- reconnect with nature by hiking and exploring, or just lying barefoot in the grass, perhaps drawing or journaling what you see.

- reconnect with the heart, energy, and soul through imagery, breath, meditation, gratitude, and prayer.

There is nothing broken to fix; we must just reconnect and rebalance the pieces of ourselves and our lives. We must reprioritize our time based on what offers us meaning, value, and joy.

Although no two healing paths are the same, Molly's story offers a glimpse of possibility. Molly is a middle-aged woman with lifelong anxiety and depression who has been in counseling and on psychiatric medications for over twenty years. She arrived in my office after suffering from a stroke and fearing that her cocktail of medications may have played a role. "This stroke was a wake-up call," she told me. "I don't exercise. I eat bad food. All I want to do is sleep and my body is falling apart."

Molly was unable to mentally focus and concentrate, and was terrified of losing the job she loathed. Feeling overly emotional and weak, she was petrified to head down the same path as her mother, who had spent years in and out of psychiatric hospitals, loading up on shock treatments and medications.

Molly had already started walking daily and eating better on her own. Because of thyroid issues, I suggested a gluten-free elimination trial, and shifting over to primarily whole organic foods. She discovered gluten made her angry and irritable, and she felt much better without it. We added turmeric and fish oil for inflammation and mood. Molly's breath was shallow and restricted on exhalation, so she started a daily breathing and mindfulness routine, simply noticing her breath, body sensations, emotions, and thoughts—especially the self-critical, self-sabotaging ones. When the stories sucked her in, she would tap on them to reframe and reduce her reactivity to them.

Taking care of herself was novel, as Molly and her siblings had been forced to raise themselves since mom was often absent or emotionally unavailable. As her emotional resilience grew, we tapered Molly slowly off her medications. The emotional ups and downs, and physical sensations of the medication withdrawal, stirred up fears of "being like mom and needing medications to survive."

We tapped and did EMDR around these fears. Auricular acupuncture helped calm her physical and emotional withdrawal. She was stunned by how alive she started to feel. Eight months later, Molly was at a new job that she enjoyed much more than her previous sedentary desk job. She had lost weight and felt more energetic, confident, and assured. She was back to being the gregarious, vivacious Molly who had been lost so many years ago under the influence of medications.

As she slowly reemerged, she expressed joy at noticing the beautiful foliage of fall for the first time. "For twenty-two years I was under a cloud of pharmaceuticals. Now I am getting to start over and do and see everything fresh," she told me. She was excited to go on her annual trip to Florida. "I have been going for twenty years, but this will be the first time I will actually be able to see and feel the ocean."

By daring to come off the medications Molly had been told she would need forever, and taking a leap of faith in her body's own ability to heal, she reconnected with her breath, and reconnected with the parts of her brain severed by childhood traumas. She became aware and able to create space around the critical and false stories of her mind. She reconnected with her love for nature and dirt, and the joy of moving her body in yoga and digging in her organic vegetable garden. She also reconnected with her passion for music and the support, love, and protection of her guardian angel.

By balancing and reconnecting breath, mind, body, environment, and soul, Molly transformed depression's urgent call into an opportunity for growth and renewal. This does not mean she does not still fall into the hole of despair when old scars rip off—especially when she forgets to keep practicing her skills and gets lost in the old tapes in her head insisting she is incapable, not good enough, and needs medication to function. But each time this happens, she can now pull herself out more quickly and easily, sometimes on her own and sometimes with help.

The poet Rumi wrote, "The wound is the place where the light enters you." Shifting our perceptions and shining a light of kindness, attention, and forgiveness on our broken places has the potential to alchemize our individual and collective suffering and flaws into compassion, resilience, and grace.

In Japan there is a word, *wabi-sabi,* which means seeing beauty in the flawed and imperfect. Here in the United States, we tend to judge and conceal imperfections, replacing old broken objects—and sometimes people—for shiny new ones. How we treat our used objects unfortunately parallels how we treat the flaws and imperfections of ourselves and others. We cover outer wrinkles with layers of concealer and makeup, designer clothes, endless dieting, and even surgery while burying inner wounds with alcohol, drugs, food, shopping, distraction, and busyness. Judging perceived flaws and cracks as mere imperfections, we fail to notice the potential for mystery and beauty.

If we dare to listen, depression alerts us to the presence of these untended, buried wounds in need of healing. It may be the critical voice of a parent or teacher berating you; the angry hand smacked across the face or belt across the rump; the bullies who teased or punched you in the schoolyard; the sad, faraway look in your mother's face when you tried to tell her something important; the unwanted touch of a teacher, neighbor, or boss; the loss of a beloved parent, grandparent, or pet; the voice of a loved one telling you to shake it off and suck it up when you felt hurt, angry, or scared; and all the other times you were unheard, unseen, invalidated, and told directly or indirectly that you were not good enough. These life events leave a trail of scars.

In our culture, we are often taught to bury these scars, to "just get over it," to cover it up, yet when left uncared for, they can become infected and putrid, seeping out through the cracks in self-sabotaging or harmful ways—as the studies on the effects of adverse childhood events have profoundly demonstrated. Although summoning up the courage to seek help for these wounds of life may be the first step to healing, all too often the healers turned to for help instead label these imperfections—and ourselves—as pathologically broken. This disempowering rebuke adds yet another scar to the tapestry.

The 500-year-old Japanese art form *kintsukuroi* mends broken pottery using a lacquer laced with gold, creating a work of beauty and art out of flawed everyday objects. This art form invites us to consider and understand the environment from which the cracks of our being have emerged, and to honor with kindness and compassion the resilience of the being that has withstood life's battery. It offers an opportunity to distill gold and meaning from these raw experiences. How we tell our stories to ourselves and others becomes our own personal mythology. These stories have the power to transform the ugly to become the beautiful. We can cast ourselves as the victim, perpetrator, or survivor. Which role we focus on will not only change our perception of our powerlessness or strength but, as we have seen, change our physiology and health.

Remember the psychologist Ellen Langer, who conducted the study on the hotel maids? She discovered that by simply reframing the perceived amount of exercise these women carried out on a daily basis—by changing their stories about themselves—they became fitter, thinner, and stronger.

Langer carried out another mind-changing study proving the power of how changing our perceptions and stories changes our physical and emotional well-being. She transported a group of seventy-year-old men "back in time" to 1959. These men spent a long weekend at a monastery, which had been meticulously transformed into a time warp. All the books, magazines, music, and TV shows were from 1959, when the men had been twenty-two years younger. They were instructed to speak, live, and act as if it was truly the late 1950s. After five days of reliving this earlier period, the men not only looked and acted younger, but showed astonishing improvement in their dexterity, strength, flexibility, vision, hearing, memory, and cognition. The old saying "aging is a state of mind" appears to be literally true.

As we have seen again and again throughout this book, our perceptions of what is worthy, acceptable, beautiful, and possible influence how we see the world and ourselves, which in turn influences our body, mind, and health. If we believe aging means we cannot run as far, lift as much, or remember as quickly, those beliefs manifest as fissures in our body and physiology. If we believe our doctor when she tells us that we are broken and cannot heal without a lifetime of medications, it fractures our sense of ourselves and our power.

When we judge ourselves as less than and focus on our flaws and imperfections while shamefully attempting to conceal them from others, it requires a tremendous amount of energy and deception, and keeps us small and powerless. This depletes our bodies and keeps us stuck in the depressed, broken view of ourselves and the world. It prevents the inner wounds from healing, and worse, keeps us from believing that it is even possible to heal, or that we are worthy of it.

On the other hand, if we can acknowledge and honor our flaws with the kindness and compassion we did not get when the wounds were first inflicted, we can begin to heal the tenderness. We can begin to see depression not as an oppressive threat from which we are helpless to escape, caused by our irreparable brokenness, but rather a call to pay attention to the wounds we have ignored and find meaning in them.

In Nikita Gill's poem "Kintsugi," she wrote, "On the days when you feel ashamed of your scars, your mind only registering how ugly you are rather than the beauty they prove of you having survived, remember that there is an entire art form dedicated to filling the cracks of broken things with lacquered gold." Remember the broken bowl filled with gold was made stronger and more beautiful for having been broken and repaired.

Just like the bowls glued back together with gold, depression and illness alert us that our system is out of balance and our wounds need tending, so that we can be stronger, kinder, and more resilient. Maybe we need slower, deeper breaths to provide nourishment to oxygen-deprived cells of the body, and to downshift a lifetime of chronic stress responses. Maybe we need to acknowledge our negative, self-defeating, self-critical thoughts and intentionally choose to spend more time offering ourselves compassion and kindness.

Maybe we need to spend more time focusing on what we have with gratitude, rather than what we lack. Maybe we need to listen to the messages of the body rather than resist, avoid, or ignore them. Maybe we need to move the body rather than in an office or on a couch, or like the maids, reframe the exercise we are actually getting as we engage in our daily routine. Maybe we need to get to bed earlier and establish better sleep habits so that we receive our nightly dose of therapy and have the energy to function efficiently.

Maybe we need to get outside and reconnect with the natural world around us, breathe in some phytoncides, and reduce our exposures to the toxins in our bathrooms and kitchen cabinets. Maybe we need to remember how to listen to the heart to guide us toward purpose, meaning, compassion, and connection. All of these shifts serve to restore energy and balance to our lives, pulling us out of dark moods and distress, and leading us toward health, happiness, and vitality. Each small step ripples outward, influencing not just you, but those around you.

We all have the power to slowly, patiently, kindly, and diligently shift our relationship with these beliefs and stories. We may never get rid of the thoughts telling us we are broken, flawed, and not enough, but we can learn to step away and acknowledge these as old stories of a scared, helpless child who knew no better. We can change the thoughts and emotions from dragons to shmoos.

Let these truths resonate through your cells and your being, feeding the Wolf of Hope and Possibility. These new thoughts, even if you do not yet believe them, shift the expression of your genes, rewire your brain, and change your body and physiology.

All the suggestions in this book may feel overwhelming, but start where you are. Change requires intention and commitment. I challenge you to set the intention to make one change this week. Write it down and post it where you can see it. Imagine what it would feel like with all your senses to follow through. See yourself having accomplished it. Feel it in your body. Breathe it into your heart.

Share your intention with others so they can support you and hold you accountable. Notice when thoughts arise that tell you that this is pointless, that you do not have the time, that it is not possible. Recognize the thoughts as old stories fueling the Wolf of Fear. Do not lob insults at the thoughts or the wolf. Acknowledge with kindness the old stories of fears, then place your hands over your heart as you breathe into the fear. As you breathe out, invite it to release.

As we have learned, just a few minutes of our day practicing the skills in this book can radically shift your health and vitality. Eight minutes of focusing on the breath and seven minutes of focusing on the heart, daily, can change the structure and function of the brain to increase our capacities for attention, focus, and compassion for ourselves and others. Add in eight minutes of exercise, ideally outdoors when you can, and you have a powerful triple-strength antidepressant that balances your nervous system and reduces your reactivity to stress. Mix this in with paying attention to what foods and personal care products you throw into your grocery basket, and you have the power to change your mood and your life.

With empowerment comes responsibility. It can be a difficult road to travel alone. It works best if you have a therapist, a therapy group, or even just a group of friends to join you on the journey, online or in person. By traveling together, we make the journey easier and more fun. An interesting study was done in which people were asked to assess how tall a mountain in the distance was and how difficult it would be to climb. Those looking at the mountain in the presence of others, or even while just thinking about a friend, saw it as smaller and more surmountable than those looking at it alone.

Just by reading this book, you have become part of a larger community of like-minded individuals who are determined to take back their power over their lives and bodies. You do this first by recognizing it is possible, and then by setting the intention to take daily actions to incorporate these skills and ideas into your life.

We must listen to the wisdom of our bodies and hearts. We must venture outside our self-created confines. We must offer kindness to our wounded selves, our wounded neighbors, community, and planet. We must reconnect the pieces of our bodies and lives with the golden balm of compassion, creating a work of beauty and meaning from the pain and suffering we have endured and survived. We must restore inner and outer balance.

By doing this we heal ourselves, our loved ones, and the planet. The inner critic in your head may say this sounds grandiose and impossible, yet science is pointing us toward this truth. As I heal, you heal. As you heal, so do those around you. We depend on each other.

Restoring balance is possible if we lean in and take the first steps. It is time to nourish the Wolf of Hope, Love, and Joy. She has been malnourished for far too long. Change starts with you. What one simple action can you take today, this week, this month, to create a ripple effect that benefits your mood and helps us all?

Notes

INTRODUCTION: THE UNRAVELING OF TRUTH

Chabris, C. F., and D. J. Simons. 2010. *The Invisible Gorilla: Thinking Clearly in a World of Illusions.* London: HarperCollins.

Chabris, C. F., and D. J. Simons. 2010. "The Invisible Gorilla." Video. https://tinyurl.com/2d29jw3.

Hampton, L. M., M. Daubresse, H. Chang, G. Alexander, and D. Budnitz. 2014. "Emergency Department Visits by Adults for Psychiatric Medication Adverse Events." *JAMA Psychiatry* 71(9): 1006–14. doi:10.1001/jamapsychiatry.2014.436.

Morris, Z. S., S. Wooding, and J. Grant. 2011. "The Answer Is 17 Years, What Is the Question: Understanding Time Lags in Translational Research." *Journal of the Royal Society of Medicine* 104(12): 510–20. doi:10.1258/jrsm.2011.110180.

1. DEBUNKING THE MYTH OF NEUROCHEMICAL IMBALANCE

Andrews, P. W., A. Bharwani, K. R. Lee, M. Fox, and J. A. Thomson Jr. 2015. "Is Serotonin an Upper or a Downer? The Evolution of the Serotonergic System and Its Role in Depression and the Antidepressant Response." *Neuroscience and Biobehavioral Reviews* 51, 164–88. doi:10.1016/j.neubiorev.2015.01.018. (This review of available evidence suggests it may be more likely that depression is related to higher, not lower, levels of serotonin.)

Belmaker, R. H., and Galila Agam. 2008. "Major Depressive Disorder." *New England Journal of Medicine* 358, 55–68. doi:10.1056/NEJMra073096. (References discussion on the lack of evidence "to identify the purported [neurochemical] deficiency reliably.")

Brach, T. 2012. Tara Brach blog. "Accepting Absolutely Everything." https://tinyurl.com/y39sje8k.

Celia, Frank. 2017. "Pharma Ups the Ante on DTC Advertising." Pharmaceutical Commerce, April 4, 2017. https://tinyurl.com/y4ce9ktd. (References the dramatic increase in spending on DTC advertisements.)

Coppen, A. 1967. "The Biochemistry of Affective Disorders." *British Journal of Psychiatry* 113(504): 1237–64. doi:10.1192/bjp.113.504.1237.

Davies, D., and M. Shepherd. 1955. "Reserpine in the Treatment of Anxious and Depressed Patients." *The Lancet* 266(6881): 117–20. doi:10.1016/s0140-6736(55)92118-8. (This study showed reserpine acts as antidepressant despite decreasing instead of increasing serotonin levels.)

France, C., P. Lysaker, and R. Robinson. 2007. "The 'Chemical Imbalance' Explanation for Depression: Origins, Lay Endorsement, and Clinical Implications." *Professional Psychology: Research and Practice* 38(4): 411–20. doi:10.1037/0735-7028.38.4.411.

Gaynes, Bradley N., Diane Warden, Madhukar H. Trivedi, Stephen R. Wisniewski, Maurizio Fava, and John Rush. 2009. "What Did STAR*D Teach Us? Results From a Large-Scale, Practical, Clinical Trial for Patients with Depression." *Psychiatric Services*, November 1, 2009. doi:10.1176/ps.2009.60.11.1439. (References the discussion on how virtually any drug with any mechanism of action has similar effect sizes on reducing depression.)

Kemp, Joshua J., James L. Lickel, and Brett J. Deacon. 2014. "Effects of a Chemical Imbalance Causal Explanation on Individuals' Perceptions of Their Depressive Symptoms." *Behaviour Research and Therapy* 56, 47–52. doi:10.1016/j.brat .2014.02.009.

Kuhn, R. 1958. "The Treatment of Depressive States with G 22355 (Imipramine Hydrochloride)." *American Journal of Psychiatry* 115(5): 459–64. doi:10.1176 /ajp.115.5.459.

Lacasse, Jeffrey R., and Jonathan Leo. 2005. "Serotonin and Depression: A Disconnect between the Advertisements and the Scientific Literature." *PLoS Medicine*, November 8, 2005. doi:10.1371/journal.pmed.0020392. (References discussion on how television ads for antidepressants effectively pathologized depression and promoted the neurochemical imbalance narrative.)

Lacasse, Jeffrey R., and Jonathan Leo. 2015. "Challenging the Narrative of Chemical Imbalance: A Look at the Evidence." In *Critical Thinking in Clinical Diagnosis and Assessment*, edited by B. Probst. New York: Springer, 275–82. https://tinyurl .com/y5aqewa4. (References discussion about responses by psychiatrists regarding neurochemical imbalance theory.)

Lieberman, J., Robert Golden, Scott Stroup, and Joseph McEvoy. 2000. "Drugs of the Psychopharmacological Revolution in Clinical Psychiatry." *Psychiatric Services*, October 1, 2000. doi:10.1176/appi.ps.51.10.1254.

Mendels, J., and A. Frazer. 1974. "Brain Biogenic Amine Depletion and Mood." *Archives of General Psychiatry* 30(4): 447–51. doi:10.1001/archpsyc.1974.01760100019004. (This study showed that reserpine, a medication that depletes levels of serotonin, only causes depression in about six percent of those taking it, contrary to the pillars of the neurochemical imbalance theory.)

Moncrieff, Joanna. 2008. "The Creation of the Concept of an Antidepressant: An Historical Analysis." *Social Science & Medicine* 66(2008): 2346–55. doi:10.1016/j.socscimed.2008.01.047.

Moncrieff, Joanna. 2009. *The Myth of the Chemical Cure: A Critique of Psychiatric Drug Treatment.* Basingstoke, UK: Palgrave Macmillan. pp. 122–25.

Moncrieff, Joanna, and David Cohen. 2006. "Do Antidepressants Cure or Create Abnormal Brain States?" *PLoS Medicine,* June 6, 2006. doi:10.1371/journal.pmed.0030240.

Pies, Ronald W. 2011. "Doctor, Is My Mood Disorder Due to a Chemical Imbalance?" *Psychiatric Times,* August 12, 2011. https://tinyurl.com/y3btgs77.

Pies, Ronald W. 2011. "Psychiatry's New Brain-Mind and the Legend of the 'Chemical Imbalance.'" *Psychiatric Times,* July 11, 2011. https://tinyurl.com/yxra9hw6.

Schildkraut, J. J. 1965. "The Catecholamine Hypothesis of Affective Disorders: A Review of Supporting Evidence." *American Journal of Psychiatry* 122(5): 509–22. doi:10.1176/ajp.122.5.509.

Valenstein, E. S. 2002. *Blaming the Brain: The Truth about Drugs and Mental Health.* New York: Free Press. pp. 24, 95, 180, 241. (References the "veritable chemical lobotomy" and the Eli Lilly handout.)

Whitaker, R. 2015. *Anatomy of an Epidemic: Magic Bullets, Psychiatric Drugs, and the Astonishing Rise of Mental Illness in America.* New York: Broadway Books. pp. 43–44, 60–74. (References the discussions on the history of mental illness, Roland Kuhn, James Maas, and the lack of evidence supporting association between depression and serotonin levels.)

2. THE POWER OF PLACEBO

Beecher, Henry K. 1955. "The Powerful Placebo." *Journal of the American Medical Association* 159(17): 1602–6. doi:10.1001/jama.1955.02960340022006.

Center for Drug Evaluation and Research. 1998. Application Number 20822 Administrative Documents/Correspondence. https://tinyurl.com/yxb6w6ht.

Cipriani, A., T. A. Furukawa, G. Salanti, A. Chaimani, L. Z. Atkinson, Y. Ogawa, S. Leucht, et al. 2018. "Comparative Efficacy and Acceptability of 21 Antidepressant Drugs for the Acute Treatment of Adults with Major Depressive Disorder: A Systematic Review and Network Meta-Analysis." *Lancet* 391(10128): 1357–66. doi:10.1016/S0140-6736(17)32802-7.

Cipriani, Andrea, Xinyi Zhou, Cinzia Del Giovane, Sarah E. Hetrick, Bin Qin, and Craig Whittington. 2016. "Comparative Efficacy and Tolerability of Antidepressants for Major Depressive Disorder in Children and Adolescents: A Network Meta-Analysis." *Lancet* 388(10047): 881–90. doi:10.1016/S0140-6736(16)30385-3. (This study found that only fluoxetine had any advantage over placebo for depressed adolescents.)

Doshi, Peter. 2015. "No Correction, No Retraction, No Apology, No Comment: Paroxetine Trial Reanalysis Raises Questions about Institutional Responsibility." *BMJ* 351. doi:10.1136/bmj.h4629. (Despite the FDA's conclusion that Study 329 was "a failed trial," the published article indicating otherwise was never retracted, and all those involved continue to hold high positions with AACAP.)

Ebrahim, S., S. Bance, A. Athale, C. Malachowski, and J. P. Ioannidis. 2016. "Meta-Analyses with Industry Involvement Are Massively Published and Report No Caveats for Antidepressants." *Journal of Clinical Epidemiology* 70, 155–63. doi:10.1016/j.jclinepi.2015.08.021. (References discussion about how the majority of published meta-analyses are written by authors financed by drug companies.)

Fournier, J. C., R. J. DeRubeis, S. D. Hollon, S. Dimidjian, J. D. Amsterdam, R. C. Shelton, and J. Fawcett. 2010. "Antidepressant Drug Effects and Depression Severity: A Patient-Level Meta-Analysis." *Journal of the American Medical Association* 303(1): 47–53. doi:10.1001/jama.2009.1943. (References meta-analysis concluding the effect size of antidepressants "nonexistent to negligible.")

Gaynes, Bradley N., Diane Warden, Madhukar H. Trivedi, Stephen R. Wisniewski, Maurizio Fava, and John Rush. 2009. "What Did STAR*D Teach Us? Results From a Large-Scale, Practical, Clinical Trial for Patients with Depression." *Psychiatric Services,* November 1, 2009. doi:10.1176/ps.2009.60.11.1439.

Greenberg, G. 2011. *Manufacturing Depression: The Secret History of a Modern Disease.* New York: Simon and Schuster. pp. 269–74. (References discussion on introduction of SSRIs to the market.)

Greenberg, R. P., R. F. Bornstein, M. D. Greenberg, and S. Fisher. 1992. "A Meta-Analysis of Antidepressant Outcome under 'Blinder' Conditions." *Journal of Consulting and Clinical Psychology* 60(5): 664–69. doi:10.1037//0022-006x.60.5.664.

Insel, T. R. 2009. "Disruptive Insights in Psychiatry: Transforming a Clinical Discipline." *Journal of Clinical Investigation,* April 1, 2009. doi:10.1172/JCI38832.

Jureidini, Jon N., Leemon B. McHenry, and Peter R. Mansfield. 2008. "Clinical Trials and Drug Promotion: Selective Reporting of Study 329." *International Journal of Risk & Safety in Medicine* 20(2008): 73–81. doi:10.3233/JRS-2008-0426. (Study finding that the majority of trials shift primary outcomes to make results appear more positive.)

Kaptchuk, T. J., E. Friedlander, J. M. Kelley, M. N. Sanchez, E. Kokkotou, J. P. Singer, M. Kowalczykowski, et al. 2010. "Placebos without Deception: A Randomized

Controlled Trial in Irritable Bowel Syndrome." *PLoS One* 5(12): e15591. doi:10.1371 /journal.pone.0015591.

Keller, Martin B., Neal D. Ryan, Michael Strober, Rachel G. Klein, Stan P. Kutcher, Boris Birmaher, Owen R. Hagino, et al. 2001. "Efficacy of Paroxetine in the Treatment of Adolescent Major Depression: A Randomized, Controlled Trial." *Journal of the American Academy of Child and Adolescent Psychiatry* 40(7): 762–72. https://tinyurl.com /yxhpuq4v. (The original publication of Study 329.)

Khan, Arif, James Faucett, Pesach Lichtenberg, Irving Kirsch, and Walter A. Brown. 2012. "A Systematic Review of Comparative Efficacy of Treatments and Controls for Depression." *PLoS One* 7(7): e41778. doi:10.1371/journal.pone.0041778.

Khan, M. A. 2000. "Symptom Reduction and Suicide Risk in Patients Treated with Placebo in Antidepressant Clinical Trials." *JAMA Psychiatry* 57(4): 311–17. doi:10.1001/archpsyc.57.4.311.

Khin, N. A., Y. F. Chen, Y. Yang, P. Yang, and T. P. Laughren. 2011. "Exploratory Analyses of Efficacy Data from Major Depressive Disorder Trials Submitted to the US Food and Drug Administration in Support of New Drug Applications." *Journal of Clinical Psychiatry* 72(4): 464–72. doi:10.4088/JCP.10m06191.

Kirsch, Irving, and Guy Sapirstein. 1998. "Listening to Prozac but Hearing Placebo: A Meta-Analysis of Antidepressant Medication." *Prevention & Treatment* 1:0002a. https://tinyurl.com/yxcludxp.

Kirsch, Irving, Brett J. Deacon, Tania B. Huedo-Medina, Alan Scoboria, Thomas J. Moore, and Blair T. Johnson. 2008. "Initial Severity and Antidepressant Benefits: A Meta-Analysis of Data Submitted to the Food and Drug Administration." *PLoS Medicine,* February 26, 2008. doi:10.1371/journal.pmed.0050045. (This study concluded that there seems "little evidence to support the use of antidepressants to any but the most severely depressed.")

Kirsch, Irving, Thomas J. Moore, Alan Scoboria, and Sarah S. Nicholls. 2002. "The Emperor's New Drugs: An Analysis of Antidepressant Medication Data Submitted to the U.S. Food and Drug Administration." *Prevention & Treatment* 5:23. https:// tinyurl.com/q2te8k9.

Kirsch, Irving. 2010. *The Emperor's New Drugs: Exploding the Antidepressant Myth.* New York: Basic Books. pp. 14, 18, 38.

Kocsis, James H., Alan J. Gelenberg, Barbara O. Rothbaum, Daniel N. Klein, Madhukar H. Trivedi, Rachel Manber, Martin B. Keller, et al. 2009. "Cognitive Behavioral Analysis System of Psychotherapy and Brief Supportive Psychotherapy for Augmentation of Antidepressant Nonresponse in Chronic Depression: The REVAMP Trial." *JAMA Psychiatry* 66(11): 1178–88. doi:10.1001/archgenpsychiatry.2009.144.

Kondro, Wayne. 2004. "Drug Company Experts Advised Staff to Withhold Data about SSRI Use in Children." *CMAJ* 170(5): 783. doi:10.1503/cmaj.1040213. (References the internal memo leaked from GSK to the *Canadian Medical Association Journal*.)

Locher, Cosima, Helen Koechlin, Sean R. Zion, Christoph Werner, Daniel S. Pine, Irving Kirsch, Ronald C. Kessler, and Joe Kossowsky. 2017. "Efficacy and Safety of Selective Serotonin Reuptake Inhibitors, Serotonin-Norepinephrine Reuptake Inhibitors, and Placebo for Common Psychiatric Disorders Among Children and Adolescents: A Systematic Review and Meta-Analysis." *JAMA Psychiatry,* August 30, 2017. doi:10.1001/jamapsychiatry.2017.2432. (2017 review that determined that none of the antidepressant medications [ADMs] offered any clinical advantage over placebo, yet increased suicidality and side effects.)

Mojtabai, R., and M. Olfson. 2010. "National Trends in Psychotropic Medication Polypharmacy in Office-Based Psychiatry." *Archives of General Psychiatry* 67(1): 26–36. doi:10.1001/archgenpsychiatry.2009.175.

Moseley, J. Bruce, Kimberly O'Malley, Nancy J. Petersen, Terri J. Menke, Baruch A. Brody, David H. Kuykendall, John C. Hollingsworth, et al. 2002. "A Controlled Trial of Arthroscopic Surgery for Osteoarthritis of the Knee." *New England Journal of Medicine* 347, 81–88. doi:10.1056/NEJMoa013259.

National Institute of Mental Health. n.d. "Antidepressant Medications for Children and Adolescents: Information for Parents and Caregivers." https://tinyurl.com/yc7thzhn.

Pigott, H E., A. M. Leventhal, G. S. Alter, and J. J. Boren. 2010. "Efficacy and Effectiveness of Antidepressants: Current Status of Research." *Psychotherapy and Psychosomatics* 79, 267–279. doi:10.1159/000318293. (References discussion about how pharmaceutical companies may conduct multiple trials in order to get two that meet clinical significance.)

Rabkin, J. G., J. S. Markowitz, J. Stewart, P. McGrath, W. Harrison, F. M. Quitkin, and D. F. Klein. 1986. "How Blind Is Blind? Assessment of Patient and Doctor Medication Guesses in a Placebo-Controlled Trial of Imipramine and Phenelzine." *Psychiatry Research* 19(1): 75–86. doi:10.1016/0165-1781(86)90094-6.

Reeves, R. R., M. E. Ladner, R. H. Hart, and R. S. Burke. 2007. "Nocebo Effects with Antidepressant Clinical Drug Trial Placebos." *General Hospital Psychiatry* 29(3): 275–77. doi:10.1016/j.genhosppsych.2007.01.010. (References the case study of Mr. A.)

Restoring Study 329. 2016. "Restoring Study 329: Scientific Integrity Through Data Based Medicine." https://study329.org. (References discussion about GSK's failed trials for use of Paxil in depressed kids, yet successful marketing attempts to suggest it was effective and safe.)

Rush, A. John, Madhukar H. Trivedi, Jonathan W. Stewart, Andrew A. Nierenberg, Maurizio Fava, Benji T. Kurian, Diane Warden, et al. 2011. "Combining Medications to Enhance Depression Outcomes (CO-MED): Acute and Long-Term Outcomes of a Single-Blind Randomized Study." *American Journal of Psychiatry,* July 1, 2011. doi:10.1176 /appi.ajp.2011.10111645.

Rush, A. J., M. H. Trivedi, S. R. Wisniewski, A. A. Nierenberg, J. W. Stewart, D. Warden, G. Niederehe, et al. 2006. "Acute and Longer-Term Outcomes in Depressed Outpatients Requiring One or Several Treatment Steps: A STAR*D Report. *American Journal of Psychiatry* 163(11): 1905–17. doi:10.1176/ajp.2006.163.11.1905.

Sifferlin, Alexandra. 2018. "These Antidepressants Are Most Effective, Study Says." *Time,* February 21, 2018. https://tinyurl.com/yxerydlp.

Sinyor, M., A. J. Levitt, A. H. Cheung, A. Schaffer, A. Kiss, Y. Dowlati, and K. L. Lanctôt. 2010. "Does Inclusion of a Placebo Arm Influence Response to Active Antidepressant Treatment in Randomized Controlled Trials? Results from Pooled and Meta-Analyses." *Journal of Clinical Psychiatry* 71(3): 270–79. doi:10.4088/JCP.08r04516blu.

Turner, Erick H., Annette M. Matthews, Eftihia Linardatos, Robert A. Tell, and Robert Rosenthal. 2008. "Selective Publication of Antidepressant Trials and Its Influence on Apparent Efficacy." *New England Journal of Medicine* 358, 252–60. doi:10.1056 /NEJMsa065779.

United States *v.* GlaxoSmithKline. 2011. U.S. District Court for the District of Massachusetts. CA No. 11-10398-RWZ. https://tinyurl.com/y584ybmz.

Valenstein, Elliot S. 2002. *Blaming the Brain: The Truth about Drugs and Mental Health.* New York: Free Press. p. 177.

Whitaker, Robert. 2015. *Anatomy of an Epidemic: Magic Bullets, Psychiatric Drugs, and the Astonishing Rise of Mental Illness in America.* New York: Broadway Books. p. 155.

Whittington, Craig J., Tim Kendall, Peter Fonagy, David Cottrell, Andrew Cotgrove, and Ellen Boddington. 2004. "Selective Serotonin Reuptake Inhibitors in Childhood Depression: Systematic Review of Published versus Unpublished Data." *Lancet* 363, 1341–45. https://tinyurl.com/y5em7dpf.

Zimmerman, M., M. A. Posternak, and I. Chelminski. 2002. "Symptom Severity and Exclusion from Antidepressant Efficacy Trials." *Journal of Clinical Psychopharmacology* 22(6): 610–14. doi:10.1097/00004714-200212000-00011. (References the fact that 70 percent of people started on ADMs are mildly to moderately depressed and unlikely to be helped by ADMs.)

3. The Cost of a Quick Fix

Andrade, Chittaranjan. 2017. "Antidepressant Exposure during Pregnancy and Risk of Autism in the Offspring, 1: Meta-Review of Meta-Analyses." *Journal of Clinical*

Psychiatry 78(8): e1052–56. doi:10.4088/JCP.17f11916. (Review of six studies found increased risk of autism in offspring of women on ADMs during pregnancy.)

Andrews, Paul W., J. Anderson Thomson Jr., Ananda Amstadtre, and Michael C. Neale. 2012. "Primum Non Nocere: An Evolutionary Analysis of Whether Antidepressants Do More Harm than Good." *Frontiers in Psychology,* April 24, 2012. doi:10.3389 /fpsyg.2012.00117.

Andrews, Paul W., Susan G. Kornstein, Lisa J. Halberstadt, Charles O. Gardner, and Michael C. Neale. 2011. "Blue Again: Perturbational Effects of Antidepressants Suggest Monoaminergic Homeostasis in Major Depression." *Frontiers in Psychology* 2:159. doi:10.3389/fpsyg.2011.00159. https://tinyurl.com/y4wpucl9. (References discussion on how SSRIs drastically shift serotonin levels, leading to imbalance and an increased risk of relapse.)

Bérard, Anick, Jin-Ping Zhao, and Odile Sheehy. 2017. "Antidepressant Use during Pregnancy and the Risk of Major Congenital Malformations in a Cohort of Depressed Pregnant Women: An Updated Analysis of the Quebec Pregnancy Cohort." *BMJ Open,* January 12, 2017. doi:10.1136/bmjopen-2016-013372. (2017 study concluding that ADMs increase the risk of potential fetal malformations.)

Boseley, S. 1999. "They Said It Was Safe." *Guardian,* October 29, 2009. https://tinyurl .com/yyqkyfbr. (References discussion about Eli Lilly's tactics to bury data regarding the risks of agitation, suicidal ideation, and even psychosis caused by fluoxetine, including reference to internal memos documenting the very issues they continue to refute, and their flawed meta-analysis designed to refute evidence of these risks.)

Boukhris, Takoua, Odile Sheehy, and Laurent Mottron. 2016. "Antidepressant Use during Pregnancy and the Risk of Autism Spectrum Disorder in Children." *JAMA Pediatrics* 170(2): 117–24. doi:10.1001/jamapediatrics.2015.3356. (Study finding an 87 percent increased risk for autism associated with use of ADMs during pregnancy.)

Brauser, Deborah. 2014. "Antidepressants Blunt Sexual Function, Feelings of Love." *Medscape,* October 20, 2014. https://tinyurl.com/y28fswvh.

Breggin, Peter R. 2004. "Suicidality, Violence and Mania Caused by Selective Serotonin Reuptake Inhibitors (SSRIs): A Review and Analysis." *International Journal of Risk & Safety in Medicine* 16, 31–49. https://tinyurl.com/y3zv6fcg. (References discussion about documents disclosed during litigation with Eli Lilly revealing increased risk of activation symptoms and suicidality on fluoxetine, and later notes a 1995 study finding a 3.5-fold greater risk of suicidality for those on SSRIs.)

Cartwright, Claire, Kerry Gibson, John Read, Ondria Cowan, and Tamsin Dehar. 2016. "Long-Term Antidepressant Use: Patient Perspectives of Benefits and Adverse Effects." *Dovepress* 2016, 1401–7. doi:10.2147/PPA.S110632. (References discussion on side effects of ADMs, including weight gain and emotional numbing.)

Carvalho, Andre F., Manu Sharma, Andre Russowsky Brunoni, and Eduard Vieta. 2016. "The Safety, Tolerability and Risks Associated with the Use of Newer Generation Antidepressant Drugs: A Critical Review of the Literature." *Psychotherapy and Psychosomatics* 85(5): 270–88. doi:10.1159/000447034. (References discussion on SSRIs and cardiovascular risks.)

Cole, Jonathan O. 1964. "Therapeutic Efficacy of Antidepressant Drugs: A Review." *JAMA* 190(5): 448–55. doi:10.1001/jama.1964.03070180046007. (Early studies suggested most depressions are "self-limited.")

Cosgrove, L. 2011. "Antidepressants and Breast and Ovarian Cancer Risk: A Review of the Literature and Researchers' Financial Associations with Industry." *PLoS One,* April 6, 2011. doi:10.1371/journal.pone.0018210. (Study found increased risk of breast and ovarian cancer for those on ADMs.)

Donavan, Stuart, Richard Madeley, Andrew Clayton, Min Beeharry, Sheron Jones, Chris Kirk, Keith Waters, et al. 2000. "Deliberate Self-Harm and Antidepressant Drugs: Investigation of a Possible Link." *British Journal of Psychiatry* 177, 551–56. https://tinyurl.com/y6j8zxc6. (Study found four- to sixfold increased risk of self-harm on fluoxetine.)

Downing, Nicholas S., Nilay D. Shah, Jenerius A. Aminawung, Alison M. Pease, Jean-David Zeitoun, Harlan M. Krumholz, and Joseph S. Ross. 2017. "Postmarket Safety Events Among Therapeutics Approved by the FDA." *JAMA* 317(18): 1854–63. doi:10.1001/jama.2017.5150.

Eli Lilly. n.d. "Prozac (Fluoxetine Hydrochloride) Capsules Label." https://tinyurl .com/y54vkfrv.

El-Mallakh, Rif S., Yonglin Gao, and R. Jeannie Roberts. 2011. "Tardive Dysphoria: The Role of Long-Term Antidepressant Use in Inducing Chronic Depression." *Medical Hypotheses* 2011. doi:10.1016/j.mehy.2011.01.020. (References studies dating back to the 1990s that first raised the possibility that ADMs may act over time as pro-depressants.)

Fava, G. A., A. Gatti, C. Belaise, J. Guidi, and E. Offidani. 2015. "Withdrawal Symptoms after Selective Serotonin Reuptake Inhibitor Discontinuation: A Systematic Review." *Psychotherapy and Psychosomatics* 84(2): 72–81. doi:10.1159/000370338. (Review found three-quarters of those who choose to taper off meds experience withdrawal.)

Fava, Giovanni A. 1994. "Do Antidepressant and Antianxiety Drugs Increase Chronicity in Affective Disorders?" *Psychotherapy and Psychosomatics* 61, 125–31. https:// tinyurl.com/yxzn26so.

Ferguson, J. M. 2001. "SSRI Antidepressant Medication: Adverse Effects and Tolerability." *Primary Care Companion to the Journal of Clinical Psychiatry* 3(1): 22–27. doi:10.4088/pcc.v03n0105. (References discussion on side effects, including sexual dysfunction and weight gain.)

Frankenfield, Diane L., Susan P. Baker, W. Robert Lange, Yale H. Caplan, and John E. Smialek. 2004. "Fluoxetine and Violent Death in Maryland." *Forensic Science International* 64(2–3): 107–17. doi:10.1016/0379-0738(94)90220-8.

Gafoor, Rafael, Helen P. Booth, and Martin C. Gulliford. 2018. "Antidepressant Utilisation and Incidence of Weight Gain During 10 Years' Follow-Up: Population Based Cohort Study." *BMJ* 361. doi:10.1136/bmj.k1951. (2018 study finding that ADMs increase weight gain by 21 percent.)

Gartlehner, G., R. A. Hansen, L. C. Morgan, K. Thaler, L. Lux, M. Van Noord, and U. Mager. 2011. "Comparative Benefits and Harms of Second-Generation Antidepressants for Treating Major Depressive Disorder: An Updated Meta-Analysis." *Annals of Internal Medicine* 155(11): 772–85. doi:10.7326/0003-4819-155-11-201112060-00009.

Geffen, E. C., S. W. Wal, R. V. Hulten, M. C. Groot, A. C. Egberts, and E. R. Heerdink. 2007. "Evaluation of Patients' Experiences with Antidepressants Reported by Means of a Medicine Reporting System." *European Journal of Clinical Pharmacology* 63(12): 1193–99. doi:10.1007/s00228-007-0375-4.

Gibson, Jack E., Richard B. Hubbard, Christopher J. P. Smith, Laila J. Tata, John R. Britton, and Andrew W. Fogarty. 2009. "Use of Self-Controlled Analytical Techniques to Assess the Association between Use of Prescription Medications and the Risk of Motor Vehicle Crashes." *American Journal of Epidemiology* 169(6): 761–68. doi:10.1093/aje/kwn364.

GlaxoSmithKline. 2006. "Important Prescribing Information." https://tinyurl.com/y4c67x53.

Goldberg, David, Martin Privett, Bedirhan Ustun, Greg Simon, and Michael Linden. 1998. "The Effects of Detection and Treatment on the Outcome of Major Depression in Primary Care: A Naturalistic Study in 15 Cities." *British Journal of General Practice* 48, 1840–44. https://tinyurl.com/yxuz52jr. (This study found that those who remain on ADMs have increased risk of chronic severe illness.)

Grigoriadis, Sophie, Emily H. VonderPorten, Lana Mamisashvili, George Tomlinson, Cindy-Lee Dennis, Gideon Koren, Meir Steiner, et al. 2014. "Prenatal Exposure to Antidepressants and Persistent Pulmonary Hypertension of the Newborn: Systematic Review and Meta-Analysis." *BMJ* 348. doi:10.1136/bmj.f6932.

Hammad, Tarek A. 2006. "Suicidality in Pediatric Patients Treated With Antidepressant Drugs." *Archives of General Psychiatry* 63, 332–39. https://tinyurl.com/y4ruet8l.

Hengartner, M P., and W. Rössler. 2018. "Antidepressant Use Prospectively Relates to a Poorer Long-Term Outcome of Depression: Results from a Prospective Community Cohort Study over 30 Years." *Psychotherapy and Psychosomatics* 87:181–83. doi:10.1159/000488802. (A researcher at the NIMH in the 1970s declared that most episodes of depression "run their course and terminate with virtually complete recovery without specific intervention.")

Hilzenrath, David S. 2016. "FDA Depends on Industry Funding; Money Comes with 'Strings Attached.'" POGO, December 1, 2018. https://tinyurl.com/y4dx9jbd.

Hughes, Shannon, David Cohen, and Rachel Jaggi. 2014. "Differences in Reporting Serious Adverse Events in Industry-Sponsored Clinical Trial Registries and Journal Articles on Antidepressant and Antipsychotic Drugs: A Cross-Sectional Study." *BMJ Open* 4(7): e005535. doi:10.1136/bmjopen-2014-005535.

Huybrechts, Krista F., Brian T. Bateman, Kristin Palmsten, Rishi J. Desai, Elisabetta Patorno, Chandrasekar Gopalakrishnan, Raisa Levin, et al. 2015. "Antidepressant Use Late in Pregnancy and Effects on Newborn." *JAMA* 313(21): 2142–51. doi:10.1001/jama.2015.5605. (References discussion about increased risk of PPHN when ADMs are taken during last trimester of pregnancy.)

Jakobsen, Janus Christian, Kiran Kumar Katakam, Anne Schou, Signe Gade Hellmuth, Sandra Elkjær Stallknecht, Katja Leth-Møller, Maria Iversen, et al. 2017. "Selective Serotonin Reuptake Inhibitors versus Placebo in Patients with Major Depressive Disorder: A Systematic Review with Meta-Analysis and Trial Sequential Analysis." *BMC Psychiatry*, February 8, 2017. https://tinyurl.com/ha8hmnm.

Jung, Woo-Young, Sae-Heon Jang, Sung-Gon Kim, Young-Myo Jae, Bo-Geum Kong, Ho-Chan Kim, Byeong-Moo Choe, Jeong-Gee Kim, and Choong-Rak Kim. 2016. "Times to Discontinue Antidepressants Over 6 Months in Patients with Major Depressive Disorder." *Psychiatry Investigation* 13(4): 440–46. doi:10.4306/pi.2016.13.4.440.

Jureidini, John, Leemon McHenry, and Peter R. Mansfield. 2008. "Clinical Trials and Drug Promotion: Selective Reporting of Study 329." *The International Journal of Risk & Safety in Medicine* 203233(1): 73–81. doi:10.3233/JRS-2008-0426. (References a discussion about how GSK deleted all side effects except for headaches from the final draft of a published paper, conveniently leaving out worsening depression, emotional liability, and hostility as possible consequences.)

Le Noury, Joanna, John M. Nardo, David Healy, Jon Jureidini, Melissa Raven, Catalin Tufanaru, and Elia Abi-Jaoude. 2015. "Restoring Study 329: Efficacy and Harms of Paroxetine and Imipramine in Treatment of Major Depression in Adolescence." *BMJ* 351. doi:10.1136/bmj.h4320. (References a discussion about how increased risk of suicidality and other psychiatric symptoms among adolescents on paroxetine were removed from a published study.)

Levinson-Castiel, Rachel, Paul Merlob, Nehama Linder, Lea Sirota, and Gil Klinger. 2006. "Neonatal Abstinence Syndrome After In Utero Exposure to Selective Serotonin Reuptake Inhibitors in Term Infants." *Archives of Pediatric & Adolescent Medicine* 160(2): 173–76. doi:10.1001/archpedi.160.2.173.

Llamas, Michelle. 2019. "SSRIs Taken During Pregnancy Increase Autism Risk." DrugWatch. https://tinyurl.com/y2kscllt. (Study found a 200 percent increased risk of autism for offspring of women on sertraline or paroxetine during pregnancy.)

Mauney, Matt. 2008. "SSRIs and Birth Defects." DrugWatch. https://tinyurl.com /ybgssy7g. (References the birth-defect lawsuits settled by GSK in 2010.)

Merikangas, Kathleen R., Robert Jin, Jian-Ping He, Ronald C. Kessler, Sing Lee, Nancy A. Sampson, Maria Carmen Viana, et al. 2011. "Prevalence and Correlates of Bipolar Spectrum Disorder in the World Mental Health Survey Initiative." *JAMA Psychiatry* 68(3): 241–51. doi:10.1001/archgenpsychiatry.2011.12. (Americans have the highest rate of bipolar diagnosis among eleven countries surveyed in this study.)

Mosholder, Andrew D., and Mary Willy. 2006. "Suicidal Adverse Events in Pediatric Randomized, Controlled Clinical Trials of Antidepressant Drugs Are Associated with Active Drug Treatment: A Meta-Analysis." *Journal of Child and Adolescent Psychopharmacology* 16:1–2. doi:10.1089/cap.2006.16.25.

Ostrow, Laysha, Lauren Jessell, Manton Hurd, Sabrina M. Darrow, and David Cohen. 2017. "Discontinuing Psychiatric Medications: A Survey of Long-Term Users." *Psychiatric Services,* July 17, 2017. doi:10.1176/appi.ps.201700070. (Despite the challenges of withdrawal symptoms, the majority of those who discontinue ADMs are grateful to have done so.)

Patten, Scott B. 2004. "The Impact of Antidepressant Treatment on Population Health: Synthesis of Data from Two National Data Sources in Canada." *Population Health Metrics* 2:9. doi:10.1186/1478-7954-2-9. (WHO study determined those on meds fared worse over time.)

Pigott, H. Edmund, Allan M. Leventhal, Gregory S. Alter, and John J. Boren. 2010. "Efficacy and Effectiveness of Antidepressants: Current Status of Research." *Psychotherapy and Psychosomatics* 79(5): 267–79. doi:10.1159/000318293. (References discussion on side effects of ADMs, including doubling the risk of diabetes. Also addresses poor outcomes of the STAR*D trial.)

Posternak, M. A., and I. Miller. 2001. "Untreated Short-Term Course of Major Depression: A Meta-Analysis of Outcomes from Studies Using Wait-List Control Groups." *Journal of Affective Disorders* 66(2–3): 139–46. doi:10.1016/s0165-0327(00)00304-9. (Meta-analysis found that 85 percent of depressed patients recovered from depression without interventions and that those started on ADMs fared worse over time.)

Posternak, Michael A., David A. Solomon, Andrew C. Leon, Timothy I. Mueller, Tracie Shea, Jean Endicott, and Martin B. Keller. 2006. "The Naturalistic Course of Unipolar Major Depression in the Absence of Somatic Therapy." *Journal of Nervous and Mental Disorders* 194, 324–29. https://tinyurl.com/yxttw5kz. (Study found that those started on ADMs fared worse over time.)

Preda, Adrian, Rebecca W. MacLean, Carolyn M. Mazure, and Malcolm B. Bowers Jr. 2001. "Antidepressant-Associated Mania and Psychosis Resulting in Psychiatric Admissions." *Journal of Clinical Psychiatry* 62, 30–33. https://tinyurl.com

/y4t3kcr6. (Study finding that 8 percent of psychiatric admissions are likely due to ADM-induced mania.)

Price, J., V. Cole, and G. M. Goodwin. 2009. "Emotional Side-Effects of Selective Serotonin Reuptake Inhibitors: Qualitative Study." *British Journal of Psychiatry* 195(3): 211–17. doi:10.1192/bjp.bp.108.051110.

Ramsey, Lydia, and Lauren F. Friedman, 2016. "The Government Agency in Charge of Approving Drugs Gets a Surprising Amount of Money from the Companies that Make Them." *Business Insider,* August 17, 2016. https://tinyurl.com/ybv9aj8j. (Three-quarters of the FDA's budget is funded by pharmaceutical companies they are supposed to oversee.)

Reefhuis, Jennita, Owen Devine, Jan M. Friedman, Carol Louik, and Margaret A. Honein. 2015. "Specific SSRIs and Birth Defects: Bayesian Analysis to Interpret New Data in the Context of Previous Reports." *BMJ* 351. doi:10.1136/bmj.h3190. (CDC study finding increased risk of birth defects for women on paroxetine and fluoxetine.)

Richardson, Kathryn, Chris Fox, Ian Maidment, Nicholas Steel, Yoon K. Loke, Antony Arthur, Phyo K Myint, et al. 2018. "Anticholinergic Drugs and Risk of Dementia: Case-Control Study." *BMJ* 361. doi:10.1136/bmj.k1315.

Roest, Annelieke M., Peter De Jonge, Craig D. Willams, and Ymkje Anna de Vries. 2015. "Reporting Bias in Clinical Trials Investigating the Efficacy of Second-Generation Antidepressants in the Treatment of Anxiety Disorders: A Report of 2 Meta-Analyses." *JAMA Psychiatry* 72. doi:10.1001/jamapsychiatry.2015.15.

Rosenbaum, J. F., M. Fava, S. L. Hoog, R. C. Ascroft, and W. B. Krebs. 1988. "Discontinuation-Emergent Signs and Symptoms (DESS) Scale." *Biological Psychiatry* 44(2): 77–87. https://tinyurl.com/y3kvkbvh. doi:10.1016/s0006-3223(98)00126-7.

Rush, A. John, Madhukar Trivedi, Thomas J. Carmody, Melanie M. Biggs, Kathy Shores-Wilson, Hisham Ibrahim, and M. Lynn Crismon. 2004. "One-Year Clinical Outcomes of Depressed Public Sector Outpatients: A Benchmark for Subsequent Studies." *Biological Psychiatry* 56(1): 46–53. https://tinyurl.com/y5hjdb8s. doi:10.1016/j.biopsych.2004.04.005. (Another study demonstrating that those on ADMs fare worse over time.)

Salvi, Virginio, Ilaria Grua, Giancarlo Cerveri, Claudio Mencacci, and Francesco Barone-Adesi. 2017. "The Risk of New-Onset Diabetes in Antidepressant Users: A Systematic Review and Meta-Analysis." *PLoS One,* July 31, 2017. doi:10.1371/journal.pone.0182088.

Sharma, Tarang, Louise Schow Guski, Nanna Freund, and Peter C. Gøtzsche. 2016. "Suicidality and Aggression during Antidepressant Treatment: Systematic Review and Meta-Analyses Based on Clinical Study Reports." *BMJ* 352. doi:10.1136/bmj.i65. (Data indicates that for adolescents and young adults, ADMs double the risk of suicidality and aggression.)

Smoller, Jordan W., Matthew Allison, Barbara B. Cochrane, J. David Curb, Roy H. Perlis, Jennifer G. Robinson, Milagros C. Rosal, et al. 2009. "Antidepressant Use and Risk of Incident Cardiovascular Morbidity and Mortality Among Postmenopausal Women in the Women's Health Initiative Study." *JAMA Internal Medicine* 169(22): 2128–39. doi:10.1001/archinternmed.2009.436.

Tarn, Derjung M., Debora A. Paterniti, Richard L. Kravitz, John Heritage, Honghu Liu, Sue Kim, and Neil S. Wenger. 2008. "How Much Time Does It Take to Prescribe a New Medication?" *Patient Counselling and Health Education* 72(2): 311–19. doi:10.1016/j.pec.2008.02.019.

Teicher, M., C. Glod, and J. O. Cole. 1990. "Emergence of Intense Suicidal Preoccupation during Fluoxetine Treatment." *American Journal of Psychiatry* 147(2): 207–10. doi:10.1176/ajp.147.2.207. (Case study at Harvard evaluating six patients who became violently suicidal on fluoxetine.)

U.S. Food and Drug Administration. 2011. "FDA Drug Safety Communication: Abnormal Heart Rhythms Associated with High Doses of Celexa (Citalopram Hydrobromide)." https://tinyurl.com/y5x9zl3d.

Valenstein, M., H. M. Kim, D. Ganoczy, J. F. McCarthy, K. Zivin, K. L. Austin, K. Hoggatt, et al. "Higher-Risk Periods for Suicide among VA Patients Receiving Depression Treatment: Prioritizing Suicide Prevention Efforts." *Journal of Affective Disorders* 112(1–3): 50–58. doi:10.1016/j.jad.2008.08.020. (Study found that for the first four months after starting a new ADM, the risk of suicide was doubled, just like in younger populations.)

Vedantam, Shankar. 2004. "FDA Urged Withholding Data on Antidepressants: Makers Were Dissuaded From Labeling Drugs as Ineffective in Children." *Washington Post,* September 10, 2004. https://tinyurl.com/3qroho.

Whitaker, R. 2017. "Antidepressants/Depression." Mad in America, April 12, 2015. https://tinyurl.com/y5xqn6ds.

Wu, C. S., S. S. Gau, and M. S. Lai. 2014. "Long-Term Antidepressant Use and the Risk of Type 2 Diabetes Mellitus: A Population-Based, Nested Case-Control Study in Taiwan." *Journal of Clinical Psychiatry* 75(1): 31–38. doi:10.4088/JCP .13m08421. (References a discussion on how the risk of diabetes is greatest in those on ADMs under age forty.)

4. Getting to the Roots

American Institute of Stress. 2017. "What Is Stress?" https://tinyurl.com/yxd69cp4.

Anda, Robert F. David W. Brown, Vincent J. Felitti, J. Douglas Bremner, Shanta R. Dube, and Wayne H. Giles. 2007. "Adverse Childhood Experiences and Prescribed Psychotropic Medications in Adults." *American Journal of Preventive Medicine*

32(5): 389–94. doi:10.1016/j.amepre.2007.01.005. (This study documents the link between ACE scores and rates of prescribed psychiatric medications.)

Arana, G. W., R. Baldessarini, and M. Ornsteen. 1985. "The Dexamethasone Suppression Test for Diagnosis and Prognosis in Psychiatry. Commentary and Review." *Archives of General Psychiatry* 42(12): 1193–204. doi:10.1001/archpsyc.1985.01790350067012.

Bowers, Mallory E., and Rachel Yehuda. 2016. "Intergenerational Transmission of Stress in Humans." *Neuropsychopharmacology* 41(1): 232–44. doi:10.1038/npp.2015.247.

Cosgrove, Lisa, and Sheldon Krimsky. 2012. "A Comparison of DSM-IV and DSM-5 Panel Members' Financial Associations with Industry: A Pernicious Problem Persists." *PLoS Medicine,* March 13, 2012. doi:10.1371/journal.pmed.1001190.

Crum, Alia J., Modupe Akinolab, Ashley Martinb, and Sean Fath. 2017. "The Role of Stress Mind-Set in Shaping Cognitive, Emotional, and Physiological Responses to Challenging and Threatening Stress." *Anxiety, Stress, & Coping* 2017. https://tinyurl.com/y4py5vu5. doi:10.1080/10615806.2016.1275585.

Danese, Andrea, Carmine M. Pariante, Avshalom Caspi, Alan Taylor, and Richie Poulton. 2007. "Childhood Maltreatment Predicts Adult Inflammation in a Life-Course Study." *Proceedings of the National Academy of Sciences USA* 104(4): 1319–24. doi:10.1073/pnas.0610362104.

Dube, Shanta R., Robert F. Anda, Vincent J. Felitti, Daniel P. Chapman, David F. Williamson, and Wayne H. Giles. 2001. "Childhood Abuse, Household Dysfunction, and the Risk of Attempted Suicide Throughout the Lifespan: Findings From the Adverse Childhood Experiences Study." *JAMA* 286(24): 3089–96. doi:10.1001/jama.286.24.3089. (This study documents the links between ACE scores and depression, suicide, and other mental health issues.)

Esernio-Jenssen, Debra, Angelo Giardino, Randell Alexander, Jonathan D. Thackeray, and David Chadwick. 2014. *Chadwick's Child Maltreatment: Sexual Abuse and Psychological Maltreatment,* Volume 2, 4th edition. St. Louis: STM Learning.

Felitti, Vincent J., Robert F. Anda, Dale Nordenberg, David F. Williamson, Alison M. Spitz, Valerie Edwards, Mary P. Koss, and James S. Marks. 1998. "Relationship of Childhood Abuse and Household Dysfunction to Many of the Leading Causes of Death in Adults." *American Journal of Preventive Medicine* 14(4): 245–58. doi:10.1016/S0749-3797(98)00017-8. (This is the original ACE study.)

Felitti, Vincent. 2018. "Adverse Childhood Experiences and Their Repressed Relationship to Adult Well-Being, Disease and Death." Lecture presented at Close-Up on the Effects of Childhood Trauma on the Family Conference, Akron, Ohio, April 2018.

Frances, Allen J., and Thomas Widiger. 2011. "Psychiatric Diagnosis: Lessons from the DSM-IV Past and Cautions for the DSM-5 Future." *Annual Review of*

Clinical Psychology 8, 109–130. https://tinyurl.com/y563z5t3. doi:10.1146 /annurev-clinpsy-032511-143102.

Goldstein, Ellen, Ninad Athale, Andrés F. Sciolla, and Sheryl L. Catz. 2017. "Patient Preferences for Discussing Childhood Trauma in Primary Care." *Permanente Journal* 21:16–055. doi:10.7812/TPP/16-055.

Greenberg, Rebecca. 2018. "Suicide Deaths Climb Dramatically in U.S., Nearly Double for Women." *Psychiatric News*, June 28, 2018. doi:10.1176/appi.pn.2018.7a24.

Hedegaard, Holly, Sally C. Curtin, and Margaret Warner. 2018. "National Center for Health Statistics." CDC NCHS Data Brief No. 309, June 2018. https://tinyurl .com/y6forxwh.

Horwitz, Allan, Jerome C. Wakefield, and Lorenzo Lorenzo-Luaces. 2016. "History of Depression." In *The Oxford Handbook of Mood Disorders,* edited by Robert J. DeRubeis and Daniel R. Strunk. New York: Oxford. pp. 1–24. doi:10.1093/oxfordhb /9780199973965.013.2.

Kandel, Eric R. 1998. "A New Intellectual Framework for Psychiatry." *American Journal of Psychiatry,* April 1, 1998. doi:10.1176/ajp.155.4.457.

Keller, A., K. Litzelman, L. E. Wisk, T. Maddox, E. R. Cheng, P. D. Creswell, and W. P. Witt. "Does the Perception That Stress Affects Health Matter? The Association with Health and Mortality." *Health Psychology* 31(5): 677–84. doi:10.1037/a0026743.

Kendler, Kenneth S., Charles O. Gardner, and Carol A. Prescott. 2002. "Toward a Comprehensive Developmental Model for Major Depression in Women." *American Journal of Psychiatry,* July 1, 2002. doi:10.1176/appi.ajp.159.7.1133. (This study followed twins for nine years and confirms that the likelihood of depression is not associated with genetics but a history of childhood trauma.)

Khandaker, Golam M., Rebecca M. Pearson, Stanley Zammit, Glyn Lewis, and Peter B. Jones. 2014. "Association of Serum Interleukin 6 and C-Reactive Protein in Childhood With Depression and Psychosis in Young Adult Life: A Population-Based Longitudinal Study." *JAMA Psychiatry* 71(10): 1121–28. doi:10.1001/jamapsychiatry .2014.1332.

Lê-Scherban, Félice, Xi Wang, Kathryn H. Boyle-Steed, and Lee M. Pachter. 2018. "Intergenerational Associations of Parent Adverse Childhood Experiences and Child Health Outcomes." *Pediatrics* 141:6. https://tinyurl.com/y2ml8pcb.

McClinton Appollis, T., C. Lund, P. J. de Vries, and C. Mathews. 2015. "Adolescents' and Adults' Experiences of Being Surveyed about Violence and Abuse: A Systematic Review of Harms, Benefits, and Regrets." *American Journal of Public Health* 105(2): e32–45. doi:10.2105/AJPH.2014.302293.

McGonigal, Kelly. 2015. *The Upside of Stress: Why Stress Is Good for You, and How to Get Good at It.* New York: Avery.

Nanni, Valentina, Rudolf Uher, and Andrea Danese. 2012. "Childhood Maltreatment Predicts Unfavorable Course of Illness and Treatment Outcome in Depression: A Meta-Analysis." *American Journal of Psychiatry,* February 1, 2012. doi:10.1176/appi .ajp.2011.11020335.

Qato, Dima Mazen, Katharine Ozenberger, and Mark Olfson. 2018. "Prevalence of Use of Prescription Medication With Depression as a Potential Adverse Effect." *JAMA* 319(22): 2289–98. doi:10.1001/jama.2018.6741.

Raison, Charles L., and Andrew H. Miller. 2003. "When Not Enough Is Too Much: The Role of Insufficient Glucocorticoid Signaling in the Pathophysiology of Stress-Related Disorders." *American Journal of Psychiatry* 160(9): 1554–65. https:// tinyurl.com/y2ct2w2m.

Solomon, Andrew. 2016. "History." In *The Noonday Demon: An Atlas of Depression,* 285–34. New York: Scribner. (References a discussion on Hippocrates' description of melancholia.)

University of California, Los Angeles. n.d. "Grand Challenges: Understanding, Preventing and Treating the World's Greatest Health Problem." https://tinyurl.com /y4kqlgyd.

Varnekar, Vrinda. n.d. "The Thomas Theorem of Sociology Explained with Examples." PsycholoGenie. https://tinyurl.com/y3brfv4a.

Whitfield, Charles L. 2003. *The Truth about Depression: Choices in Healing Mental Illness.* Deerfield Beach, FL: Health Communications. (This book discusses the hundreds of studies linking ACE scores and mental illness.)

Winfrey, Oprah. 2018. "Treating Childhood Trauma." *60 Minutes,* March 11, 2018. https://tinyurl.com/y8pr6agr.

Yang, Bao-Zhu, Huiping Zhang, Wenjing Ge, Natalie Weder, Heather Douglas-Palumberi, Francheska Perepletchikova, Joel Gelernter, and Joan Kaufman. 2013. "Child Abuse and Epigenetic Mechanisms of Disease Risk." *American Journal of Preventive Medicine* 44(2): 101–7. doi:10.1016/j.amepre.2012.10.012.

Yehuda, R., and L. M. Bierer. 2008. "Transgenerational Transmission of Cortisol and PTSD Risk." *Progress in Brain Research* 167:121–35. doi:10.1016/S0079-6123(07)67009-5.

PART 2. IS THERE ANOTHER WAY?

Kirksey, Kellie N. 2018. "Journey Series." In *Poetry, Prose and Miscellaneous Musings* 18:1. Xlibris.

5. CALL OF THE IMAGINATION

Apostolo, João Luís Apóstolo, and Katharine Kolcaba. 2008. "The Effects of Guided Imagery on Comfort, Depression, Anxiety, and Stress of Psychiatric Inpatients with Depressive Disorders." *Archives of Psychiatric Nursing* 23(6): 403–11. doi:10.1016/j.apnu.2008.12.003. (This study demonstrates how imagery improved depression for psychiatric inpatients.)

Cleveland Clinic Wellness. n.d. "Stress Free Now: The Science of Guided Imagery." https://tinyurl.com/yxlxh7qu.

Krpan, Katherine M., Ethan Kross, Marc G. Berman, Patricia J. Deldin, Mary K. Askren, and John Jonides. 2013. "An Everyday Activity as a Treatment for Depression: The Benefits of Expressive Writing for People Diagnosed with Major Depressive Disorder." *Journal of Affective Disorders* 150(3): 1148–51. doi:10.1016/j.jad.2013.05.065.

McTaggart, Lynne. 2013. *The Intention Experiment: Using Your Thoughts to Change Your Life and the World.* New York: Atria.

McTaggart, Lynne. 2017. *The Power of Eight: The Miraculous Healing Power of Small Groups.* New York: Atria.

Muraven, M., and R. F. Baumeister. "Self-regulation and Depletion of Limited Resources: Does Self-control Resemble a Muscle?" *Psychological Bulletin* 126(2): 247–59. doi:10.1037/0033-2909.126.2.247.

Naparstek, Belleruth. 1995. *Staying Well with Guided Imagery.* New York: Wellness Central. pp. 19–20. (References the benefits of guided imagery and study on how perceptions shift response to poison ivy.)

O'Craven, K. M., and N. Kanwisher. 2000. "Mental Imagery of Faces and Places Activates Corresponding Stimulus-Specific Brain Regions." *Journal of Cognitive Neuroscience* 12(6): 1013–23. doi:10.1162/08989290051137549.

Parnell, Laurel. 2014. "Proceedings of Transforming Trauma with EMDR." Omega Institute, Rhinebeck, NY.

Ranganathan, Vinoth, Vlodek Siemionow, Jing Z. Liu, Vinod Sahga, and Guang H. Yue. 2004. "From Mental Power to Muscle Power—Gaining Strength by Using the Mind." *Neuropsychologia* 42(7): 944–56. doi:10.1016/j.neuropsychologia.2003.11.018.

Statistic Brain Research Institute. "New Years Resolution Statistics." 2018. https://tinyurl.com/yxakgfkk.

Stone, Jon, and Michael Smollin. 1971. *The Monster at the End of This Book.* New York: Golden Books.

Young, Kathy. n.d. "Intentionality vs. Resolution." Be Intentional. https://tinyurl.com/y3k73k2e.

6. The Breath as an Anchor

Brown, Richard P., and Patricia Gerbarg. 2012. *The Healing Power of the Breath: Simple Techniques to Reduce Stress and Anxiety, Enhance Concentration, and Balance Your Emotions.* Boston: Shambhala. (References discussion on *pranayama* and research on its healing effects on mind and body.)

Janakiramaiah, N., B. Gangadhar, P. Naga, M. Harish, D. Subbakrishna, and A. Vedamurthachar. 2000. "Antidepressant Efficacy of Sudarshan Kriya Yoga (SKY) in Melancholia: A Randomized Comparison with Electroconvulsive Therapy (ECT) and Imipramine." *Journal of Affective Disorders* 57(1–3): 255–59. doi:10.1016 /s0165-0327(99)00079-8. (Study found yogic breathing as efficacious as an antidepressant.)

Kean, Sam. 2017. "The Last Breath." In *Caesar's Last Breath: Decoding the Secrets of the Air around Us,* 1–10. New York: Little, Brown and Company.

Koch, Christof. 2016. "Sleeping with Half a Brain." *Scientific American,* September 1, 2016. https://tinyurl.com/y2xy77jy.

Ma, Xiao, Zi-Qi Yue, Zhu-Qing Gong, Hong Zhang, Nai-Yue Duan, Yu-Tong Shi, Gao-Xia Wei, and You-Fa Li. 2017. "The Effect of Diaphragmatic Breathing on Attention, Negative Affect and Stress in Healthy Adults." *Frontiers in Psychology* 8, 874. doi:10.3389/fpsyg.2017.00874.

Priya, Mithuna. 2016. "What Is the Average Number of Breaths in an Average Lifetime?" Quora, August 23, 2016. https://tinyurl.com/y4upmm3r.

Salyers, Michelle P., Candice Hudson, Gary Morse, Angela L. Rollins, Maria Monroe-DeVita, Cynthia Wilson, and Leah Freeland. 2011. "BREATHE: A Pilot Study of a One-Day Retreat to Reduce Burnout Among Mental Health Professionals." *Psychiatric Services* 6(2): 214–17. doi:10.1176/appi.ps.62.2.214.

Schünemann, H. J., J. Dorn, B. J. Grant, W. Winkelstein Jr., and M. Trevisan. 2000. "Pulmonary Function Is a Long-term Predictor of Mortality in the General Population: 29-Year Follow-up of the Buffalo Health Study." *Chest* 118(3): 656–64. doi:10.1378 /chest.118.3.656. (Study found that breathing patterns predict longevity.)

Siegel, Daniel J. 2011. "Minding the Brain." In *Mindsight: The New Science of Personal Transformation,* 14–22. New York: Bantam Books.

Vranich, Belisa. 2016. "How Bad Is It, Doc?" In *Breathe: The Simple, Revolutionary 14-day Program to Improve Your Mental and Physical Health,* 22–29. New York: St. Martin's Griffin. (References data on the benefits of breathing and how nine out of ten people breathe incorrectly.)

Werntz, D. A., R. G. Bickford, and D. Shannahoff-Khalsa. 1987. "Selective Hemispheric Stimulation by Unilateral Forced Nostril Breathing." *Human Neurobiology* 6(3): 165–71. https://tinyurl.com/yycltsuc.

7. THE MIND AS MASTER STORYTELLER

Brach, Tara. 2018. "Transforming Two Fears: FOF and FOMO." Podcast. https://tinyurl .com/y28lqycv.

Carmody, James, Sybil Crawford, Elena Salmoirago-Blotcher, Katherine Leung, Linda Churchill, and Nicholas Olendzki. 2012. "Mindfulness Training for Coping with Hot Flashes: Results of a Randomized Trial." *Menopause* 18(6): 611–20. doi:10.1097/gme.0b013e318204a05c.

Creswell, J. D., A. A. Taren, E. K. Lindsay, C. M. Greco, P. J. Gianaros, A. Fairgrieve, A. L. Marsland, et al. 2016. "Alterations in Resting-State Functional Connectivity Link Mindfulness Meditation With Reduced Interleukin-6: A Randomized Controlled Trial." *Biological Psychiatry* 80(1): 53–61. doi:10.1016/j.biopsych.2016.01.008.

Epel, Elissa, Jennifer Daubenmier, Judith T. Moskowitz, Susan Folkman, and Elizabeth Blackburn. 2011. "Can Meditation Slow Rate of Cellular Aging? Cognitive Stress, Mindfulness, and Telomeres." *Annals of the New York Academy of Sciences,* 2011. doi:10.1111/j.1749-6632.2009.04414.x.

Gotink, R. A., R. Meijboom, M. W. Vernooij, M. Smits, and M. G. Hunink. 2016. "8-Week Mindfulness Based Stress Reduction Induces Brain Changes Similar to Traditional Long-Term Meditation Practice: A Systematic Review." *Brain and Cognition* 108, 32–41. doi:10.1016/j.bandc.2016.07.001.

Greeson, Jeffrey M. 2009. "Mindfulness Research Update: 2008." *Complementary Health Practice Review* 14(1): 10–18. doi:10.1177/1533210108329862.

Hanh, Thich Nhat. 1988. *The Sun My Heart: Reflections on Mindfulness, Concentration, and Insight.* Berkeley, CA: Parallax Press.

Harris, Dan. 2018. "Susan Piver: Buddhist Wisdom for Modern Relationships." *Ten Percent Happier.* Podcast. https://tinyurl.com/yxcg8cot.

Hernández, Quintana, Ibáñez Fernández, García Rodríguez Jr, and JR Hernández. 2014. "Efectos de un programa de intervención neuropsicológica basado en mindfulness sobre la enfermedad de Alzheimer: ensayo clínico aleatorizado a doble ciego." [Effects of a Neuropsychology Program Based on Mindfulness on Alzheimer's Disease: Randomized Double-Blind Clinical Study.] *Revista Espanola de Geriatria y Gerontologia* 49(4): 165–72. doi:10.1016/j.regg.2014.03.002.

Hilton, L., S. Hempel, B. A. Ewing, E. Apaydin, L. Xenakis, S. Newberry, B. Colaiaco, et al. 2017. "Mindfulness Meditation for Chronic Pain: Systematic Review and Meta-Analysis." *Annals of Behavioral Medicine* 51(2): 199–213. doi:10.1007/s12160-016-9844-2.

Hölzel, B. K., J. Carmody, M. Vangel, C. Congleton, S. M. Yerramsetti, T. Gard, and S. W. Lazar. 2011. "Mindfulness Practice Leads to Increases in Regional Brain Gray Matter Density." *Psychiatry Research* 191(1): 36–43. doi:10.1016/j.pscychresns.2010.08.006.

Kabat-Zinn, J., E. Wheeler, T. Light, A. Skillings, M. J. Scharf, T. G. Cropley, D. Hosmer, and J. D. Bernhard. 1998. "Influence of a Mindfulness Meditation-Based Stress Reduction Intervention on Rates of Skin Clearing in Patients with Moderate to Severe

Psoriasis Undergoing Phototherapy (UVB) and Photochemotherapy (PUVA)." *Psychosomatic Medicine* 60(5): 625–32. doi:10.1097/00006842-199809000-00020.

Keng, S. L., M. J. Smoski, and C. J. Robins. 2011. "Effects of Mindfulness on Psychological Health: A Review of Empirical Studies." *Clinical Psychology Review* 31(6): 1041–56. doi:10.1016/j.cpr.2011.04.006.

Khoury, B., T. Lecomte, G. Fortin, M. Masse, P. Therien, V. Bouchard, M. A. Chapleau, et al. 2013. "Mindfulness-Based Therapy: A Comprehensive Meta-Analysis." *Clinical Psychology Review* 33(6): 763–71. doi:10.1016/j.cpr.2013.05.005.

Kuyken, W., F. C. Warren, R. S. Taylor, B. Whalley, C. Crane, G. Bondolfi, R. Hayes, et al. 2016. "Efficacy of Mindfulness-Based Cognitive Therapy in Prevention of Depressive Relapse: An Individual Patient Data Meta-Analysis From Randomized Trials." *JAMA Psychiatry* 73(6): 565–74. doi:10.1001/jamapsychiatry.2016.0076.

Lazar, S. W., C. E. Kerr, R. H. Wasserman, J. R. Gray, D. N. Greve, M. T. Treadway, M. McGarvey, et al. 2005. "Meditation Experience Is Associated with Increased Cortical Thickness." *Neuroreport* 16(17): 1893–97. doi:10.1097/01.wnr.0000186598.66243.19.

Luders, Eileen, Nicolas Cherbuin, and Christian Gaser. 2016. "Estimating Brain Age Using High-Resolution Pattern Recognition: Younger Brains in Long-Term Meditation Practitioners." *NeuroImage* 134, 508–13. https://tinyurl.com/y4vb9ame. doi:10.1016/j.neuroimage.2016.04.007.

MacKenzie, Meagan B., Kayleigh A. Abbott, and Nancy L. Kocovski. 2018. "Mindfulness-Based Cognitive Therapy in Patients with Depression: Current Perspectives." *Neuropsychiatric Disease and Treatment* 14, 1599–1605. doi:10.2147/NDT.S160761.

Martin, Ralph. 2006. *The Fulfillment of All Desire: A Guidebook for the Journey to God Based on the Wisdom of the Saints,* 121. Steubenville, OH: Emmaus Road.

Menke, Andreas, Dominik Lehrieder, Jasmin Fietz, Carolin Leistner, Catherina Wurst, Saskia Stonawski, Jannika Reitz, et al. 2018. "Childhood Trauma Dependent Anxious Depression Sensitizes HPA Axis Function." *Psychoneuroendocrinology* 98, 22–29. doi:10.1016/j.psyneuen.2018.07.025.

Mrazek, M. D., J. Smallwood, and J. W. Schooler. 2012. "Mindfulness and Mind-Wandering: Finding Convergence through Opposing Constructs." *Emotion* 12(3): 442–48. doi:10.1037/a0026678. (This study found that even eight minutes of mindfulness can improve memory and focus.)

Orsillo, Susan, and Lizabeth Roemer. 2011. *The Mindful Way through Anxiety.* New York: Guilford Press, 196–98.

Panahi, Faeze, and Mahbobeh Faramarzi. 2016. "The Effects of Mindfulness-Based Cognitive Therapy on Depression and Anxiety in Women with Premenstrual Syndrome." *Depression Research and Treatment,* 2016. doi:10.1155/2016/9816481.

Pickert, Kate. 2014. "The Art of Being Mindful: Finding Peace in a Stressed-Out, Digitally Dependent Culture May Just Be a Matter of Thinking Differently." *Time*, February 3, 2014, 40–46.

Ray, Indranill Basu, Arthur R. Menezes, Pavan Malur, Aimee E. Hiltbold, John P. Reilly, and Carl J. Lavie. 2014. "Meditation and Coronary Heart Disease: A Review of the Current Clinical Evidence." *Ochsner Journal* 14(4): 696–703. https://tinyurl.com/yxf9ukj8.

Rosenkranz, M. A., R. J. Davidson, D. G. Maccoon, J. F. Sheridan, N. H. Kalin, and A. Lutz. 2013. "A Comparison of Mindfulness-Based Stress Reduction and an Active Control in Modulation of Neurogenic Inflammation." *Brain, Behavior, and Immunity* 27(1): 174–84. doi:10.1016/j.bbi.2012.10.013.

Rubia, K. 2009. "The Neurobiology of Meditation and Its Clinical Effectiveness in Psychiatric Disorders." *Biological Psychology* 82(1): 1–11. doi:10.1016/j.biopsycho.2009.04.003.

Santarnecchi, Emiliano, Sicilia D'Arista, Eutizio Egiziano, Concetta Gardi, Roberta Petrosino, Giampaolo Vatti, Mario Reda, and Alessandro Rossi. 2014. "Interaction between Neuroanatomical and Psychological Changes after Mindfulness-Based Training." *PLoS One* 9(10): e108359. https://tinyurl.com/yxm6ku6h.

Segal, Z. V., S. Kennedy, M. Gemar, K. Hood, R. Pedersen, and T. Buis. 2006. "Cognitive Reactivity to Sad Mood Provocation and the Prediction of Depressive Relapse." *Archives of General Psychiatry* 63(7): 749–55. doi:10.1001/archpsyc.63.7.749.

Taren, A. A., P. J. Gianaros, C. M. Greco, E. K. Lindsay, A. Fairgrieve, K. W. Brown, R. K. Rosen, et al. 2015. "Mindfulness Meditation Training Alters Stress-Related Amygdala Resting State Functional Connectivity: A Randomized Controlled Trial." *Social Cognitive and Affective Neuroscience* 10(12): 1758–68. doi:10.1093/scan/nsv066.

Teasdale, J. D., Z. V. Segal, J. M. Williams, V. A. Ridgeway, J. M. Soulsby, and M. A. Lau. 2000. "Prevention of Relapse/Recurrence in Major Depression by Mindfulness-Based Cognitive Therapy." *Journal of Consulting and Clinical Psychology* 68(4): 615–23. doi:10.1037//0022-006x.68.4.615.

Williams, Mark, John Teasdale, Zindel Segal, and Jon Kabat-Zinn. 2007. *The Mindful Way through Depression: Freeing Yourself from Chronic Unhappiness.* New York: Guilford Press.

8. The Body as Navigator

de Jong, Marasha, Sara W. Lazar, Kiran Hug, Wolf E. Mehling, Britta K. Hölzel, Alexander T. Sack, Frenk Peeters, et al. 2016. "Effects of Mindfulness-Based Cognitive Therapy on Body Awareness in Patients with Chronic Pain and Comorbid Depression." *Frontiers in Psychology* 7, 967. doi:10.3389/fpsyg.2016.00967.

Kraft, T. L., and S. D. Pressman. 2012. "Grin and Bear It: The Influence of Manipulated Facial Expression on the Stress Response." *Psychological Science* 23(11): 1372–78. doi:10.1177/0956797612445312.

Michalak, J., J. Mischnat, and T. Teismann. 2014. "Sitting Posture Makes a Difference—Embodiment Effects on Depressive Memory Bias." *Clinical Psychology and Psychotherapy* 21(6): 519–24. doi:10.1002/cpp.1890.

Online Etymology Dictionary. 2019. s.v. "emotion." https://tinyurl.com/y6tf2slx.

Pert, Candace B. 1997. *Molecules of Emotion: Why You Feel the Way You Feel.* New York: Scribner, 187–89.

Strack, F., L. L. Martin, and S. Stepper. 1988. "Inhibiting and Facilitating Conditions of the Human Smile: A Nonobtrusive Test of the Facial Feedback Hypothesis." *Journal of Personality and Social Psychology* 54(5): 768–77. doi:10.1037//0022-3514.54.5.768.

Thera, Nyanaponika. 2010. "The Anger-Eating Demon." *Wisdom Quarterly: American Buddhist Journal,* December 31, 2010. https://tinyurl.com/y3wqso5f.

Veenstra, L., I. K. Schneider, and S. L. Koole. 2017. "Embodied Mood Regulation: The Impact of Body Posture on Mood Recovery, Negative Thoughts, and Mood-Congruent Recall." *Cognition & Emotion* 31(7): 1361–76. doi:10.1080/02699931.2016.1225003.

Weintraub, Amy. 2004. *Yoga for Depression: A Compassionate Guide to Relieve Suffering through Yoga.* New York: Broadway Books. p. 80.

Williams, Mark, John Teasdale, Zindel Segal, and Jon Kabat-Zinn. 2007. *The Mindful Way through Depression: Freeing Yourself from Chronic Unhappiness.* New York: Guilford Press.

9. Moving the Body

Alderman, B. L., R. L. Olson, C. J. Brush, and T. J. Shors. 2016. "MAP Training: Combining Meditation and Aerobic Exercise Reduces Depression and Rumination While Enhancing Synchronized Brain Activity." *Translational Psychiatry* 6, e726. doi:10.1038/tp.2015.225.

Babyak, M., J. A. Blumenthal, S. Herman, P. Khatri, M. Doraiswamy, K. Moore, W. E. Craighead, et al. 2000. "Exercise Treatment for Major Depression: Maintenance of Therapeutic Benefit at 10 Months." *Psychosomatic Medicine* 62(5): 633–8. doi:10.1097/00006842-200009000-00006. (The SMILE studies found exercise more effective than ADMs at reducing depression and preventing relapses.)

Basso, Julia C., and Wendy A. Suzuki. 2017. "The Effects of Acute Exercise on Mood, Cognition, Neurophysiology, and Neurochemical Pathways: A Review." *Brain Plasticity* 2, 127–152. https://tinyurl.com/y2sm4zk7. doi:10.3233/BPL-160040.

Brown, Robert S., Donald E. Ramirez, and John M. Taub. 1978. "The Prescription of Exercise for Depression." *The Physician and Sportsmedicine* 6(12): 34–45. doi:10.1080/00913847.1978.11710794.

Chu, I. H., W. L. Wu, I. M. Lin, Y. K. Chang, Y. J. Lin, and P. C. Yang. 2017. "Effects of Yoga on Heart Rate Variability and Depressive Symptoms in Women: A Randomized Controlled Trial." *Journal of Alternative and Complementary Medicine* 23(4): 310–16. doi:10.1089/acm.2016.0135.

Diaz, Keith M., Virginia J. Howard, Brent Hutto, Natalie Colabianchi, John E. Vena, Monika M. Safford, Steven N. Blair, and Steven P. Hooker. 2017. "Patterns of Sedentary Behavior and Mortality in U.S. Middle-Aged and Older Adults: A National Cohort Study." *Annals of Internal Medicine* 167(7): 465–75. doi:10.7326/M17-0212. (This study concludes that excessive sedentary behaviors increase the risk of obesity, heart disease, diabetes, cancer, depression, and death.)

Doyne, Elizabeth J., Deborah J. Ossip-Klein, Eric D. Bowman, Kent M. Osborn, Ilona B. McDougall-Wilson, and Robert A. Neimeyer. 1987. "Running Versus Weight Lifting in the Treatment of Depression." *Journal of Consulting and Clinical Psychology* 55(5): 748–54. https://tinyurl.com/y66yrfxe.

Farmer, M. E., B. Z. Locke, E. K. Mościcki, A. L. Dannenberg, D. B. Larson, and L. S. Radloff. 1988. "Physical Activity and Depressive Symptoms: The NHANES I Epidemiologic Follow-up Study." *American Journal of Epidemiology* 128(6): 1340–51. doi:10.1093/oxfordjournals.aje.a115087. (This study found that lack of exercise doubles the risk of depression.)

Greist, John H., Marjorie H. Klein, Roger R. Eischens, John Faris, Alan S. Gurman, and William P. Morgan. 1979. "Running as Treatment for Depression." *Comprehensive Psychiatry* 20(1): 41–54. doi:10.1016/0010-440x(79)90058-0.

Harvey, Samuel B., Simon Øverland, Stephani L. Hatch, Simon Wessely, Arnstein Mykletun, and Matthew Hotopf. 2017. "Exercise and the Prevention of Depression: Results of the HUNT Cohort Study." *American Journal of Psychiatry* 175(1): 28–36. doi:10.1176/appi.ajp.2017.16111223. (The HUNT study demonstrates that one hour of exercise weekly can reduce risk of depression.)

Hoffman, Erik. n.d. Mapping the Brains Activity after Kriya Yoga." HAA International Retreat Center. https://tinyurl.com/yydur2vt.

Janakiramaiah, N., B. N. Gangadhar, P. J. Naga Venkatesha Murthy, M. G. Harish, D. K. Subbakrishna, and A. Vedamurthachar. 2000. "Antidepressant Efficacy of Sudarshan Kriya Yoga (SKY) in Melancholia: A Randomized Comparison with Electroconvulsive Therapy (ECT) and Imipramine." *Journal of Affective Disorders* 57(1–3): 255–59. doi:10.1016/s0165-0327(99)00079-8.

Keeney, Bradford. 2007. *Shaking Medicine: The Healing Power of Ecstatic Movement.* Rochester, VT: Destiny.

Kim, Youngwon, and Gregory J. Welk. 2015. "Characterizing the Context of Sedentary Lifestyles in a Representative Sample of Adults: A Cross-Sectional Study from the Physical Activity Measurement Study Project." *BMC Public Health* 15, 1218. doi:10.1186/s12889-015-2558-8.

Mandolesi, Laura, Arianna Polverino, Simone Montuori, Francesca Foti, Giampaolo Ferraioli, Pierpaolo Sorrentino, and Giuseppe Sorrentino. 2018. "Effects of Physical Exercise on Cognitive Functioning and Well-Being: Biological and Psychological Benefits." *Frontiers in Psychology* 9, 509. doi:10.3389/fpsyg.2018.00509. (References research demonstrating that exercise changes the structure and function of the brain.)

Martinsen, E., A. Hoffart, and O. Solberg. 1989. "Comparing Aerobic with Nonaerobic Forms of Exercise in the Treatment of Clinical Depression: A Randomized Trial." *Comprehensive Psychiatry* 30(4): 324–31. doi:10.1016/0010-440x(89)90057-6.

Prathikanti, Sudha, Renee Rivera, Ashly Cochran, Jose Gabriel Tungol, Nima Fayaz-manesh, and Eva Weinmann. 2017. "Treating Major Depression with Yoga: A Prospective, Randomized, Controlled Pilot Trial." *PLoS One,* March 16, 2017. doi:10.1371/journal.pone.0173869.

Ross, Alyson, and Sue Thomas. 2010. "The Health Benefits of Yoga and Exercise: A Review of Comparison Studies." *Journal of Alternative and Complementary Medicine* 16:1. doi:10.1089/acm.2009.0044.

Scutti, Susan. 2017. "Yes, Sitting Too Long Can Kill You, Even If You Exercise." CNN Health, September 12, 2017. https://tinyurl.com/y7umjdza.

Smith, Jonathan C. 1975. "Meditation as Psychotherapy: A Review of the Literature." *Psychological Bulletin* 82(4): 558–64. doi.org/10.1037/h0076888. (References a study comparing yoga to meditation and a combination of both.)

Sturt, David, and Todd Norstrom. 2015. "Is Sitting the New Smoking?" *Forbes,* January 13, 2015. https://tinyurl.com/yxlyw32a.

Suzuki, Wendy. 2017. "The Brain-Changing Benefits of Exercise." TED Ed. Video. https://tinyurl.com/y3hkskwd.

van der Kolk, Bessel. 2014. *The Body Keeps the Score: Mind, Brain and Body in the Transformation of Trauma.* New York: Viking. (References research on the benefits of yoga for depression and PTSD.)

Vollbehr, Nina K., H. J. Rogier Hoenders, Agna A. Bartels-Velthuis, and Brian D. Ostafin. 2017. "The Effects of Yoga for Depression." Center for Integrative Psychiatry, Groningen, Netherlands. https://tinyurl.com/yygu7wgv.

10. Nourishing the Body

Akbaraly, T. N., E. J. Brunner, J. E. Ferrie, M. G. Marmot, M. Kivimaki, and A. Singh-Manoux. 2009. "Dietary Pattern and Depressive Symptoms in Middle Age." *British Journal of Psychiatry* 195(5): 408–13. doi:10.1192/bjp.bp.108.058925.

Al-Karawi, D., D. A. Al Mamoori, and Y. Tayyar. 2015. "The Role of Curcumin Administration in Patients with Major Depressive Disorder: Mini Meta-Analysis of Clinical Trials." *Phytotherapy Research* 30(2): 175–83. doi:10.1002/ptr.5524.

Bădescu, S. V., C. Tătaru, L. Kobylinska, E. L. Georgescu, D. M. Zahiu, A. M. Zăgrean, and L. Zăgrean. 2016. "The Association between Diabetes Mellitus and Depression." *Journal of Medicine and Life* 9(2): 120–25. https://tinyurl.com/y24fkuvv.

Bested, A. C., A. C. Logan, and E. M. Selhub. 2013. "Intestinal Microbiota, Probiotics and Mental Health: From Metchnikoff to Modern Advances: Part II—Contemporary Contextual Research." *Gut Pathogens* 5(1): 3. doi:10.1186/1757-4749-5-3.

Buettner, Dan. 2015. *The Blue Zones Solution: Eating and Living Like the World's Healthiest People*. Washington, DC: National Geographic.

Coppen, A., and C. Bolander-Gouaille. 2005. "Treatment of Depression: Time to Consider Folic Acid and Vitamin B_{12}." *Journal of Psychopharmacology* 19(1): 59–65. doi:10.1177/0269881105048899.

Ferdman, Roberto A. 2015. "The Most American Thing There Is: Eating Alone." *Washington Post*, August 18, 2015. https://tinyurl.com/yykqzfe7.

Gangwisch, J. E., L. Hale, L. Garcia, E. Malaspina, M. G. Opler, M. E. Payne, R. C. Rossom, and D. Lane. 2015. "High Glycemic Index Diet as a Risk Factor for Depression: Analyses from the Women's Health Initiative." *American Journal of Clinical Nutrition* 102(2): 454–63. doi:10.3945/ajcn.114.103846.

Glerup, H., K. Mikkelsen, L. Poulsen, E. Hass, S. Overbeck, J. Thomsen, P. Charles, and E. F. Eriksen. 2001. "Commonly Recommended Daily Intake of Vitamin D Is Not Sufficient If Sunlight Exposure Is Limited." *Journal of Internal Medicine* 247(2): 260–68. doi:10.1046/j.1365-2796.2000.00595.x.

Grosso, Giuseppe, Fabio Galvano, Stefano Marventano, Michele Malaguarnera, Claudio Bucolo, Filippo Drago, and Filippo Caraci. 2014. "Omega-3 Fatty Acids and Depression: Scientific Evidence and Biological Mechanisms." *Oxidative Medicine and Cellular Longevity*, March 18, 2014. doi:10.1155/2014/313570.

Hallahan, B., J. R. Hibbeln, J. M. Davis, and M. R. Garland. 2007. "Omega-3 Fatty Acid Supplementation in Patients with Recurrent Self-Harm: Single-Centre Double-Blind Randomised Controlled Trial." *British Journal of Psychiatry* 190, 118–22. doi:10.1192/bjp.bp.106.022707. (This study showed that omega-3 reduced depressive symptoms, suicidality, and perception of stress.)

Harris, Herbert W., Pranay Jaiswal, Valerie Holmes, Richard H. Weisler, and Ashwin A. Patkar. 2013. "Vitamin D Deficiency and Psychiatric Illness." *Current Psychiatry* 12(4): 18–27. https://tinyurl.com/yxnzhjvp.

Holick, M. F. 2007. "Vitamin D Deficiency." *New England Journal of Medicine* 357(3): 266–81. doi:10.1056/NEJMra070553.

International Food Information Council Foundation. 2012. "2012 Food and Health Survey: Consumer Attitudes toward Food Safety, Nutrition and Health." May 23, 2012. https://tinyurl.com/yycq66d5.

Isaak, C. K., and Y. L. Siow. 2013. "The Evolution of Nutrition Research." *Canadian Journal of Physiology and Pharmacology* 91(4): 257–67. doi:10.1139/cjpp-2012 -0367.

Jacka, Felice N., A. Mykletun, M. Berk, I. Bjelland, and G. S. Tell. 2011. "The Association between Habitual Diet Quality and the Common Mental Disorders in Community-Dwelling Adults: The Hordaland Health Study." *Psychosomatic Medicine* 73(6): 483–90. doi:10.1097/PSY.0b013e318222831a. (This study found the SAD diet is associated with a 50 percent increased risk of depression.)

Jacka, Felice N., Adrienne O'Neil, Rachelle Opie, Catherine Itsiopoulos, Sue Cotton, Mohammedreza Mohebbi, David Castle, et al. 2017. "A Randomised Controlled Trial of Dietary Improvement for Adults with Major Depression (the 'SMILES' Trial)." *BMC Medicine,* January 30, 2017. https://tinyurl.com /yybvaglv. (The SMILES trial found that nutritional education improved depressive symptoms.)

Jacka, Felice N., Nicolas Cherbuin, Kaarin J. Anstey, Perminder Sachdev, and Peter Butterworth. 2015. "Western Diet Is Associated with a Smaller Hippocampus: A Longitudinal Investigation." *BMJ Medicine,* September 8, 2015. https://tinyurl. com/y3anln7e.

Jacka, Felice N., S. Overland, R. Stewart, G. S. Tell, I. Bjelland, and A. Mykletun. 2009. "Association between Magnesium Intake and Depression and Anxiety in Community-Dwelling Adults: The Hordaland Health Study." *Australian and New Zealand Journal of Psychiatry* 43(1): 45–52. doi:10.1080/00048670802534408.

Khalid, S., C. M. Williams, and S. A. Reynolds. 2017. "Is There an Association between Diet and Depression in Children and Adolescents? A Systematic Review." *British Journal of Nutrition* 116(12): 2097–2108. doi:10.1017/S0007114516004359.

Kim, J., and J. Kim. 2018. "Green Tea, Coffee, and Caffeine Consumption Are Inversely Associated with Self-Report Lifetime Depression in the Korean Population." *Nutrients* 10(9): e1201. doi:10.3390/nu10091201.

LaChance, Laura R., and Drew Ramsey. 2018. "Antidepressant Foods: An Evidence-Based Nutrient Profiling System for Depression." *World Journal of Psychiatry* 8(3): 97–104. doi:10.5498/wjp.v8.i3.97.

Lansdowne, A. T., and S. C. Provost. 1998. "Vitamin D$_3$ Enhances Mood in Healthy Subjects during Winter." *Psychopharmacology (Berl.)* 135(4): 319–23. doi:10.1007/ s002130050517.

Larrieu, T., and S. Layé. 2018. "Food for Mood: Relevance of Nutritional Omega-3 Fatty Acids for Depression and Anxiety." *Frontiers in Physiology* 9, 1047. doi:10.3389/fphys.2018.01047.

Lewis, M. D., J. R. Hibbeln, J. E. Johnson, Y. H. Lin, D. Y. Hyun, and J. D. Loewke. 2011. "Suicide Deaths of Active Duty U.S. Military and Omega-3 Fatty Acid Status: A Case Control Comparison." *Journal of Clinical Psychiatry* 72(12): 1585–90. doi:10.4088/JCP.11m06879.

Liang, S., X. Wu, and F. Jin. 2018. "Gut-Brain Psychology: Rethinking Psychology from the Microbiota-Gut-Brain Axis." *Frontiers in Integrative Neuroscience* 12, 33. doi:10.3389/fnint.2018.00033.

Liu, Lu, and Gang Zhu. 2018. "Gut-Brain Axis and Mood Disorder." *Frontiers in Psychiatry* 9, 233. doi:10.3389/fpsyt.2018.00223.

Lopresti, A. L., and P. D. Drummond. 2016. "Efficacy of Curcumin, and a Saffron/Curcumin Combination for the Treatment of Major Depression: A Randomised, Double-Blind, Placebo-Controlled Study." *Journal of Affective Disorders* 207, 188–96. doi:10.1016/j.jad.2016.09.047.

Lu, K., M. A. Gray, C. Oliver, D. T. Liley, B. J. Harrison, C. F. Bartholomeusz, K. L. Phan, and P. J. Nathan. 2004. "The Acute Effects of L-Theanine in Comparison with Alprazolam on Anticipatory Anxiety in Humans." *Human Psychopharmacology* 19(7): 457–65. doi:10.1002/hup.611.

Mocking, R. J., I. Harmsen, J. Assies, M. Koeter, H. Ruhé, and A. Schene. 2016. "Meta-Analysis And Meta-Regression of Omega-3 Polyunsaturated Fatty Acid Supplementation for Major Depressive Disorder." *Translational Psychiatry* 6, e756. doi:10.1038/tp.2016.29. (Analysis suggests higher concentrations of EPA are most beneficial for depression.)

New Hampshire Department of Health and Human Services. 2014. "How Much Sugar Do You Eat? You May Be Surprised!" https://tinyurl.com/y5zyzyyp.

Nobre, A. C., A. Rao, and G. N. Owen. 2008. "L-Theanine, a Natural Constituent in Tea, and Its Effect on Mental State." *Asia Pacific Journal of Clinical Nutrition* 17(Suppl. 1): 167–8. https://tinyurl.com/y85c4ntm.

Opie, R. S., C. Itsiopoulos, N. Parletta, A. Sanchez-Villegas, T. N. Akbaraly, A. Ruusunen, and F. N. Jacka. 2017. "Dietary Recommendations for the Prevention of Depression." *Nutritional Neuroscience* 20(3): 161–71. doi:10.1179/1476830515Y.0000000043.

Papanikolaou, Yanni, James Brooks, Carroll Reider, and Victor L. Fulgoni. 2014. "U.S. Adults Are Not Meeting Recommended Levels for Fish and Omega-3 Fatty Acid Intake: Results of an Analysis Using Observational Data from NHANES 2003–2008." *Nutrition Journal* 13, 31. doi:10.1186/1475-2891-13-31.

Penckofer, Sue, Joanne Kouba, Mary Byrn, and Carol Estwing Ferrans. 2010. "Vitamin D and Depression: Where Is All the Sunshine?" *Issues in Mental Health Nursing* 31(6): 385–93. doi:10.3109/01612840903437657.

Plourde, M., and S. C. Cunnane. 2007. "Extremely Limited Synthesis of Long Chain Polyunsaturates in Adults: Implications for Their Dietary Essentiality and Use as Supplements." *Applied Physiology, Nutrition, and Metabolism* 32(4): 619–34. doi:10.1139/H07-034.

Pollan, Michael. 2009. *In Defense of Food: An Eater's Manifesto.* New York: Turtleback Books.

Pollan, Michael. 2013. *Food Rules: An Eater's Manual.* New York: Penguin. pp. 103, 111, 119.

Private Label Manufacturers Association. 2016. "How America's Eating Habits Are Changing." https://tinyurl.com/yxslgaga.

Sánchez-Villegas, A., M. Delgado-Rodríguez, A. Alonso, J. Schlatter, F. Lahortiga, L. Serra, and M. Martínez-González. 2009. "Association of the Mediterranean Dietary Pattern with the Incidence of Depression: The Seguimiento Universidad de Navarra/University of Navarra Follow-up (SUN) Cohort." *Archives of General Psychiatry* 66(10): 1090–98. doi:10.1001/archgenpsychiatry.2009.129.

Sanmukhani, J., V. Satodia, J. Trivedi, T. Patel, D. Tiwari, B. Panchal, A. Goel, and C. B. Tripathi. 2013. "Efficacy and Safety of Curcumin in Major Depressive Disorder: A Randomized Controlled Trial." *Phytotherapy Research* 28(4): 579–85. doi:10.1002/ptr.5025. (This study found curcumin as effective as fluoxetine.)

Sender, Ron, Shai Fuchs, and Ron Milo. 2016. "Revised Estimates for the Number of Human and Bacteria Cells in the Body." *PLoS Biology* 14(8): e1002533. doi:10.1371/journal.pbio.1002533.

Serefko, A., A. Szopa, P. Wlaź, G. Nowak, M. Radziwoń-Zaleska, M. Skalski, and E. Poleszak. 2013. "Magnesium in Depression." *Pharmacological Reports: PR* 65(3): 547–54. https://tinyurl.com/y583eswb.

Tan, Z. S., W. S. Harris, A. S. Beiser, R. Au, J. J. Himali, S. Debette, A. Pikula, et al. 2012. "Red Blood Cell Omega-3 Fatty Acid Levels and Markers of Accelerated Brain Aging." *Neurology* 78(9): 658–64. doi:10.1212/WNL.0b013e318249f6a9. (This study found that low omega-3s are associated with lower brain volumes and cognitive impairment.)

Tarleton, Emily K., Benjamin Littenberg, Charles D. MacLean, Amanda G. Kennedy, and Christopher Daley. 2017. "Role of Magnesium Supplementation in the Treatment of Depression: A Randomized Clinical Trial." *PLoS One,* June 27, 2017. doi:10.1371/journal.pone.0180067.

U.S. Centers for Disease Control and Prevention. 2017. "Only 1 in 10 Adults Get Enough Fruits or Vegetables." Press release. November 16, 2017. https://tinyurl.com/yb9wcqb6.

Zhang, Zhiying, Victor L. Fulgoni III, Penny M. Kris-Etherton, and Susan Hazels Mitmesser. 2018. "Dietary Intakes of EPA and DHA Omega-3 Fatty Acids among US Childbearing-Age and Pregnant Women: An Analysis of NHANES 2001–2014." *Nutrients* 10(4): 416. doi:10.3390/nu10040416.

11. Restoring the Body with Sleep

Anderson, Clare, and Charlotte R. Platten. 2010. "Sleep Deprivation Lowers Inhibition and Enhances Impulsivity to Negative Stimuli." *Behavioural Brain Research* 217(2): 463–66. doi:10.1016/j.bbr.2010.09.020.

Asaad, Tarek. 2015. "Sleep in Ancient Egypt." In *Sleep Medicine: A Comprehensive Guide to Its Development, Clinical Milestones and Advances in Treatment,* edited by Sudhansu Chokroverty and Michel Billiard, 159–65. New York: Springer. doi:10.1007/978-1-4939-2089-1_2.

Barbera, J. 2008. "Sleep and Dreaming in Greek and Roman Philosophy." *Sleep Medicine* 9(8): 906–10. doi:10.1016/j.sleep.2007.10.010.

Bhadra, U., N. Thakkar, P. Das, and M. Pal. 2017. "Evolution of Circadian Rhythms: From Bacteria to Human." *Sleep Medicine* 35, 49–61. doi:10.1016/j.sleep.2017.04.008.

Cartwright, Rosalind D. 2008. *The Twenty-Four Hour Mind: The Role of Sleep and Dreaming in Our Emotional Lives.* Amsterdam: Elsevier.

Chung, K. H., C. Y. Li, S. Y. Kuo, T. Sithole, W. W. Liu, and M. H. Chung. 2015. "Risk of Psychiatric Disorders in Patients with Chronic Insomnia and Sedative-Hypnotic Prescription: A Nationwide Population-Based Follow-up Study." *Journal of Clinical Sleep Medicine* 11(5): 543–51. doi:10.5664/jcsm.4700. (Study found the use of hypnotics increased the risk of depression, anxiety, and bipolar disorders.)

Ferracioli-Oda, Eduardo, Ahmad Qawasmi, and Michael H. Bloch. 2013. "Meta-Analysis: Melatonin for the Treatment of Primary Sleep Disorders." *PLoS One* 8(5): e63773. doi:10.1371/journal.pone.0063773.

Frisher, Martin, Nicholas Gibbons, James Bashford, Steve Chapman, and Scott Weich. 2016. "Melatonin, Hypnotics and Their Association with Fracture: A Matched Cohort Study." *Age and Ageing* 45(6): 801–6. doi:10.1093/ageing/afw123.

Hansen, B. T., K. M. Sønderskov, I. Hageman, P. T. Dinesen, and S. D. Østergaard. 2017. "Daylight Savings Time Transitions and the Incidence Rate of Unipolar Depressive Episodes." *Epidemiology* 28(3): 346–53. doi:10.1097/EDE.0000000000000580.

Huedo-Medina, Tania B., Irving Kirsch, Jo Middlemass, Markos Klonizakis, and A. Niroshan Siriwardena. 2012. "Effectiveness of Non-Benzodiazepine Hypnotics in Treatment of Adult Insomnia: Meta-analysis of Data Submitted to the Food and

Drug Administration." *BMJ* 345. doi:10.1136/bmj.e8343. (Analysis found that use of hypnotics amounts to about 20 minutes of additional sleep.)

Johnson, Rebecca L., Steven Foster, Tieraona Low Dog, and David Kiefer. 2014. *National Geographic Guide to Medicinal Herbs: The World's Most Effective Healing Plants.* Washington, DC: National Geographic. pp. 52–55, 145–147.

Kamphuis, J., P. Meerlo, J. Koolhaas, and M. Lancel. 2012. "Poor Sleep as a Potential Causal Factor in Aggression and Violence." *Sleep Medicine* 13(4): 327–34. doi:10.1016/j.sleep.2011.12.006.

Kasper, S., W. Müller, H. Volz, H. Möller, E. Koch, and A. Dienel. 2018. "Silexan in Anxiety Disorders: Clinical Data and Pharmacological Background." *World Journal of Biological Psychiatry* 19(6): 412–20. doi:10.1080/15622975.2017.1331046.

Kripke, D. F., R. D. Langer, and L. E. Kline. 2012. "Hypnotics' Association with Mortality or Cancer: A Matched Cohort Study." *BMJ Open* 2(1): e000850. doi:10.1136/bmjopen-2012-000850.

Lam, Raymond W., Anthony J. Levitt, Robert D. Levitan, Erin E. Michalak, Amy H. Cheung, Rachel Morehouse, Rajamannar Ramasubbu, et al. 2016. "Bright Light Treatment and Fluoxetine for Nonseasonal Depression." *JAMA Psychiatry* 73(1): 56–63. doi:10.1001/jamapsychiatry.2015.2235.

Lin, Han-Ting, Chi-Huang Lai, Huey-Jen Perng, Chi-Hsiang Chung, Chung-Ching Wang, Wei-Liang Chen, and Wu-Chien Chien. 2018. "Insomnia as an Independent Predictor of Suicide Attempts: A Nationwide Population-Based Retrospective Cohort Study." *BMC Psychiatry* 18, 117. doi:10.1186/s12888-018-1702-2.

McCall, W. V., R. M. Benca, P. B. Rosenquist, M. A. Riley, L. McCloud, J. C. Newman, D. Case, et al. 2017. "Hypnotic Medications and Suicide: Risk, Mechanisms, Mitigation, and the FDA." *American Journal of Psychiatry* 174(1): 18–25. doi:10.1176/appi.ajp.2016.16030336.

Moloney, Mairead Eastin, Thomas R. Konrad, and Catherine R. Zimmer. 2011. "The Medicalization of Sleeplessness: A Public Health Concern." *American Journal of Public Health* 101(8): 1429–33. doi:10.2105/AJPH.2010.300014. (References a discussion on the rise of prescription hypnotics.)

National Center for Complementary and Integrative Health. 2017. "National Health Interview Survey: Most Used Natural Products." https://tinyurl.com/y475w6pm.

National Center for Complementary and Integrative Health. 2017. "National Health Interview Survey: Wellness-Related Use of Natural Product Supplements, Yoga, and Spinal Manipulation Among Adults." https://tinyurl.com/y3qecqg4.

National Institutes of Health Consensus Development Program. 2005. "NIH Insomnia Conference on Manifestations and Management of Chronic Insomnia in Adults: Panel Statement." 2005. https://tinyurl.com/y5zqqold.

National Sleep Foundation. 2006. "2006 Sleep in America Poll." https://tinyurl.com/y5d46kwy.

Nutt, David, Sue Wilson, and Louise Paterson. 2008. "Sleep Disorders as Core Symptoms of Depression." *Dialogues in Clinical Neuroscience* 10(3): 329–36. https://tinyurl.com/gvzbyc2.

Physicians for Human Rights. 2007. *Leave No Marks: Enhanced Interrogation Techniques and the Risk of Criminality.* Washington, DC: Physicians for Human Rights. https://tinyurl.com/y3godvdy.

Rössler, Wulf, Jules Angst, Vladeta Ajdacic-Gross, Helene Haker, Sofian Berrouiguet, Mariam Ujeyl, Nicholas Glozier, and Michael P. Hengartner. 2018. "Sleep Disturbances and Suicidality: A Longitudinal Analysis from a Representative Community Study Over 30 Years." *Frontiers in Psychiatry* 9, 320. doi:10.3389/fpsyt.2018.00320.

Salter, Shanah, and Sonya Brownie. 2010. "Treating Primary Insomnia—The Efficacy of Valerian and Hops." *Australian Family Physician* 39(6): 433–37. https://tinyurl.com/y27eqxvl.

Suh, Sooyeon. 2015. "Cognitive Behavioral Therapy for Insomnia: Is It Effective in Treating Symptoms of Comorbid Psychiatric and Medical Disorders? A Review." *Sleep Medicine Research* 6(1): 10–15. doi:10.17241/smr.2015.6.1.10.

Taveras, Elsie M., Sheryl L. Rifas-Shiman, Kristen L. Bub, Matthew W. Gillman, and Emily Oken. 2017. "Prospective Study of Insufficient Sleep and Neurobehavioral Functioning Among School-Age Children." *Academic Pediatrics* 17(6): 625–32. doi:10.1016/j.acap.2017.02.001.

Terman, M., and J. S. Terman. 2006. "Controlled Trial of Naturalistic Dawn Simulation and Negative Air Ionization for Seasonal Affective Disorder." *American Journal of Psychiatry* 163(12): 2126–33. doi:10.1176/ajp.2006.163.12.2126.

U.S. Centers for Disease Control and Prevention. 2011. "Effect of Short Sleep Duration on Daily Activities—United States, 2005–2008." *Morbidity and Mortality Weekly Report* 60(8): 239–42. https://tinyurl.com/y4dypmw4.

Walker, Matthew. 2018. *Why We Sleep: Unlocking the Power of Sleep and Dreams.* New York: Scribner. pp. 52, 138–47, 195–216, 269. (Referenced frequently, including referral to a study finding that sleep deprivation leads to more car crashes than alcohol and drugs, and data about the sleep cycle.)

Weich, S., H. L. Pearce, P. Croft, S. Singh, I. Crome, J. Bashford, and M. Frisher. 2014. "Effect of Anxiolytic and Hypnotic Drug Prescriptions on Mortality Hazards: Retrospective Cohort Study." *BMJ* 348, g1996. doi:10.1136/bmj.g1996.

Winsler, A., A. Deutsch, R. D. Vorona, P. A. Payne, and M. Szklo-Coxe. 2014. "Sleepless in Fairfax: The Difference One More Hour of Sleep Can Make for Teen Hopelessness, Suicidal Ideation, and Substance Use." *Journal of Youth and Adolescence* 44(2): 362–78. doi:10.1007/s10964-014-0170-3.

Xie, L., H. Kang, Q. Xu, M. J. Chen, Y. Liao, M. Thiyagarajan, J. O'Donnell, et al. 2013. "Sleep Drives Metabolite Clearance from the Adult Brain." *Science* 342(6156): 373–77. doi:10.1126/science.1241224.

Ye, Yuan-yuan, Ni-ka Chen, Jia Chen, Juan Liu, Ling Lin, Ya-zhen Liu, Ying Lang, Xun-jun Li, et al. 2016. "Internet-Based Cognitive-Behavioural Therapy for Insomnia (ICBT-i): A Meta-analysis of Randomised Controlled Trials." *BMJ Open* 6(11): e010707. doi:10.1136/bmjopen-2015-010707.

12. Environment as Sustenance or Poison

"The Age of the Thing." 1994. *The Economist*, January 25, 1994, 47.

Aitbali, Yassine, Saadia Ba-M'hamed, Najoua Elhidar, Ahmed Nafis, Nabila Soraa, and Mohamed Bennis. 2018. "Glyphosate Based Herbicide Exposure Affects Gut Microbiota, Anxiety and Depression-Like Behaviors in Mice." *Neurotoxicology and Teratology* 67, 44–49. doi:10.1016/j.ntt.2018.04.002.

Alcock, I., M. White, B. Wheeler, L. Fleming, and M. Depledge. 2014. "Longitudinal Effects on Mental Health of Moving to Greener and Less Green Urban Areas." *Environmental Science and Technology* 48(2): 1247–55. doi:10.1021/es403688w.

Banyan, Leyla, Peir Hossain Koulivand, and Ali Gorji. 2014. "Garlic: A Review of Potential Therapeutic Effects." *Avicenna Journal of Phytomedicine* 4(1): 1–14. https://tinyurl.com/y9bys9wl.

Barker, S. B., and A. R. Wolen. 2008. "The Benefits of Human-Companion Animal Interaction: A Review." *Journal of Veterinary Medical Education* 35(4): 487–95. doi:10.3138/jvme.35.4.487.

Bassil, K. L., C. Vakil, M. Sanborn, D. C. Cole, J. S. Kaur, and K. J. Kerr. 2007. "Cancer Health Effects of Pesticides: Systematic Review." *Canadian Family Physician* 53(10): 1704–11. https://tinyurl.com/y4qvrfeg. (Review found that children exposed to pesticide-treated lawns at increased risk of leukemia, brain tumors, asthma, and behavioral issues, and adults at increased risk of cancers and lymphoma.)

Baudry, Julia, Karen E. Assmann, Mathilde Touvier, Benjamin Allès, Louise Seconda, Paule Latino-Martel, and Khaled Ezzedine. 2018. "Association of Organic Food Consumption With Cancer Risk." *JAMA Internal Medicine* 178(12): 1597–1606. doi:10.1001/jamainternmed.2018.4357.

Beard, J. D., D. M. Umbach, J. A. Hoppin, M. Richards, M. C. Alavanja, A. Blair, D. P. Sandler, and F. Kamel. 2014. "Pesticide Exposure and Depression among Male Private Pesticide Applicators in the Agricultural Health Study." *Environmental Health Perspectives* 122(9): 984–91. doi:10.1289/ehp.1307450.

Berman, M. G., E. Kross, K. M. Krpan, M. K. Askren, A. Burson, P. J. Deldin, S. Kaplan, et al. 2012. "Interacting with Nature Improves Cognition and Affect for Individuals with Depression." *Journal of Affective Disorders* 140(3): 300–5. doi:10.1016/j.jad.2012.03.012.

Beseler, Cheryl, Lorann Stallones, Jane A. Hoppin, Michael C. R. Alavanja, Aaron Blair, Thomas Keefe, and Freya Kamel. 2007. "Depression and Pesticide Exposures in Female Spouses of Licensed Pesticide Applicators in the Agricultural Health Study Cohort." *Journal of Occupational and Environmental Medicine* 48(10): 1005–13. doi:10.1097/01.jom.0000235938.70212.dd.

Beyer, Kirsten M., Andrea Kaltenbach, Aniko Szabo, Sandra Bogar, F. Javier Nieto, and Kristen M. Malecki. 2014. "Exposure to Neighborhood Green Space and Mental Health: Evidence from the Survey of the Health of Wisconsin." *International Journal of Environmental Research and Public Health* 11(3), 3453–72. doi:10.3390/ijerph110303453.

Blaser, Martin J. 2014. *Missing Microbes: How the Overuse of Antibiotics Is Fueling Our Modern Plagues.* New York: Henry Holt. (References the fact that the average American child receives seventeen prescriptions for antibiotics by his or her eighteenth birthday.)

Carr, Teresa. 2017. "Too Many Meds? America's Love Affair with Prescription Medication." *Consumer Reports,* August 3, 2017. https://tinyurl.com/yazbazp3.

Carson, Rachel. 1966. *Silent Spring.* Greenwich, CT: Fawcett.

Carwile, Jenny L., Henry T. Luu, Laura S. Bassett, Daniel A. Driscoll, Caterina Yuan, Jennifer Y. Chang, Xiaoyun Ye, et al. 2009. "Polycarbonate Bottle Use and Urinary Bisphenol A Concentrations." *Environmental Health Perspectives* 117(9): 1368–72. doi:10.1289/ehp.0900604.

Cederberg, Henna, Alena Stančáková, Nagendra Yaluri, Shalem Modi, Johanna Kuusisto, and Markku Laakso. 2015. "Increased Risk of Diabetes with Statin Treatment Is Associated with Impaired Insulin Sensitivity and Insulin Secretion: A 6 Year Follow-up Study of the METSIM Cohort." *Diabetologia* 58(5): 1109–17. https://tinyurl.com/y2b4dmf2. doi:10.1007/s00125-015-3528-5.

Chen, C. J., K. J. Kumar, Y. T. Chen, N. W. Tsao, S. C. Chien, S. T. Chang, F. H. Chu, and S. Y. Wang. 2015. "Effect of Hinoki and Meniki Essential Oils on Human Autonomic Nervous System Activity and Mood States." *Natural Product Communications* 10(7): 1305–8. https://tinyurl.com/y3nw8hku.

Chevalier, G. 2015. "The Effect of Grounding the Human Body on Mood." *Psychological Reports* 116(2): 534–42. doi:10.2466/06.PR0.116k21w5.

Chevalier, Gaétan, Stephen T. Sinatra, James L. Oschman, Karol Sokal, and Pawel Sokal. 2012. "Earthing: Health Implications of Reconnecting the Human Body to the Earth's Surface Electrons." *Journal of Environmental and Public Health* 2012, 291541. doi:10.1155/2012/291541.

The Conservation Volunteers. n.d. "Green Gym: Exercise to Make a Difference." www.tcv.org.uk/greengym.

Culver A. L., I. S. Ockene, R. Balasubramanian, B. C. Olendzki, D. M. Sepavich, J. Wactawski-Wende, J. E. Manson, et al. 2012. "Statin Use and Risk of Diabetes Mellitus in Postmenopausal Women in the Women's Health Initiative." 172(2): 144–52. doi:10.1001/archinternmed.2011.625.

Dethlefsen, L., S. Huse, M. L. Sogin, and D. A. Relman. 2008. "The Pervasive Effects of an Antibiotic on the Human Gut Microbiota, as Revealed by Deep 16S rRNA Sequencing." *PLoS Biology* 6(11): e280. doi:10.1371/journal.pbio.0060280.

Diamond, D. M., and U. Ravnskov. 2015. "How Statistical Deception Created the Appearance that Statins are Safe and Effective in Primary and Secondary Prevention of Cardiovascular Disease." *Expert Review of Clinical Pharmacology* 8(2): 201–10. doi:10.1586/17512433.2015.1012494.

Environmental Defence. 2011. "Report: Heavy Metal Hazard: The Health Risks of Hidden Heavy Metals in Face Makeup." https://tinyurl.com/y27uubsp.

Environmental Working Group. 2009. "Pollution in Minority Newborns." https://tinyurl.com/yxcpwfls.

Environmental Working Group. 2013. "EWG's Skin Deep Cosmetics Database." www.ewg.org/skindeep.

Environmental Working Group. 2013. "New FDA Rule for Antibacterial Soap Is Important Step, More Action Needed." Press release. https://tinyurl.com/y3cufnzw.

Environmental Working Group. 2018. "EWG's 2018 Shopper's Guide to Pesticides in Produce." www.ewg.org/foodnews.

Environmental Working Group. 2018. "Personal Care Products Safety Act Would Improve Cosmetics Safety." https://tinyurl.com/y3zb2n93.

Environmental Working Group. n.d. "Exposures Add Up—Survey Results." https://tinyurl.com/y6g8655n.

Gibson, Megan. 2015. "Birth Control Pills, Carl Djerassi and a History of Pregnancy Prevention." *Time,* February 2, 2015. https://tinyurl.com/y2rhc89q.

Gill, N. S. 2018. "About the Giant and Invincible Antaeus in Mythology." Thought Co., January 23, 2018. www.thoughtco.com/antaeus-112058.

Halden, R. U., A. E. Lindeman, A. E. Aiello, D. Andrews, W. A. Arnold, P. Fair, R. E. Fuoco, et al. 2017. "The Florence Statement on Triclosan and Triclocarban." 125(6): 064501. doi:10.1289/EHP1788.

Hertel, Johannes, Johanna König, Georg Homuth, Sandra Van der Auwera, Katharina Wittfeld, Maik Pietzner, Tim Kacprowski, et al. 2017. "Evidence for Stress-like Alterations in the HPA-Axis in Women Taking Oral Contraceptives." *Scientific Reports* 7:1. doi:10.1038/s41598-017-13927-7.

Houlden, V., S. Weich, J. Porto, S. Jarvis, and K. Rees. 2018. "The Relationship between Greenspace and the Mental Well-Being of Adults: A Systematic Review." *PLoS One* 13(9): e0203000. doi:10.1371/journal.pone.0203000.

Houlihan, Jane, Sonya Lunder, and Anila Jacob. 2011. "Timeline: BPA from Invention to Phase-Out." Environmental Working Group. https://tinyurl.com/y6r7n6s4.

Hudson, James B. 2012. "Applications of the Phytomedicine *Echinacea purpurea* (Purple Coneflower) in Infectious Diseases." *Journal of Biomedicine and Biotechnology* 2012, 769896. doi:10.1155/2012/769896.

Imhann, F., A. Vich Vila, M. J. Bonder, A. G. Lopez Manosalva, D. P. Y. Koonen, J. Fu, C. Wijmenga, et al. 2017. "The Influence of Proton-Pump Inhibitors and Other Commonly Used Medication on the Gut Microbiota." *Gut Microbes* 8(4): 351–58. doi:10.1080/19490976.2017.1284732.

Kellert, Stephen R., and David J. Case. 2014. "The Nature of Americans." https://natureofamericans.org.

Klepeis, Neil E., William C. Nelson, Wayne R. Ott, John P. Robinson, Andy M. Tsang, Paul Switzer, Joseph V. Behar, et al. 2001. "The National Human Activity Pattern Survey (NHAPS): A Resource for Assessing Exposure to Environmental Pollutants." *Journal of Exposure Science and Environmental Epidemiology* 11, 231–52. doi:10.1038/sj.jea.7500165.

Komori, T., R. Fujiwara, M. Tanida, J. Nomura, and M. Yokoyama. 1995. "Effects of Citrus Fragrance on Immune Function and Depressive States." *Neuroimmunomodulation* 2(3):174–80. doi:10.1159/000096889.

Li, Qing. 2018. *Forest Bathing: How Trees Can Help You Find Health and Happiness.* New York: Viking. pp. 76, 91.

Lurie, I., X. Y. Yang, K. Haynes, R. Mamtani, and B. Boursi. 2015. "Antibiotic Exposure and the Risk for Depression, Anxiety, or Psychosis: A Nested Case-Control Study." *Journal of Clinical Psychiatry* 76(11): 1522–8. doi:10.4088/JCP.15m09961.

Manisha, Deb, and Shyamapada Mandal. 2011. "Honey: Its Medicinal Property and Antibacterial Activity." *Asian Pacific Journal of Tropical Biomedicine* 1(2): 154–60. doi:10.1016/S2221-1691(11)60016-6.

Manoogian, Jack. 2016. "There Are Only 12 Quiet Places Left in the U.S. (and This Man Will Only Tell Us 3 of Them)." The Inertia, June 21, 2016. https://tinyurl.com/yyuzhewl.

McDade, Thomas W., Julienne Rutherford, Linda Adair, and Christopher W. Kuzawa. 2009. "Early Origins of Inflammation: Microbial Exposures in Infancy Predict Lower Levels of C-Reactive Protein in Adulthood." *Proceedings of the Royal Society B* 278:1684. doi:10.1098/rspb.2009.1795.

McDonald, L. C. 2017. "Effects of Short- and Long-Course Antibiotics on the Lower Intestinal Microbiome as They Relate to Traveller's Diarrhea." *Journal of Travel Medicine* 24(Suppl. 1): S35–38. doi:10.1093/jtm/taw084.

Muldoon, M. F., S. B. Manuck, and K. A. Matthews. 1990. "Lowering Cholesterol Concentrations and Mortality: A Quantitative Review of Primary Prevention Trials."

BMJ 301(6747): 309–14. doi:10.1136/bmj.301.6747.309. (This review reveals that low levels of cholesterol are associated with increased mortality, depression, violence, and suicide.)

Myrick, Jessica Gail. 2015. "Emotion Regulation, Procrastination, and Watching Cat Videos Online: Who Watches Internet Cats, Why, and to What Effect?" *Computers in Human Behavior* 52, 168–176. doi:10.1016/j.chb.2015.06.001.

National Cancer Institute. 2011. "Diethylstilbestrol (DES) and Cancer." https://tinyurl.com/yyoavhf3.

National Institutes of Health. 2018. "Oral Contraceptives and Cancer Risk." https://tinyurl.com/znjf8pf.

National Park Service. n.d. "NPS Healthy Parks Healthy People US." www.nps.gov/orgs/1735.

Nature Rx. 2015. "Nature Rx Part 1." YouTube. Video. www.youtube.com/watch?v=Bf5TgVRGND4.

NHS Shetland. n.d. "Nature Prescriptions Calendar." https://tinyurl.com/yd7zkcrq.

Nicolopoulou-Stamati, Polyxeni, Sotirios Maipas, Chrysanthi Kotampasi, Panagiotis Stamatis, and Luc Hens. 2016. "Chemical Pesticides and Human Health: The Urgent Need for a New Concept in Agriculture." *Frontiers in Public Health* 4, 148. doi:10.3389/fpubh.2016.00148.

O'Connor, Anahad. 2014. "BPA in Cans and Plastic Bottles Linked to Quick Rise in Blood Pressure." *New York Times,* December 8, 2014. https://tinyurl.com/y5p8ts9t.

Ober, A. Clinton. 2000. "Grounding the Human Body to Neutralize Bio-Electric Stress from Static Electricity and EMFs." *ESD Journal.* https://tinyurl.com/y5qsvz2n.

Ober, Clinton, Stephen T. Sinatra, and Martin Zucker. 2014. *Earthing: The Most Important Health Discovery Ever!* Laguna Beach, CA: Basic Health Publications. p. 3.

Oliver, Mary. 2004. *Wild Geese: Selected Poems.* Eastburn, UK: Bloodaxe Books.

Park Rx America. n.d. "Find Your Park." https://parkrxamerica.org.

Pendergrass, Drew C., and Michelle Y. Raji. 2017. "The Bitter Pill: Harvard and the Dark History of Birth Control." *Harvard Crimson,* September 28, 2017. https://tinyurl.com/y3avlxlf.

Perera, F., E. L. R. Nolte, Y. Wang, A. E. Margolis, A. M. Calafat, S. Wang, W. Garcia, et al. "Bisphenol A Exposure and Symptoms of Anxiety and Depression among Inner City Children at 10–12 Years of Age." *Environmental Research* 151, 195–202. doi:10.1016/j.envres.2016.07.028.

Praag, Cassandra D., Gould van Praag, Sarah N. Garfinkel, Oliver Sparasci, Alex Mees, Andrew O. Philippides, Mark Ware, et al. 2017. "Mind-Wandering and Alterations to Default Mode Network Connectivity When Listening to Naturalistic Versus Artificial Sounds." *Scientific Reports* 7. doi:10.1038/srep45273.

Qato, D. M., K. Ozenberger, and M. Olfson. 2018. "Prevalence of Prescription Medications With Depression as a Potential Adverse Effect Among Adults in the United States." *Journal of the American Medical Association* 319(22): 2289–98. doi:10.1001/jama.2018.6741.

Ravnskov, Uffe, David M. Diamond, Rokura Hama, Tomohito Hamazaki, Björn Hammarskjöld, Niamh Hynes, Malcolm Kendrick, et al. 2016. "Lack of an Association or an Inverse Association between Low-Density-Lipoprotein Cholesterol and Mortality in the Elderly: A Systematic Review." *BMJ Open* 6:6. doi:10.1136/bmjopen-2015-010401. (Low levels of cholesterol are associated with increased mortality.)

Reuters. 2018. "Monsanto Ordered to Pay $289 Million in Roundup Cancer Trial." *New York Times,* August 10, 2018. https://tinyurl.com/yd4ajufg.

Richardson, Harriet. 2015. "Pine Trees." Historic Hospitals. https://tinyurl.com/y2ss5r74.

Roberts, James R., and Catherine J. Karr. 2012. "Pesticide Exposure in Children." *Pediatrics* 130(6): e1765–88. doi:10.1542/peds.2012-2758. (Children's levels of pesticide in the blood are ten times higher than the levels of original application.)

Savage, Jessica H., Elizabeth C. Matsui, Robert A. Wood, and Corinne A. Keet. 2012. "Urinary Levels of Triclosan and Parabens Are Associated with Aeroallergen and Food Sensitization." *Journal of Allergy and Clinical Immunology* 130(2): 453–60. doi:10.1016/j.jaci.2012.05.006.

Seaman, Greg. 2009. "Lawn Care Chemicals: How Toxic Are They?" EarthEasy, January 28, 2009. https://tinyurl.com/y5p8andh.

Sehested, Thomas S., Emil L. Fosbøl, Peter W. Hansen, Mette G. Charlot, Christian Torp-Pedersen, and Gunnar H. Gislason. 2018. "Proton-Pump Inhibitor Use Increases the Associated Risk of First-Time Ischemic Stroke. A Nationwide Cohort Study." *Circulation* 134(Suppl. 1). https://tinyurl.com/y6mq9r92.

Sehulster, Lynne, and Raymond Y. W. Chinn. 2003. "Guidelines for Environmental Infection Control in Health-Care Facilities: Recommendations of CDC and the Healthcare Infection Control Practices Advisory Committee (HICPAC)." U.S. Centers for Disease Control and Prevention. https://tinyurl.com/y4596cmb. (CDC has not found any evidence that use of antimicrobials improves health or prevents disease.)

Selhub, Eva M., and Alan C. Logan. 2014. *Your Brain on Nature: The Science of Nature's Influence on Your Health, Happiness, and Vitality.* New York: HarperCollins. pp. 11–15, 24–28, 56–57, 132. (References data throughout this chapter, including information on MRI studies showing how nature changes activity in brain.)

Seuss, Dr. 1999. *The Lorax.* New York: Random House.

Skovlund, C. W., L. S. Mørch, L. V. Kessing, and Ø. Lidegaard. 2016. "Association of Hormonal Contraception with Depression." *JAMA Psychiatry* 73(11): 1154–62. doi:10.1001/jamapsychiatry.2016.2387.

Skovlund, C. W., L. S. Mørch, L. V. Kessing, T. Lange, and Ø. Lidegaard. 2017. "Association of Hormonal Contraception With Suicide Attempts and Suicides." *American Journal of Psychiatry* 175(4): 336–42. doi:10.1176/appi.ajp.2017 .17060616.

Stigsdotter, U. K., O. Ekholm, J. Schipperijn, M. Toftager, F. Kamper-Jørgensen, and T. B. Randrup. 2010. "Health Promoting Outdoor Environments—Associations between Green Space, and Health, Health-Related Quality of Life and Stress Based on a Danish National Representative Survey." *Scandinavian Journal of Public Health* 38(4): 411–17. doi:10.1177/1403494810367468.

Stoiber, Tasha. 2018. "New Round of EWG Testing Finds Glyphosate in Kids' Breakfast Foods from Quaker Oats, General Mills." Environmental Working Group. https://tinyurl.com/y7ex6kft.

Strand, Daniel S., Daejin Kim, and David A. Peura. 2017. "25 Years of Proton-Pump Inhibitors: A Comprehensive Review." *Gut and Liver* 11(1): 27–37. doi:10.5009/ gnl15502.

Taylor, Richard. 2017. "Fractal Patterns in Nature and Art Are Aesthetically Pleasing and Stress-Reducing." Smithsonian.com, March 31, 2017. https://tinyurl.com/yxhtxj5v.

Thompson, Catharine Ward, Jenny Roe, Peter Aspinall, Richard Mitchell, Angela Clow, and David Miller. 2012. "More Green Space Is Linked to Less Stress in Deprived Communities: Evidence from Salivary Cortisol Patterns." *Landscape and Urban Planning* 105(3): 221–29. doi:10.1016/j.landurbplan.2011.12.015.

Thompson, J., K. Boddy, K. Stein, R. Whear, J. Barton, and M. Depledge. 2011. "Does Participating in Physical Activity in Outdoor Natural Environments Have a Greater Effect on Physical and Mental Well-Being Than Physical Activity Indoors? A Systematic Review." *Environmental Science and Technology* 45(5): 1761–72. doi:10.1021 /es102947t.

Tippett, Krista. 2012. "Gordon Hempton: Silence and the Presence of Everything." *On Being.* Podcast. https://tinyurl.com/y6yeatho.

Tollefson, Jeff. 2016. "Why the Historic Deal to Expand US Chemical Regulation Matters." *Nature,* May 25, 2016. https://tinyurl.com/y5gzmgrt.

U.S. Centers for Disease Control and Prevention. 2017. "Antibiotic Use in the United States, 2017: Progress and Opportunities." https://tinyurl.com/yyx2c5po.

U.S. Centers for Disease Control and Prevention. 2017. "National Center for Health Statistics: Therapeutic Drug Use." https://tinyurl.com/y76w7h3v.

U.S. Centers for Disease Control and Prevention. 2019. "National Report on Human Exposure to Environmental Chemicals." https://tinyurl.com/y6hbg9dt. (CDC found 100 percent of study participants tested positive for pesticides in the blood.)

U.S. Centers for Disease Control and Prevention. n.d. "DES History." https://tinyurl .com/y6yqt7u2.

U.S. Environmental Protection Agency. 2018. "Chemicals Evaluated for Carcinogenic Potential." https://tinyurl.com/y42nfop8.

U.S. Food and Drug Administration. 2016. "Safety and Effectiveness of Consumer Antiseptics; Topical Antimicrobial Drug Products for Over-the-Counter Human Use. Final Rule." *Federal Register* 81(172): 61106–30. https://tinyurl.com/y6cxqv8z. (FDA has found no evidence that antimicrobial agents offer any advantage over soap and water.)

Ulrich, R. S. 1984. "View through a Window May Influence Recovery from Surgery." *Science* 224(4647): 420–1. doi:10.1126/science.6143402.

Vom Saal, Frederick S., and John Peterson Myers. 2008. "Bisphenol A and Risk of Metabolic Disorders." *JAMA* 300(11): 1353–55. https://tinyurl.com/y4kby42r. doi:10.1001/jama.300.11.1353.

Westhoff, Carolyn L., Stephen Heartwell, Sharon Edwards, Mimi Zieman, Gretchen Stuart, Carrie Cwiak, Anne Davis, et al. 2007. "Oral Contraceptive Discontinuation: Do Side Effects Matter?" *American Journal of Obstetrics and Gynecology* 196(4): 412.e1–7. doi:10.1016/j.ajog.2006.12.015. (One of the most common reasons for discontinuation of the pill is depression and mood lability.)

World Health Organization. 2011. "What Are Reproductive Health (RH) Essential Medicines?" https://tinyurl.com/y3ejk4ct.

World Health Organization. 2015. "International Agency for Research on Cancer Monographs Volume 112: Evaluation of Five Organophosphate Insecticides and Herbicides." https://tinyurl.com/y3c8fb4g.

Xie, Yan, Benjamin Bowe, Tingting Li, Hong Xian, Yan Yan, and Ziyad Al-Aly. 2017. "Risk of Death among Users of Proton-Pump Inhibitors: A Longitudinal Observational Cohort Study of United States Veterans." *BMJ Open,* July 1, 2017. doi:10.1136/bmjopen-2016-015735.

Zareifopoulos, N., and G. Panayiotakopoulos. 2017. "Neuropsychiatric Effects of Antimicrobial Agents." *Clinical Drug Investigation* 37(5): 423–37. doi:10.1007/s40261-017-0498-z.

13. Heart, Energy, and Soul as Conductors and Synthesizers

Brainy Quote. n.d. "Ralph Waldo Emerson." https://tinyurl.com/yybajbyg.

Cacioppo, John T., Louise C. Hawkley, John M. Ernst, Mary Burleson, Gary G. Berntson, Bita Nouriani, and David Spiegel. 2006. "Loneliness within a Nomological Net: An Evolutionary Perspective." *Journal of Research in Personality* 40, 1054–85. https://tinyurl.com/yy4fs7sz. doi:10.1016/j.jrp.2005.11.007. (This study showed how feelings of isolation plummet mood and self-esteem.)

Chanda, M. L., and D. J. Levitin. 2013. "The Neurochemistry of Music." *Trends in Cognitive Sciences* 17(4): 179–93. doi:10.1016/j.tics.2013.02.007.

Childre, Doc, and Deborah Rozman. 2007. *Transforming Depression: The HeartMath Solution to Feeling Overwhelmed, Sad, and Stressed.* Oakland, CA: New Harbinger. (This book references research on the heart's electromagnetic field and heart rate variability, and offers tools for creating greater coherence within the heart, mind, and body.)

Childre, Doc, Howard Martin, Deborah Rozman, and Rollin McCraty. 2016. *Heart Intelligence.* Cardiff, CA: Waterfront Press. pp. 53–57, 114–17. (This book references research on the heart's electromagnetic field, the influence of emotions on the intuitive nature of the heart, and the power of group intentions to change reality.)

Church, D., G. Yount, and A. J. Brooks. 2012. "The Effect of Emotional Freedom Techniques on Stress Biochemistry: A Randomized Controlled Trial." *Journal of Nervous and Mental Disease* 200(10): 891–96. doi:10.1097/NMD.0b013e31826b9fc1.

Church, Dawson. 2013. "Clinical EFT as an Evidence-Based Practice for the Treatment of Psychological and Physiological Conditions." *Psychology* 4(8): 645–54. doi:10.4236/psych.2013.48092.

Cuypers, K., S. Krokstad, T. L. Holmen, M. Skjei Knudtsen, L. O. Bygren, and J. Holmen. 2012. "Patterns of Receptive and Creative Cultural Activities and Their Association with Perceived Health, Anxiety, Depression and Satisfaction with Life among Adults: The HUNT Study, Norway." *Journal of Epidemiology and Community Health* 66(8): 698–703. doi:10.1136/jech.2010.113571.

Darley, John M., and C. Daniel Batson. 1973. "From Jerusalem to Jericho: A Study of Situational and Dispositional Variables in Helping Behavior. *Journal of Personality and Social Psychology* 27(1): 100–8. https://tinyurl.com/y35jbb7d.

Eden, Donna, and David Feinstein. 2008. *Energy Medicine: Balancing Your Body's Energies for Optimal Health, Joy, and Vitality.* New York: Tarcher/Putnam. p. 3.

EMDR Institute. n.d. "History of EMDR." www.emdr.com/history-of-emdr.

Emmons, R. A., and M. E. McCullough. 2003. "Counting Blessings versus Burdens: An Experimental Investigation of Gratitude and Subjective Well-being in Daily Life." *Journal of Personality and Social Psychology* 84(2): 377–89. doi:10.1037//0022-3514.84.2.377.

Emoto, Masaru. 2005. *The Hidden Messages in Water.* New York: Atria Books.

Fang, J., Z. Jin, Y. Wang, K. Li, J. Kong, E. E. Nixon, Y. Zeng, et al. 2009. "The Salient Characteristics of the Central Effects of Acupuncture Needling: Limbic-Paralimbic-Neocortical Network Modulation." *Human Brain Mapping* 30(4): 1196–206. doi:10.1002/hbm.20583.

Fikowski, Megan M., R. Nick Cochran, and Brian W Haas. 2016. "Altruistic Behavior: Mapping Responses in the Brain." *Neuroscience and Neuroeconomics* 5, 65–75. doi:10.2147/NAN.S87718.

Fowler, James H., and Nicholas A Christakis. 2008. "Dynamic Spread of Happiness in a Large Social Network: Longitudinal Analysis over 20 Years in the Framingham Heart Study." *BMJ* 337. doi:10.1136/bmj.a2338.

Goleman, Daniel, and Richard J. Davidson. 2017. *Altered Traits: Science Reveals How Meditation Changes Your Mind, Brain, and Body.* New York: Avery.

Grinberg-Zylberbaum, J., M. Delaflor, L. Attie, and A. Goswami. 1994. "The Einstein-Podolsky-Rosen Paradox in the Brain: The Transferred Potential." *Physics Essays* 7(4): 422–28. https://tinyurl.com/y67fdqmc. (References the study of how the brains of former strangers who meditated together for twenty minutes became entrained.)

Hansen, E., E. Sund, M. Skjei Knudtsen, S. Krokstad, and T. L. Holmen. 2015. "Cultural Activity Participation and Associations With Self-Perceived Health, Life-Satisfaction and Mental Health: The Young HUNT Study, Norway." *BMC Public Health* 15:544. doi:10.1186/s12889-015-1873-4.

Holt-Lunstad, J., T. B. Smith, M. Baker, T. Harris, and D. Stephenson. 2015. "Loneliness and Social Isolation as Risk Factors for Mortality: A Meta-analytic Review." *Perspectives on Psychological Science* 10(2): 227–37. doi:10.1177/1745691614568352.

Homer. 2018. *The Odyssey.* Translated by Robert Fitzgerald. Newbury, UK: CSS Books.

Hopton, A., H. Macpherson, A. Keding, and S. Morley. 2014. "Acupuncture, Counselling or Usual Care for Depression and Comorbid Pain: Secondary Analysis of a Randomised Controlled Trial." *BMJ Open* 4(5): e004964. doi:10.1136/bmjopen-2014-004964.

Hui, Kathleen K. S., Ovidiu Marina, Jing Liu, Bruce R. Rosen, and Kenneth K. Kwong. 2010. "Acupuncture, the Limbic System, and the Anticorrelated Networks of the Brain." *Journal of the Autonomic Nervous System* 157(0): 81–90. doi:10.1016/j.autneu.2010.03.022.

Hutcherson, C. A., E. M. Seppala, and J. J. Gross. 2008. "Loving-Kindness Meditation Increases Social Connectedness." *Emotion* 8(5): 720–24. doi:10.1037/a0013237.

Jung, Carl G. 1989. *Memories, Dreams, Reflections.* New York: Vintage. pp. 247–52.

Kang, Yoona, Jeremy R. Gray, and John F. Dovidio. 2013. "The Nondiscriminating Heart: Lovingkindness Meditation Training Decreases Implicit Intergroup Bias." *Journal of Experimental Psychology General* 143(3): 1306–1313. doi:10.1037/a0034150.

Karns, C. M., W. E. Moore III, and U. Mayr. 2017. "The Cultivation of Pure Altruism via Gratitude: A Functional MRI Study of Change with Gratitude Practice." *Frontiers in Human Neuroscience* 11:599. doi:10.3389/fnhum.2017.00599.

Kemp, Andrew H., and Daniel S. Quintana. 2013. "The Relationship between Mental and Physical Health: Insights from the Study of Heart Rate Variability." *International Journal of Psychophysiology* 89(3): 288–96. doi:10.1016/j.ijpsycho.2013.06.018.

Kini, P., J. Wong, S. McInnis, N. Gabana, and J. W. Brown. 2016. "The Effects of Gratitude Expression on Neural Activity." *NeuroImage* 128, 1–10. doi:10.1016/j.neuroimage.2015.12.040.

Klimecki, O. M., L. Leiberg, C. Lamm, and T. Singer. 2013. "Functional Neural Plasticity and Associated Changes in Positive Affect after Compassion Training." *Cerebral Cortex* 23(7): 1552–61. doi:10.1093/cercor/bhs142. (This study found that six hours of at-home online training activated empathy circuitry in the brain.)

Kramer, Adam D. I., Jamie E. Guillory, and Jeffrey T. Hancock. 2014. "Experimental Evidence of Massive-Scale Emotional Contagion through Social Networks." *PNAS* 111(24): 8788–90. doi:10.1073/pnas.1320040111.

Leskovec, Jure, and Eric Horvitz. 2008. "Planetary-Scale Views on a Large Instant-Messaging Network." International World Wide Web Conference, April 21–25, 2008, Beijing. https://tinyurl.com/y6nw4cow.

Luberto, C. M., N. Shinday, R. Song, L. L. Philpotts, E. R. Park, G. L. Fricchione, and G. Y. Yeh. 2018. "A Systematic Review and Meta-analysis of the Effects of Meditation on Empathy, Compassion, and Prosocial Behaviors." *Mindfulness* 9(3): 708–24. doi:10.1007/s12671-017-0841-8.

MacPherson, H., S. Richmond, M. Bland, S. Brealey, R. Gabe, A. Hopton, A. Keding, et al. 2013. "Acupuncture and Counselling for Depression in Primary Care: A Randomised Controlled Trial." 10(9): e1001518. doi:10.1371/journal.pmed .1001518.

Maharaj, Marjorie E. 2016. "Differential Gene Expression after Emotional Freedom Techniques (EFT) Treatment: A Novel Pilot Protocol for Salivary mRNA Assessment." *Energy Psychology Journal.* doi:10.9769/EPJ.2016.8.1.MM.

Martin, Howard. 2017. "New World Now: The Science of Heart-Connected Living." Lecture. River's Edge, Cleveland, September 16, 2017.

McTaggart, Lynne. 2017. *The Power of Eight: The Miraculous Healing Power of Small Groups.* New York: Atria Books.

Mitchell, Alex J., Amol Vaze, and Sanjay Rao. 2009. "Clinical Diagnosis of Depression in Primary Care: A Meta-Analysis." *Lancet* 374(9690): 609–19. doi:10.1016 /S0140-6736(09)60879-5.

Morris, Steven M. 2010. "Achieving Collective Coherence: Group Effects on Heart Rate Variability Coherence and Heart Rhythm Synchronization." *Alternative Therapies* 16(4): 62–72. https://tinyurl.com/y2mzn6wu.

Nelms, J. A., and L. Castel. 2016. "A Systematic Review and Meta-Analysis of Randomized and Nonrandomized Trials of Clinical Emotional Freedom Techniques (EFT) for the Treatment of Depression." *Explore (NY)* 12(6): 416–26. doi:10.1016/j. explore.2016.08.001.

Nelson, R. D., D. I. Radin, R. Shoup, and P. A. Bancel. 2002. "Correlations of Continuous Random Data with Major World Events." https://tinyurl.com/yd85zmp.

Ostacoli, L., S. Carletto, M. Cavallo, P. Baldomir-Gago, G. Di Lorenzo, I. Fernandez, M. Hase, et al. 2018. "Comparison of Eye Movement Desensitization Reprocessing and Cognitive Behavioral Therapy as Adjunctive Treatments for Recurrent

Depression: The European Depression EMDR Network (EDEN) Randomized Controlled Trial." *Frontiers in Psychology* 9:74. doi:10.3389/fpsyg.2018.00074.

Pillemer, K., T. E. Fuller-Rowell, M. C. Reid, and N. M. Wells. 2010. "Environmental Volunteering and Health Outcomes over a 20-Year Period." *Gerontologist* 50(5): 594–602. doi:10.1093/geront/gnq007.

Radin, Dean I. 1997. "Unconscious Perception of Future Emotions: An Experiment in Presentiment." *Journal of Scientific Exploration* 11(2): 163–80. https://tinyurl.com/yxa3j7ge.

Reece, Andrew G., and Christopher M. Danforth. 2016. "Instagram Photos Reveal Predictive Markers of Depression." arXiv.org. https://arxiv.org/abs/1608.03282.

Rettner, Rachael. 2014. "Life after Brain Death: Is the Body Still 'Alive'?" Live Science, January 3, 2014. https://tinyurl.com/y3qrrbcr.

Solly, Meilan. 2018. "Canadian Doctors Will Soon Be Able to Prescribe Museum Visits as Treatment." Smithsonian.com, October 22, 2018. https://tinyurl.com/y6nju4f4.

Steptoe, A., N. Owen, S. R. Kunz-Ebrecht, and L. Brydon. 2004. "Loneliness and Neuroendocrine, Cardiovascular, and Inflammatory Stress Responses in Middle-Aged Men and Women." *Psychoneuroendocrinology* 29(5): 593–611. doi:10.1016/S0306-4530(03)00086-6.

UK Department for Digital, Culture, Media and Sport. 2018. "A Connected Society: A Strategy for Tackling Loneliness—Laying the Foundations for Change." https://tinyurl.com/y8r3xmal.

van der Kolk, B. A., J. Spinazzola, M. E. Blaustein, J. W. Hopper, E. K. Hopper, D. L. Korn, and W. B. Simpson. 2007. "A Randomized Clinical Trial of Eye Movement Desensitization and Reprocessing (EMDR), Fluoxetine, and Pill Placebo in the Treatment of Post-Traumatic Stress Disorder: Treatment Effects and Long-Term Maintenance." *Journal of Clinical Psychiatry* 68(1): 37–46. doi:10.4088/jcp.v68n0105.

Veith, Ilza, trans. 2016. *The Yellow Emperor's Classic of Internal Medicine.* Berkeley, CA: University of California Press.

Wells, Diane. 2017. "Fun Facts About the Heart You Didn't Know." Healthline, July 6, 2017. https://tinyurl.com/yazzlmlj.

Weng, Helen Y., Andrew S. Fox, Alexander J. Shackman, Diane E. Stodola, Jessica Z. K. Caldwell, Matthew C. Olson, Gregory M. Rogers, and Richard J. Davidson. 2013. "Compassion Training Alters Altruism and Neural Responses to Suffering." *Psychological Science* 24(7): 1171–80. doi:10.1177/0956797612469537. (This study found that after eight hours of training, the brain scans of novices resembled those of more experienced meditators.)

Winfrey, Oprah. 2018. "Karen Armstrong: Steps to a Compassionate Life." *Oprah's SuperSoul Conversations.* Podcast. December 25, 2018. https://tinyurl.com/y4ayye8v.

14. CONNECTING THE PIECES

Brach, Tara. 2017. "From Dragons to Schmoos—Meeting Life with Compassionate Presence." September 20, 2017. https://tinyurl.com/yyr36j49.

Church, Dawson. 2018. *Mind to Matter: The Astonishing Science of How Your Brain Creates Material Reality.* Sydney, NSW: Hay House. pp.111–13.

Gill, Nikita. 2018. Nikita Gill (@nikita_gill). Photos and videos. www.instagram.com /nikita_gill.

Grierson, Bruce. 2014. "What if Age Is Nothing but a Mind-Set?" *New York Times Magazine,* October 22, 2014. https://tinyurl.com/y6rzgcou. (References Ellen Langer's study in which she transported a group of seventy-year-old men "back in time.")

Hari, Johann. 2018. *Lost Connections: Uncovering the Real Causes of Depression and the Unexpected Solutions.* New York: Bloomsbury. pp. 10, 159–61.

Rummage, Stephen N. 2007. "Houdini's Failed Escape." https://tinyurl.com/y6qrkjx3.

Schnall, Simone, Kent D. Harber, Jeanine K. Stefanucci, and Dennis R. Proffitt. 2008. "Social Support and the Perception of Geographical Slant." *Journal of Experimental Social Psychology* 44(5): 1246–55. doi:10.1016/j.jesp.2008.04.011.

Tippett, Krista. 2017. "Carlo Rovelli: All Reality Is Interaction." *On Being.* Podcast. March 16, 2017. https://tinyurl.com/yxn3bqw6.

Index

About the Author

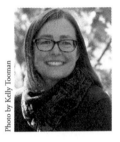

JODIE SKILLICORN, DO, is an osteopathic physician board certified in psychiatry and a diplomate of the American Board of Integrative Holistic Medicine. She integrates conventional medical training with evidence-based holistic methods that include breathwork, meditation, yoga, mindfulness-based cognitive therapy (MBCT), eye movement desensitization and reprocessing (EMDR), Emotional Freedom Technique (EFT), Mind-Body Medicine, energy medicine, nutrition, exercise, and auricular acupuncture at her private practice. She lives in Hudson, Ohio, with her husband, two kids, two cats, and dog.

Check out www.jodieskillicorn.com for more resources, information, and audio files of exercises in this book.

About North Atlantic Books